Choose to Lose
Weight-Loss Plan for Men

Books by Dr. Ron and Nancy Goor

Choose to Lose: A Food Lover's Guide
to Permanent Weight Loss

Eater's Choice: A Food Lover's Guide
to Lower Cholesterol

Eater's Choice Low-Fat Cookbook

Choose to Lose Weight-Loss Plan for Men:
A Take-Control Program for Men with
the Guts to Lose

Choose to Lose Weight-Loss Plan for Men

A Take-Control Program for Men with the Guts to Lose

Dr. Ron and Nancy Goor

HOUGHTON MIFFLIN COMPANY

Boston • New York   2000

For information about permission to reproduce selections from
this book, write to Permissions, Houghton Mifflin Company,
215 Park Avenue South, New York, New York 10003.

Library of Congress Cataloging-in-Publication Data

Goor, Ron.
  Choose to lose weight-loss plan for men : a take control
program for men with the guts to lose / Ron and Nancy Goor.
      p.   cm.
  Includes index.
  ISBN 0-395-96649-3
  1. Weight loss.   2. Men — Health and hygiene.   I. Goor, Nancy.
II. Title
RM222.2.G626   2000
613.7'0449 — dc21   99-43381   CIP

Printed in the United States of America

Choose to Lose® and Eater's Choice® are registered
trademarks of Ronald S. and Nancy M. Goor.

QUM 10 9 8 7 6 5 4 3 2 1

Before beginning this or any diet, you should
consult your physician to be sure it is safe for you.

With love to our sons,
Alex and Dan

Acknowledgments

Ron and Nancy Goor wish to thank the following people
for their contributions to the development of this book:
Robert R. Betting, Shari Bilt, R.D., Dave Bytell, M.D.,
Joseph Cejka, Alex Goor, Dan Goor, Kimra Hawk, R.D.,
Dan King, Sandy Leonard, M.S., R.D., Kathy McFalls, R.D.,
Nancy Ochsner, Mike Pierce, Robert and Muriel Rabin,
Lawrence Saladino, M.D.

Contents

Foreword

In May of 1997, 1 had an emergency angioplasty — a procedure to open a blocked artery in my heart to prevent a potentially fatal heart attack. Despite my years of medical education and after more than 20 years of practice treating patients with heart disease, I thought I had a pretty good idea of the risk factors. In fact, there were plenty of times I looked at patients, particularly men, looked at their risk factors, and felt that they were at increased risk for a heart attack. I referred them to cardiologists, and my evaluation generally turned out to be right. I thought that I had it figured out and that I was immune. At age 46 1 never expected a life-threatening heart condition. Then it happened to me.

When the shock wore off, I felt lost and scared. I knew I had to do something about my health, particularly my weight. Despite my years of medical education and practice, I didn't know where to begin with diet or weight reduction. A cardiologist friend recommended several books. I moved myself as fast as I could to the nearest bookstore. The book that caught my attention was *Choose to Lose* by Dr. Ron and Nancy Goor. I quickly realized I had found a low-fat diet program that I could follow without having to starve or feel deprived.

Ten days after my angioplasty, I started following *Choose to Lose*. I was amazed by how comprehensive it was and easy to read and what an easy program it was to follow.

Before *Choose to Lose*, I had never thought I would ever be able to lose weight. I weighed 231 pounds and as a result suffered sleep apnea. After following *Choose to Lose* for 2 months, I had lost 30 pounds. I felt so light I felt I could fly. After 6 months, I had lost 60 pounds. I no longer needed the two blood pressure medications I had been taking, and my sleep apnea cleared up. My cholesterol levels and triglyceride levels dropped.

I have become a great advocate for *Choose to Lose*. I recommend it to patients, friends, and neighbors. I tell them that *Choose to Lose* is the best investment they will make. I encourage them to buy one for someone else — their mother or father or sisters or brothers. Not only is it effective, it is safe and medically sound.

In my practice, I am interested in looking at the whole person. I try to be comprehensive so I don't just deal with the problem they come in with. If a patient comes in with pink eye and I notice they have a weight or blood pressure problem, I prescribe *Choose to Lose.* My patients have been very successful following *Choose to Lose* in both losing weight and lowering cholesterol and blood pressure. Today the wife of one of my patients called to thank me because her husband lost 30 pounds following *Choose to Lose* and felt so good. I have many, many success stories from my patients.

A while ago, I called the Goors to tell them how much *Choose to Lose* has benefited me. I told them I wanted them to write more books because I enjoyed reading *Choose to Lose* so much. They told me they were writing *Choose to Lose Weight-Loss Plan for Men* and asked me to write a foreword. I was grateful for the opportunity to tell my story because I understand so well how invulnerable young men feel. I want all the men who read this book to know that the time to do something about your health is right now and you are doing the right thing. *Choose to Lose Weight-Loss Plan for Men* makes it simple to make important lifestyle changes that will make all the difference in your health and well-being. I know.

— Lawrence P. Saladino, M. D.,
    Internal Medicine, Vienna, Virginia
    Assistant Clinical Professor of Healthcare Sciences and Medicine,
    George Washington University School of Medicine

Choose to Lose
Weight-Loss Plan for Men

1. You Are a Lucky Man

CONGRATULATIONS! You have taken the first step to becoming a lean and healthy man. Whether you have been inspired by your soaring cholesterol level, an inability to keep your buttons from popping off, energy and stamina approaching the level of a limp rag, a sense you could definitely feel better than you do, or you are just fed up with being overweight, you have made an important decision that will totally change and improve your life. The Lean You is just under the surface waiting to break out. With little effort, you can become the healthy, fit, active man you want to be. You are a lucky man.

Being a Man: The Upside

You are lucky because you are a man. Men have a tremendous advantage in fighting the battle of the bulge. Men (even fat men) are endowed with substantial muscle mass. Muscle is the tissue that burns fat. So it follows that most men can lose fat quickly. In addition, since most men have not been dieting since birth, they don't have the diet-related hangups that many women have. Many men do not even realize how overweight they are. Men who want to lose their beer belly or love handles have nature on their side.

Being a Man: The Downside

Being a man may make losing weight easier, but men who eat a high-fat, high-saturated-fat diet clog their coronary arteries faster than women do. In fact, simply being a male is a risk factor for heart disease. Men who persist in following an unhealthy lifestyle are more likely to suffer strokes or colon cancer than women. So take advantage of the upside of being a male to ensure that you never suffer the downside. You can easily reduce your risks and increase your chances for a long and healthy life. *Choose to Lose Weight-Loss Plan for Men* will show you how.

STRATEGIES FOR SUCCESS

You can capitalize on your fat-burning muscle mass to eat your way to a lean and healthy body. You can eat regular foods that you choose — you don't have to limit your diet to rabbit food. (In fact, salads are often a bad weight-loss choice.) You can eat satisfying portions so you're never hungry. You won't even have to spend half your day in a gym running around the track or lifting weights. You will be in control of your food choices, your weight, and your health. You just have to do three things:

1. Eat a low-fat diet (with an occasional high-fat splurge).
2. Eat plenty of nutritious food.
3. Exercise aerobically about 30 minutes a day (walking is great).

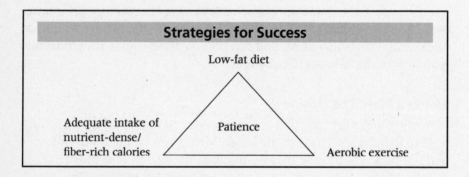

Strategies for Success

Low-fat diet

Adequate intake of nutrient-dense/ fiber-rich calories

Patience

Aerobic exercise

1. Eat a Low-Fat Diet

Let's start with Strategy #1: Eat a low-fat diet. Extensive scientific research and the experience of thousands of Choosers to Lose have shown that FAT makes you fat. The less fat you put into your body's fat stores, the less fat you will have to remove later.

But how much fat are you eating? One of the reasons you are heavier than you want to be is that you are probably eating more fat than you realize. How do you know how much fat you should eat or how much fat is in foods?

Choose to Lose Weight-Loss Plan for Men gives you a simple tool: a Fat Budget. This budget — the maximum amount of fat you can eat each day and still reach and maintain your desirable weight — is like your salary. Imagine how difficult it would be to make financial choices if you didn't know your salary. How would you know what kind of car to buy or what kind of vacation to take? Could you afford a Lexus or a Taurus, a trip to the beach or a cruise around the world? Your salary is one of the most powerful behavior modification tools in your life.

Like your salary, your Fat Budget empowers you to make choices — food choices. When you know your Fat Budget and the number of fat calories in foods,* you can decide which combination of foods you can afford to eat. No food is prohibited; no food is required.

Here's how the Fat Budget works. Say you are at the office Christmas party. Your Fat Budget is 400 fat calories a day. Instead of chug-a-lugging 3 cups of eggnog (510 fat calories) and causing a significant overdraft in your Fat Budget, you will ask, "Are 3 cups of eggnog worth 510 fat calories?" Why not spend 0 fat calories for wine or beer instead? It's your Fat Budget and your choice.

The Fat Budget even allows for splurges. Maybe 1 cup of eggnog *is* worth 170 fat calories to you. Budget it in. You don't have to give up everything. You just learn to make better choices. Eventually, your tastes may even change. Many men following *Choose to Lose* have told us that they can no longer stomach the high-fat, greasy foods they once ate with gusto. This may happen to you too.

Maximizing Fat Loss. Eating less fat is essential for weight loss, but you can't stop there. To shrink the fat stores, you must not only add less fat to them; you need to remove the fat that is already there. The next two strategies are aimed at removing the stored fat.

2. Eat Plenty of Nutrient-Dense, Fiber-Rich Carbohydrates

Strategy #2 is to eat low-fat, nutritious food to lose weight. You need to eat enough calories to keep your metabolism chugging along so you will burn fat at a maximum rate and thus help reduce your fat stores. Of course, you can't eat just any food. Not high-fat foods that add to your fat stores. And not empty calories like fat-free cakes and nonfat crackers, which only slow down your weight loss because your body burns them in preference to fat. We mean fruits, vegetables, whole grains — high-fiber, nutrient-dense carbohydrates. These foods have a lot of bulk and fill you up without filling you out. They are chock-full of vitamins and minerals too, which ensures your good health now and in the future.

---

* The Food Tables at the end of the book list fat calories for over 6000 foods.

Add low-fat meats like chicken, turkey, fish, seafood, and some lean cuts of red meats, and you'll have a full, delicious, healthy diet.

Not only will these foods rev up your metabolism, they will keep you full and satisfied so you won't build up high-fat cravings and fall off the healthy-eating wagon. They will keep your energy at an all-time high. It is the carbohydrates in foods that give you energy and stamina — the prerequisites to fulfilling the third strategy: daily aerobic exercise.

3. Exercise Aerobically Every Day

The third strategy for losing weight (and getting healthier) is daily aerobic exercise. Daily aerobic exercise is vital because it increases your energy needs. To satisfy the increased demand, the body burns fat from the fat stores and you lose weight. In addition, exercise builds and preserves muscle. Muscle is the tissue that burns fat. The more muscle you have, the higher is your capacity to burn your stockpiled fat. Before you insist that you are much too busy to run 5 miles a day or work out 2 hours each morning, rest assured that the exercise we recommend is not time-consuming or punishing. All you have to do is walk. We recommend walking for at least 30 minutes a day — the more, the better. The longer you exercise nonstop over 20 minutes, the more fat you burn and the leaner you'll become. It need not be intense. In fact, you should be able to carry on a normal conversation without becoming breathless.

Turn Your Vicious Cycle Into a Virtuous Cycle

The Vicious Cycle goes like this: You eat too much fat so you become overweight. Because you are overweight, you find it difficult to exercise and you don't make the effort. Because you aren't exercising, you lose muscle. With less muscle, you burn less fat and become fatter. You feel bad because you are fat, so you eat more fat and become even fatter.

This is the Virtuous Cycle, or *Choose to Lose* in Action: You eat a low-fat, high-carbohydrate diet, so you have lots of energy. You have lots of energy, so you find it easy to exercise. Exercising makes you feel better, so you eat healthfully. Because you are eating healthfully and exercising, you lose weight, which makes you feel better about yourself, so you continue to eat healthfully and exercise and lose weight.

Of course, if you want to do something more vigorous, like bicycling or rowing, that's fine. Strength training and stretching are not aerobic but will also add enormously to your fitness and quality of life. (See Chapter 13 for more on exercise.)

Choose to Lose for Life

You are going to be making major lifestyle changes, but it won't be difficult. *Choose to Lose Weight-Loss Plan for Men* is easy to follow and incorporate into your life — forever. The most common comment we hear from men following *Choose to Lose Weight-Loss Plan for Men* is, "Why didn't I start doing this years ago?"

Patience

You probably noticed that the word *patience* is at the center of the success triangle. Being a man and having a lot of muscle gives you an added advantage in losing weight (fat), but don't think that by next week you'll be mistaken for a skeleton. It takes time for all that excess fat to be pulled out of your body's fat stores and burned. Think about how long it took to pack your fat stores. You *will* lose weight — some Choosers to Lose have lost more than 165 pounds — and reach your goal, but don't expect to lose weight on a strict timetable.* In fact, the best policy is to focus on how much delicious low-fat food you are eating, how good you feel, how healthy you are becoming, and not on pounds at all. *Choose to Lose Weight-Loss Plan for Men* is about so much more than weight loss.

The Benefits Are Great, or Good-bye, Heartburn

Here are some of the benefits you can expect to achieve following *Choose to Lose Weight-Loss Plan for Men:*

• Reduced risks of heart disease, cancer, diabetes — you'll be so healthy your doctor will ask *you* for advice.
• Increased energy and endurance — you'll have to find younger friends to keep up with the New You.
• A more attractive you — you'll look in the mirror and like what you see.
• No more heartburn — throw away your lifetime supply of antacids.
• Increased self-esteem — you'll be in control and it will show.

---

* See Chapter 16 on "The Scale" (page 170) and "Weight-Loss Rate" (page 166) and Chapter 17 on measuring success (page 180).

• Improved sex life — you'll have more vigor and stamina, and you won't crush your partner.

Sex

A friend confided to us that the reason he started following *Choose to Lose Weight-Loss Plan for Men* was because of his sex life. He huffed and puffed so much during sex he thought he would have a heart attack. *Choose to Lose Weight-Loss Plan for Men* turned his problem around. He lost weight, gained energy, and could enjoy sex again (so did his wife).

  Choose to Lose Weight-Loss Plan for Men is great in every area. It will improve your stamina, your outlook, your love of life!

Now that you are ready to embark on *Choose to Lose Weight-Loss Plan for Men* and eat more good food than you have ever imagined, lose weight, and be in control of your life, read the next chapter to understand the scientific basis of the plan. The science makes sense. Understanding how and why the three *Choose to Lose* strategies work is a great motivator.

2. How *Choose to Lose* Works and Why

TO LOSE WEIGHT you need to reduce the amount of fat in your fat stores. The three *Choose to Lose* strategies effectively accomplish this goal. In this chapter, we will explore the scientific basis for each of the three strategies and show the unique way they work together to maximize your weight loss.

WEIGHT LOSS: ENERGY SUPPLY AND DEMAND
Your Body Needs Energy to Operate

We will start with energy because weight loss is all about how your body uses and stores energy.

Basal Metabolism. Your body needs a certain amount of energy to function — to power your heart, lungs, brain, kidneys, and other organs and keep them in good repair. The amount of energy you use when you are completely at rest is called your basal metabolism. The rate at which you burn energy when you are completely at rest is called your basal metabolic rate (BMR).

Each person has his own BMR determined partly by heredity and partly by lifestyle. Your heredity sets the upper and lower limits of your BMR. You can maximize your BMR within this range by doing daily aerobic exercise and by eating a lot of nutrient-dense, fiber-rich carbohydrates. The higher your BMR, the faster and more easily you lose weight.

Physical Activity. Unlike your basal metabolic rate, physical activity is not fixed within a range. The more exercise you do, the more energy you need to fuel it.

Total Energy Needs. Your total energy needs are the sum of your basal metabolism plus the amount of physical activity you do. The higher your BMR and the more active you are, the more energy you need.

Food Supplies Energy

Where does your body get energy to power your basal metabolism + physical activity? Just as energy stored in batteries powers machines to do work, energy stored in the food you eat powers your body.

The energy in food comes packed in three types of nutrients: fats, carbohydrates, and proteins. The amount of energy supplied by each of these nutrients is measured in calories.

Calorie Facts

A calorie is a unit of measurement of the amount of energy stored in food. The nutrients that contribute calories (energy) are carbohydrates (sugars and starches), fats, and proteins. Alcohol also contributes calories. See below for the amount of energy stored in each nutrient.

Total calories are the sum of fat, carbohydrate, and protein calories.*

> Fat Calories
> Carbohydrate Calories
> + Protein Calories
> ──────────────
> Total Calories

* If alcohol is consumed, the alcohol calories are included in the total.

Calories Per Gram	
Fat	9
Carbohydrates	4
Proteins	4
Alcohol	7

Not All Calories Are Equal

Many people believe that whether you eat fats, carbohydrates, or proteins, if you eat too much, the energy is stored and becomes fat. Not true. What is true is that the body handles carbohydrates, fats, and proteins differently and the calories from each have a totally different effect on weight gain. Each of the *Choose to Lose* strategies takes advantage of the different ways the body uses these nutrients to help you lose weight.

STRATEGY #1: EAT A LOW-FAT DIET

Fat is the villain. Fat makes you fat. Unlike carbohydrates and protein, fat is not burned off when you eat it. Almost all (97%) of the fat you eat slides right into the fat stores that pad your body. It is as if you took the hamburger you just ate and wadded it onto your belly except that it is happening from the inside.

The capacity for storing fat knows no bounds. The normal *lean* person stores about 140,000 calories of fat. Contrast this to the body's limited capacity to store carbohydrate (about 1200–1500 calories). And with fat storage, there is no upper limit. A person who weighs 300 pounds is storing about 200 pounds of fat.

Whereas it is extremely difficult to overeat carbohydrates if you are eating nutrient-dense, fiber-rich food, there are no mechanisms to protect you from overeating fat. You can overeat fat one day, and the next, and the next, and the fat stores grow larger and larger.

In short, you are overweight because you have put too much fat in cold storage.

Creating a Deficit

Each day fat from the foods you eat is added to your body's fat stores. Some is removed to furnish energy not supplied by the carbohydrates you eat. **Your weight is determined largely by how much fat you add to the fat depots versus how much you remove.**

If you eat just the amount of fat that is removed from the fat stores to furnish the energy not supplied by the carbohydrates, your weight will remain the same. If you eat more fat, the excess will go into the fat stores and you will gain weight. If you eat less fat than is required to satisfy your energy needs, then the body will have to make up the deficit by removing fat from the fat stores and you lose weight.

Strategy #1, eating a low-fat diet, ensures that you add less fat to the fat stores. The less fat you add, the less you will have to remove later.

Strategies #2 and #3 are aimed at removing the fat that already pads your frame.

STRATEGY #2: EAT PLENTY OF NUTRIENT-DENSE, FIBER-RICH CARBOHYDRATES

Carbohydrates include both sugars (simple carbohydrates) and starches (complex carbohydrates) such as potatoes, other vegetables, rice, pasta, and bread. Fiber, a nondigestible form of carbohydrate, is found in vegetables, fruits, and whole grains. Fiber is filling and helps prevent overeating.

Carbohydrate: #1 Energy Source

The body burns a mixture of the carbohydrate, fat, and protein stored in the foods you eat to produce the energy it needs. But the *primary* and preferred fuel is carbohydrate. Carbohydrate provides most of the energy to fuel the muscles and other bodily functions and, in the form of the simple sugar glucose, is the only fuel your brain can use.

Eating a lot of carbohydrates keeps your BMR chugging along at a maximum rate.

The Fate of the Carbohydrates You Eat

Each day you consume about 50–60% of your total calories as carbohydrates. Most of it is burned within a few hours of consumption to fuel your physical activity and internal functions and is not stored or converted to fat.

A small amount of carbohydrate from each meal tops up the carbohydrate stores that have been partially used up between meals. The carbohydrate is stored as glycogen — long chains of the simple sugar glucose — in the muscles and in the liver.

Glycogen in the muscle is used for short bursts of intense activity, like playing tennis, and for "fight or flight" responses, such as jumping out of the path of a speeding car. Glycogen in the liver provides a constant supply of glucose to the brain, especially between meals, when glucose lev-

---

Keep Your Carbohydrate Tank on Full

When you eat a meal, some of the carbohydrate you consume tops up the glycogen stores. If you skimp on carbohydrates because you are following a low-calorie, low-carbohydrate, and/or high-protein diet, your glycogen stores will be inadequate and you will feel it. You will have diminished energy, stamina, and endurance.

els might otherwise drop. If glucose supply to the brain falls too low, you lose consciousness — a major inconvenience.

Excess Carbohydrate Calories Don't Turn to Fat

Although scientific research has proven over and over that excess carbohydrates are burned and released as heat, people still believe that carbohydrates turn to fat. Scientific experiments have shown that only if you were to eat more than 2200 calories of pure carbohydrate in addition to your normal daily total caloric intake for 5 to 6 days in a row might the excess carbohydrates possibly turn to fat. This is called glycogen loading and is not so easy to do.

Finding the Perfect Carbohydrate Balance

You need to eat lots of carbohydrates to keep your BMR at a maximum level, fuel your activity, keep up your energy level, and fuel your brain. But you don't want to eat so much that carbohydrate alone satisfies your energy needs. How do you limit the amount of carbohydrate you eat so you eat enough to reap their many benefits without eating so much you spare the stored fat from being mobilized and burned?

Bulk Provides Brakes. The built-in safety mechanism against overeating carbohydrates is provided by eating a healthy, nutrient-dense, fiber-rich diet. The bulk provided by fruits, vegetables, and whole grains ensures that you won't eat more carbohydrates than your body can handle. Imagine eating 5 baked potatoes at one sitting. Your body would cry, "NO MORE!" before you even finished 2.

STRATEGY #3: DAILY AEROBIC EXERCISE

Daily aerobic exercise helps you to reduce fat from the fat stores in two ways.

Exercising Increases Demand for Energy

First, and most important, by exercising you increase your total energy needs. To supply the additional energy, the body draws fat from the fat stores and you lose weight. That is, of course, if you are eating a low-fat, high-fiber diet and not adding more fat to the fat stores than you are removing.

Muscle Burns Fat and Raises BMR

Second, aerobic exercise builds and preserves muscle. Muscle is the tissue in the body that burns fat. The more muscle you have, the more fat-burning capacity you have. The more muscle you have, the higher your BMR and the faster you burn fat.

If you don't exercise, the muscle is broken down and not rebuilt. Over the years the loss of muscle can become significant. Sedentary adults may lose as much as 40% of their muscle mass — and their fat-burning capacity — between the ages of 20 and 70. It is no wonder that sedentary people who eat a high-fat diet gain weight as they age.

This doesn't have to be you. By exercising you protect your muscle from being broken down.

An aside: If you have been sedentary, you are fighting the battle of the bulge with one arm tied behind your back. But it is not too late. You can reverse the negative effects of a sedentary lifestyle at any time and at any age by starting to exercise and build fat-burning muscle.

Protein: Overrated

The role of protein in our diets is greatly misunderstood. Although many people associate rippling muscles with a diet of steaks and chops, the protein you eat doesn't build bulging biceps and triceps. It is used to rebuild muscle.

We tend to think of muscle as a permanent structure, but it is constantly being broken down and rebuilt (in response to use). When muscle is broken down, protein is released and burned. Since only small amounts of muscle are broken down and rebuilt each day, you don't need much protein in your diet. Scientific research has shown that adults need only about 12–15% of their calories from protein. And no matter what we eat, we generally get that amount.

Most Americans eat more than enough protein for good health. Consuming too much protein can put stress on the kidneys. In addition, since many people equate high-quality protein with red meat, and since red meat is filled with saturated fat, by eating lots of red meat you may be raising your cholesterol level and putting your heart at risk.

PUTTING IT ALL TOGETHER FOR SUCCESS

To lose weight you need to remove more fat from the fat stores than you add. The three *Choose to Lose* strategies work together to make it happen. First, eating a low-fat diet adds less fat to the fat stores. Second, eating a high-fiber diet limits the amount of carbohydrates you eat so carbohydrates alone do not satisfy your energy needs and the body has to raid the fat stores for the balance. And third, exercising increases your energy needs, thus increasing the amount of fat you need to withdraw from your fat bank.

Defeating the System

Choose to Lose Weight-Loss Plan for Men is a great weight-loss system that really works, but you have to follow all three strategies. This is what happens if you don't:

Fat Makes Fat. If you don't eat a low-fat diet (Strategy #1), and you eat too much fat, your fat stores get larger and so do you.

Fiber-Free Is Not Self-limiting. If you eat mainly processed, fiber-free foods like nonfat cookies, fat-free ice cream, and fat-free crackers, instead of fruits, vegetables, and whole grains (Strategy #2), you consume hundreds and even thousands of empty carbohydrate calories. Because these foods provide no bulk, there is no brake on overconsuming them. Since your body has limited capacity to store carbohydrates, it burns these calories instead of burning the fat from your fat stores and your weight loss is stalled.

No Exercise Means Muscle Loss. If you don't exercise (Strategy #3), you reduce your total energy needs, you lose muscle, and your BMR slows down. With lower energy needs, you don't need to withdraw fat from the fat stores and you don't lose weight.

Choose to Lose Strategies Bring Success

By incorporating all three strategies into your life, you will be on the road to healthy, safe, and permanent weight loss.

Now, on to Chapter 3 so you can determine your Fat Budget and get going on *Choose to Lose Weight-Loss Plan for Men*.

3. Action Plan

WE KNOW YOU are eager to get started, so go for it!

Choose to Lose Weight-Loss Plan for Men is a simple system. You just need to know:

1. Your personal **Fat Budget** — the maximum number of fat calories you can eat each day and still reach and maintain your desirable and healthy weight. Your Fat Budget is 20% of the total number of calories needed to satisfy your basal metabolism at your goal weight.
2. The number of **fat calories** in foods.
3. Your **minimum total calorie intake.***

DETERMINING YOUR FAT BUDGET

Your Fat Budget is tailored to you. It is based on your height, frame size, and goal weight. If you know the weight you want to achieve, skip Step 1 below. Otherwise, if you want to determine your desirable weight according to the Metropolitan Height-Weight Tables or are just curious to see how your idea of perfection compares to those weights listed in the tables, then consult Table 1. (If you are over 6 feet 2 inches tall, you may find that the weights recommended for your size seem slightly low. Adjust accordingly.) Women who are interested in determining their Fat Budgets and don't have a copy of *Choose to Lose* will find the appropriate tables in Appendix B.

---

* You should add more nutrient-dense, fiber-rich calories to fuel your physical activity.

Step 1: Determine Your Goal Weight

Table 1 lists desirable weights according to height and frame size —
small, medium, or large. (To determine your frame size, see the box below.) Find your height along the left-hand column of Table 1. Look
across to the weight range listed under your frame size and choose the
weight within the range that is right for you. Fill in Step 1 of the worksheet on page 16. Use George's worksheet on page 21 as a guide.

How to Determine Your Frame Size

Position your left hand around your right wrist. Touch your left
thumb to the top of your middle finger. If your finger overlaps your
thumb, you have a small frame. If they just touch, your frame size
is medium. If they do not touch, you have a large frame. This
method is crude, but adequate for our purposes. (If you know you
have a smaller or larger frame than this method indicates, use your
actual frame size and ignore the results of the wrist test.)

Table 1. Desirable Weights* for Men Age 25 and Over**

HEIGHT WITHOUT SHOES		FRAME		
(FEET)	(INCHES)	SMALL	MEDIUM	LARGE
5	1	112–120	118–129	126–141
5	2	115–123	121–133	129–144
5	3	118–126	124–136	132–148
5	4	121–129	127–139	135–152
5	5	124–133	130–143	138–156
5	6	128–137	134–147	142–161
5	7	132–141	138–152	147–166
5	8	136–145	142–156	151–170
5	9	140–150	146–160	155–174
5	10	144–154	150–165	159–179
5	11	148–158	154–170	164–184
6	0	152–162	158–175	168–189
6	1	156–167	162–180	173–194
6	2	160–171	167–185	178–199
6	3	164–175	172–190	183–204
6	4	168–179	177–195	188–209
6	5	172–183	182–200	193–214
6	6	176–187	187–205	198–219

* Weight in pounds without clothing.
** Courtesy of Metropolitan Life Insurance Company, New York, 1959. For
persons between 18 and 25 years of age, subtract 1 pound for each year
under 25.

Worksheet to Determine Your Daily Fat Budget

Name _____ Date _____

STEP 1: Determine your GOAL WEIGHT
         a. Height: ____ feet _____ inches
         b. Frame (wrist method):
            Small _____ Medium _____ Large _____
         c. Weight Range (Table): _____
         d. Goal Weight: _____

STEP 2: Determine your MINIMUM DAILY TOTAL
               CALORIC INTAKE
         Minimum Daily Total Caloric Intake (Table 2): _____

STEP 3: Determine your FAT BUDGET
         20% of _____ (Minimum Daily Total Caloric
         Intake) = _____

         Fat Budget = _____

Step 2: Determine Your ⟨Minimum⟩ Daily Total Caloric Intake

Find your desirable weight in the left-hand column of Table 2. On the same line in the next column you will find your minimum daily total caloric intake. Enter this number in Step 2 of your worksheet.

This is the number of calories needed to satisfy your basal metabolism at your desirable weight. To put it another way, this is the minimum number of calories you need each day to maintain your vital functions when you are *completely* at rest. This is a MINIMUM — A FLOOR.

Yes, Eat MORE Than the Minimum Total Caloric Intake

Your body needs more than this MINIMUM total caloric intake to operate because you need additional energy to power your physical activity (basal metabolism + physical activity = total calories). How much more depends on how much physical activity you do each day. For most people, 300 to 500 total calories in addition to the minimum total caloric intake will be sufficient. But if you eat a few hundred total calories be-

Table 2. Minimum Total Caloric Intake and Fat Budget for Men, Based on Goal Weight

GOAL WEIGHT	MINIMUM DAILY TOTAL CALORIC INTAKE	FAT BUDGET (FAT CALORIES)
110	1430	286
115	1495	299
120	1560	312
125	1625	325
130	1690	338
135	1755	351
140	1820	364
145	1885	377
150	1950	390
155	2015	403
160	2080	416
165	2145	429
170	2210	442
175	2275	455
180	2340	468
185	2405	481
190	2470	494
195	2535	507
200	2600	520
205	2665	533
210	2730	546
215	2795	559
220	2860	572
225	2925	585
230	2990	598
235	3055	611
240	3120	624
245	3185	637
250	3250	650

yond even that amount as fiber-rich carbohydrates, don't worry. They will be burned off, not stored as fat.

If at the end of the day you find you have eaten below the minimum, don't run to the store for a 6-pack of Coke to boost your total calorie consumption. Not only do nutrition-free calories add nothing to your health, but your body will be busy burning all those empty high-sugar and highly processed carbohydrate calories and will leave the fat calories happily ensconced in your fat stores.

Why You Must Eat MORE Nutritious Calories Than Your Minimum Total Caloric Intake

1. To ensure that you get enough energy (calories) to fuel your basal metabolism + physical activity.
2. To keep up your BMR. If your total caloric intake falls below the minimum amount you determined, your BMR will decrease and you will lose fat more slowly.
3. To ensure that you consume enough vitamins, minerals, and fiber for long-term health.
4. To ensure that you feel full and satisfied. Hunger leads to bingeing and making poor food choices that work against your healthy-eating, fat-loss goals.

Step 3: Determine Your Fat Budget

Your Fat Budget is 20% of your minimum daily total caloric intake. To determine your Fat Budget, find your goal weight again in Table 2 and look across to the column labeled **FAT BUDGET.** Fill in Step 3 of your worksheet. Now you know your Fat Budget. Engrave it in your mind.

Your Fat Budget Is a Ceiling

Remember, your Fat Budget is a ceiling — *not* a goal. If at the end of the day you have eaten only 150 fat calories and your Fat Budget is 416, don't feel compelled to dash off to McDonald's for a cheeseburger and fries to boost your fat intake up to your Fat Budget. Instead, congratulate yourself because you will reach your fat-loss goal that much sooner. Remember too — if you eat under your Fat Budget, you can bank some of the calories you saved for a treat in the future.

Losing by Stages

If you feel that the Fat Budget for your goal weight is too restrictive, you may want to choose a Fat Budget for an intermediate weight between your actual weight and your goal weight. For example, if you weigh 230 pounds and want to weigh 160, you may want to choose a

---

Fat Calories, Not Fat Grams

Choose to Lose Weight Loss Plan for Men uses fat calories rather than fat grams for three reasons.

1. Grams are a mystery to most people; calories are familiar.
2. Since your Fat Budget is a percentage of your minimum daily total **caloric** intake, it is logical to express both in the same unit — calories. To say that out of your intake of 2500 total *calories* no more than 50 *grams* should come from fat is confusing. Change that to 500 fat calories out of 2500 total calories, and you have a clear picture. Calories are units of energy. Grams are units of weight.
3. Fat content expressed as calories is much more impressive than fat content expressed as grams, since there are 9 calories in each gram of fat. A candy bar sounds a lot less enticing at 126 fat calories than at 14 fat grams.

Fat Budget for the intermediate weight of 190. Your Fat Budget would be 494 fat calories for 190 pounds rather than 416 for 160 pounds. Adhere to the intermediate Fat Budget until you weigh 190 pounds. When you attain that weight, adopt the Fat Budget for your next goal, 160 pounds. (This will be your Fat Budget for the rest of your life.) Your weight loss may be somewhat slower this way, but if you feel more comfortable working in stages, you are more likely to follow *Choose to Lose* until you reach your final goal.

GEORGE FIGURES OUT HIS FAT BUDGET

Meet George. George may be a kindred spirit. He has decided that he isn't crazy about the way he looks or feels. He knows he eats too much junk and is out of shape. His doctor has warned him that if he doesn't do something about his cholesterol, he may not be celebrating many more birthdays. George is ready to make changes in his lifestyle. He knows it is possible because his best friend, Charlie, has already lost 40 pounds and lowered his cholesterol 60 points by following *Choose to Lose Weight-Loss Plan for Men.* George is eager to get started.

Here's how George figures out his Fat Budget. (See George's worksheet, page 21.) George is 5 feet 9 inches tall. He determines by the wrist test that he has a medium frame. To find his goal weight, he locates his height (5′9″) in the left-hand column of Table 3. Reading across to the **FRAME** column labeled **MEDIUM,** he finds that his weight range is **146–160.** George knows that he will look and feel great at 160 pounds.

Table 3				
HEIGHT WITHOUT SHOES		**FRAME**		
FEET	**INCHES**	**SMALL**	**MEDIUM**	**LARGE**
5	8	136–145	142–156	151–170
5	**9**	**140–150**	**146–160**	**155–174**
5	10	144–154	150–165	159–179

Next, George needs to determine his minimum daily caloric intake. He locates his goal weight (**160**) on Table 4. Looking across to the column labeled **MINIMUM DAILY TOTAL CALORIC INTAKE,** he finds his number: **2080.** George is pleased. He knows he must eat more than 2080 nutritious total calories if he wants to lose weight. "Wow," says George. "This makes dieting something to look forward to!"

George looks across to the column labeled **FAT BUDGET.** He finds his daily Fat Budget — **416** fat calories.

Table 4		
GOAL WEIGHT	**MINIMUM DAILY TOTAL CALORIC INTAKE**	**FAT BUDGET (FAT CALORIES)**
155	2015	403
160	**2080**	**416**
165	2145	429

A FAT BUDGET PUTS FOOD CHOICES INTO PERSPECTIVE

How does George's Fat Budget of 416 fat calories relate to food? What about your Fat Budget? How does it translate into food choices?

Here are some foods and the fat calories they contain. (Fat calories for over 6000 foods can be found in the Food Tables at the end of the book.)

Worksheet to Determine Your Daily Fat Budget

Name _____ *George* _____ Date __*5/31/00*__

STEP 1: Determine your GOAL WEIGHT
         a. Height: __*5*__ feet __*9*__ inches
         b. Frame (wrist method):
             Small _____ Medium __*x*__ Large _____
         c. Weight Range (Table): ____*146–160*____
         d. Goal Weight: ___*160*___

STEP 2: Determine your MINIMUM DAILY TOTAL
            CALORIC INTAKE
         Minimum Daily Total Caloric Intake (Table 2): _*2080*_

STEP 3: Determine your FAT BUDGET
         20% of __*2080*__ (Minimum Daily Total Caloric
            Intake) = _*416*_

         Fat Budget = ___*416*___

As you read, keep your own Fat Budget in mind. Remember, if you eat a 6-ounce bag of potato chips, your consumption of fat calories will not be 90. It will be 6 × 90 fat calories per ounce, or 540 fat calories.

The Good, the Bad, and the Ugly	
FOOD	**FAT CALORIES**
American cheese (1 oz)	80
Baked potato with skin	0
Baked potato with chili and cheese (Wendy's)	220
Belgian waffle	177
Belgian waffle + whipped topping	288
Biscuit	130
Chicken breast baked without skin	13
Chicken breast, batter-dipped and fried, with skin	166
Egg (yolk)	50

Glazed doughnut	130
Ham and cheese sandwich on buttered bread	215
Hamburger (quarter pound)	243
Hot dog (2 oz.)	150
Margarine (1 tbsp)	100
Mayonnaise (1 tbsp)	100
Milk, whole (1 cup)	75
Milk, 2% (1 cup)	45
Milk, skim (1 cup)	0
Mr. Goodbar candy bar	160
Peanut butter (1 tbsp)	70
Peanuts (1 oz)	125
Pizza (Pizza Hut, personal pan, pepperoni)	180
Potato chips (1 oz or 18 chips)	90
Ranch salad dressing (2 tbsp)	150
Sirloin steak (6 oz)	276
Spare ribs (8 oz)	616
Sweet and sour pork (Chinese restaurant)	1509
Tuna salad sandwich with mayonnaise	325

Do any of these numbers surprise you? Do you now understand why you have trouble seeing your toes?

Your Fat Budget Makes You Food-Smart

Armed with your Fat Budget, you will be able to make wise food choices. You will see the advantage of choosing a turkey sandwich with mustard on French bread (32 fat calories) over turkey on a croissant with mayonnaise (235 fat calories). Both choices are delicious, but while the turkey croissant decimates your Fat Budget, the turkey on French bread barely makes a dent. You won't eat a food just because it's there. Before you pop a handful of trail mix into your mouth, knowing that half a cup costs about 180 fat calories and your Fat Budget is 416 fat calories, you can decide if that fleeting pleasure is worth more than two-fifths of your Fat Budget.

Your Fat Budget Allows You to Splurge

Because *Choose to Lose Weight-Loss Plan for Men* is forever, you must have the option to fit high-fat favorites into your diet. (Of course, not at every meal or every day — your goal is to move away from a high-fat diet.) Your Fat Budget will help you evaluate those choices. If an urge to have a cup of Ben & Jerry's New York Super Fudge Chunk ice cream overcomes you, think it over. You determine the cost by looking it up in the Food Tables — 380 fat calories. To accommodate this overdraft, you will have to balance the fat calories with low-low-fat choices for several days, but you can have it. With *Choose to Lose Weight-Loss Plan for Men*, you never have to feel guilty or deprived.

You won't believe it now, but eventually you may find that you no longer obsess over certain foods. First of all, knowing that you can fit them into your Fat Budget makes you less frantic about eating them. Second, your tastes change. What you once thought was ambrosia may soon turn your stomach. You'll begin to taste the grease.

Having a Fat Budget and making choices will make you appreciate what you eat. You might find that pizza once a month is much more enjoyable than three times a week — because it is a treat and you really taste it.

Keeping Track

Read the next chapter to witness how George records his "perfect diet." His choices may look familiar.

4. A Day in the Life . . .

IF YOU ARE LIKE MOST MEN, you pay little attention to the health aspects of the foods you eat. You only know they are convenient or they taste good. You generally know which foods are fattening, but "how fattening?" is not a question that often crosses your mind. You may not even associate the extra fat on your body, your shortness of breath, and your elevated cholesterol count with your diet.

Turning a Negative into a Positive

Your lack of interest may prove to be a real advantage. When you start paying attention to fat calories and begin keeping track of what you eat, you are going to be able to make phenomenal changes.

The best way to get started is to look at what you are eating now.

In the following pages, you can get ideas and gain insight from the way George records and evaluates his consumption for one day. In Chapter 5, "Keeping Track," and Appendix A, we will discuss how you can start keeping track yourself.

GEORGE KEEPS TRACK

George has committed himself to *Choose to Lose Weight-Loss Plan for Men*. He is now ready to take control of his diet and keep track of every morsel he lets slip between his lips. However, he is not going to make any changes yet. He wants to see the magnitude of the damage before he begins to repair it. He wants to have a picture of how much fat he currently eats and which foods are the high-fat culprits. Writing down the times he eats will give him an idea of his eating patterns. Entering the specific amount of food he consumes will enable him to figure his fat intake exactly. He will use the Food Tables on pages 185–390 and nutrition labels to determine the fat calories of the foods he eats. He will review his food records and see if he is eating a healthy diet.

BREAKFAST: GOTTA EAT IT

George has a high-pressure job that starts early and ends late. He is supposed to be at work by 8:30 A.M., which means getting out of the house by 7:30. Instead of bothering his wife or taking the time to prepare breakfast himself, he stops off at the coffee shop near his office. He chooses a seat at the counter for quicker service.

George doesn't need a menu. He orders "the usual" — 2 eggs over easy, 2 slices of bacon, 2 pieces of buttered toast, and regular coffee. While he is waiting for the waitress, George takes his *Choose to Lose Weight-Loss Plan for Men* from his briefcase and looks up his breakfast in the Food Tables. Two fried eggs: 150 fat calories! Two slices of bacon: 56! One tablespoon of butter: 100 fat calories! George considers forgoing breakfast. However, he knows he needs to eat the way he normally eats for a few days so he can establish a baseline food record. He records his breakfast in his food record as he soberly waits to be served.

George's first entry in his food record looks like this.

George's Breakfast				
			CALORIES	
TIME	FOOD	AMOUNT	TOTAL	FAT
8:15 A.M.	Eggs	2	158	**100**
	Shortening	2 tsp	73	**73**
	Bacon	2 strips	72	**56**
	Toast	2 pieces	150	**20**
	Butter	1 tbsp	100	**100**
	Coffee	1 cup	0	**0**
	Table cream	1 tbsp	29	**26**
			Fat Calories:	**375**
			George's Fat Budget:	416

When he learned the cost, George was tempted to skip breakfast altogether. But he (or you or anyone) should *never* skip breakfast. Eating three meals a day full of low-fat, fiber-rich, nutrient-dense food is EX-TREMELY important for weight loss. Eating breakfast turns on your fat-burning motor. In addition, when you skip breakfast, it's easy to become too hungry and too weak to say no to a high-fat midmorning snack.

Eating breakfast is essential, but at 375 fat calories, the egg plate was a poor choice. George could have easily trimmed his meal by 252 fat calories by choosing poached eggs instead of fried, jelly instead of butter, 2% milk instead of cream, and by eliminating the bacon. Better still, he could take a few minutes to fix a healthy, filling breakfast — a large bowl of cold cereal with skim milk and banana slices, 2 pieces of whole-wheat toast with jelly, nonfat flavored yogurt, an orange — before he leaves for work.

For better breakfast choices, see Chapter 9, "Eating In."

Mother Knows Best

Many adults think the key to losing weight is to skip breakfast and/or lunch. Wrong. It doesn't work. Not only will your energy stores be depleted all day, causing you to be indistinguishable from a limp rag, but when you finally eat you'll lose total control. You'll tear the doors off your cupboards and refrigerator to ravage the high-fat foods inside. You'll never satisfy the emptiness you created by missing those earlier meals. If you had eaten breakfast and lunch, you would be full and have no need to binge.

Not only is it much healthier and much more satisfying to eat three well-balanced meals than to starve yourself all day, it is a more effective way to lose weight. You need to eat because your body needs fuel to keep up your BMR (see Chapter 2). Your body reacts to starvation by slowing down your metabolism, so you burn your fat more slowly. So eat and stoke the fires!

MIDMORNING SNACK

At about 10:30, Betty, the office manager, passes by George's desk with a box of doughnuts. This has become a midmorning ritual. "You get first choice," she says, cheerily pushing the box toward him. George hesitates (but not for long) and chooses a glazed doughnut. Normally he eats the doughnut with gusto. But today George first asks, "What is this glis-

tening, sinful tidbit costing me?" He looks it up in the Food Tables —
130 fat calories! He moans softly as he writes the number in his food record. He has already surpassed his Fat Budget, and it's only 10:30 in the
morning.

George's Morning Snack				
			CALORIES	
TIME	FOOD	AMOUNT	TOTAL	FAT
10:30 a.m.	Glazed doughnut	1 large	240	**130**
		Total Fat Calories:		**130**
		Accumulated Fat Calories:		**505**
		George's Fat Budget:		416

Instead of the doughnut, he could have eaten a carton of nonfat
flavored yogurt (0 fat calories), a bagel (9 fat calories) with jelly (0 fat
calories), an apple (0 fat calories), or all three (9 fat calories).

LUNCH: RELAX, CHOOSE WELL, AND ENJOY

Lunch for George is a quickly gobbled sandwich at his desk, an elegant
lunch with a client, or a hit-and-run visit to a fast-food restaurant. Since
he has a meeting after lunch, he plans to stop at a fast-food restaurant
on the way.

Fast-Food Restaurants: Limited Choices

The quickest, most convenient, and most ubiquitous restaurants are
fast-food restaurants. In fact, there are towns in which fast-food restaurants are the *only* restaurants.

Now that he has become interested in his health and weight, George
has second thoughts about the suitability of fast food. However, as he is
sticking to his typical diet on this first day, he acts normally and heads
for the sign of the golden arches. He doesn't have much time because his
meeting is scheduled for 1:30.

George looks up Big Mac and French fries in the FAST FOODS section
of the Food Tables as he waits in line. The 280 fat calories for the Big Mac
amount to two thirds of his Fat Budget, but he orders it anyway. A small

order of French fries at 90 fat calories is a better choice than a large order at 200 fat calories. George, be honest. George always gets a large order, so he writes down 200 fat calories.

One Big Mac is really not enough to eat. Every time George finishes one, he is hungry for another. But today he can't afford the second in terms of fat calories or time. He inhales his sandwich and fries, records the damage in his food records, and then rushes off to his appointment.

		George's Lunch		
			CALORIES	
TIME	**FOOD**	**AMOUNT**	**TOTAL**	**FAT**
12:30 P.M.	Big Mac	1	560	**280**
	Fries	1 large order	450	**200**
	Diet Coke	12 oz	0	**0**
		Total Fat Calories:		**480**
		Accumulated Fat Calories:		**985**
		George's Fat Budget:		416

Although George is tempted by fast-food restaurants because they are quick, relatively inexpensive, and everywhere, the price of convenience is more than his body can afford. He should weigh the cost in fat calories and health and stay away. His best choice is not to choose them at all.

Even if he comes with noble intentions, temptation abounds. A Roy Rogers cheesesteak (324 fat calories), a McChicken sandwich (261 fat calories), Long John Silver fish and fries (432 fat calories), an order of Taco Bell Nachos Supreme (220 fat calories), or even an order of fries at Burger King (190 fat calories) is hard to resist. Choose carefully at a sandwich shop or a real restaurant, or bring your lunch from home. For more on eating in and dining out, see Chapter 9, "Eating In: Best Choice" and Chapter 11, "Dining Out."

Diet Drinks: Why Waste Your Money?

After consuming 480 fat calories, George chose a diet drink. This choice is a throwback to the old diet mentality that sugar makes you fat. Unless you are a diabetic, you should not choose diet drinks. Diet drinks contain unhealthy sugar substitutes.

Regular sodas contain no fat and so are not fattening. However, regular sodas should be consumed in moderation because in excess the sugar will be burned in preference to fat and weight loss will be stalled. Both diet and regular sodas are poor choices. Choose more nutritious thirst quenchers: skim milk, 100% fruit juices, or water.

AFTERNOON SNACK

George arrives at his appointment on time. His 2-hour meeting is productive. Before he leaves, he stops by the snack room and chooses a Snickers bar from the vending machine. It is hard to imagine that such a small piece of food could be *that* high in fat. He reads the label: "Fat calories per serving: 130; serving size: one candy bar," and records it. "A high price for an energy boost," he admits to himself.

George's Afternoon Snack				
			CALORIES	
TIME	FOOD	AMOUNT	TOTAL	FAT
3:30 P.M.	Snickers bar	59 g (2 oz)	280	**130**
		Total Fat Calories:		**130**
		Accumulated Fat Calories:		**1115**
		George's Fat Budget:		416

Since George knew he was going to be on the road when a hunger attack occurred, he should have planned ahead. Packing a bag of fruit and/or a bagel makes healthy snacking as easy as peeling a banana.

DINNER: HE-MAN FARE

George returns to the office for a few hours of work. By the time he leaves work at 7:00 P.M., he is so hungry he is ready to eat his briefcase. As he drives home, he daydreams about biting into a thick steak or juicy hamburger. George's wife won't disappoint him. Although she arrives home from work several hours before he does, she isn't interested in spending time preparing dinner. Because she normally skips lunch, she is always so famished when she comes home that she immediately fills up on snack food. By the time George arrives, she is no longer hungry. For George's meal she generally throws some animal part into the broiler and a potato in the microwave. Needless to say, George's wife needs *Choose to Lose* as much as he does.

"Hi, honey!" he yells as he hangs up his coat. "What's for dinner?" George doesn't really need to ask. He smells the steak. George is ready to eat. He licks his lips as his wife sets his plate before him. Instead of just scooping up some margarine, he carefully measures out 1 tablespoon and drops it into his baked potato. For the first time he feels good about his choice. He has read that margarine is more heart-healthy than butter. "Wah?" he groans as he checks the food label. "Ninety fat calories per tablespoon?" He measures 2 tablespoons of Italian dressing and pours it over his small salad. 140 fat calories? Isn't salad diet food? George doesn't enjoy entering his dinner choices into his food record. As George puts his dinner dishes in the sink, he kicks himself for not taking a Pepcid-AC before dinner. The ads all say you can avoid heartburn if you take the pills before you eat. George assumes heartburn is a natural consequence of the digestive process.

		CALORIES		
George's Dinner				
TIME	FOOD	AMOUNT	TOTAL	FAT
8:00 P.M.	Sirloin steak	6 oz	474	**276**
	Baked potato	1 large	100	**0**
	Margarine	1 tbsp	90	**90**
	Lettuce salad	1 cup	5	**0**
	Italian salad dressing	2 tbsp	140	**140**
	Pepcid-AC	1	0	**0**
		Total Fat Calories:		**506**
		Accumulated Fat Calories:		**1621**
		George's Fat Budget:		416

George's wife is like millions of working people. They work from sunup to sundown, spend hours commuting back and forth, and when they finally arrive home, the last thing they want to do is cook. Many make dinner by zapping frozen dinners in the microwave. Some, like George's wife, choose no-fuss high-fat meats. Both alternatives are costly choices, both health-wise and money-wise. Frozen dinners often contain little food but lots of fat and additives. Red meat is not only filled with a lot of fat, but much of that fat is saturated. Saturated fat is the culprit that raises your cholesterol and clogs your coronary arteries.

Hooray for Real Food

The benefits of preparing your own meals from scratch are incalculable. Not only will you eat healthier, the food you eat will also taste delicious and you'll get a lot more to eat. *Cajun Chicken** over steamed rice, whipped sweet potatoes, and steamed broccoli will make you a lot happier than the contents of a cardboard box. Preparing dinner doesn't have to take a lot of time. Share the preparation with your significant other. Who knows? You might have the makings of a great chef.

It's Not the Potato . . .

The baked potato was an excellent choice. Chock-full of vitamins, minerals, and fiber, potatoes are both healthy and delicious. Fill that potato with butter, sour cream, or margarine, as George did, and you have reduced your potato into a receptacle for fat. Potatoes without fat *are* a treat! Eat them plain or with nonfat yogurt.

Margarine: Heart-Healthy?

Because margarine is much less saturated than butter (most margarines have 18 sat-fat calories per tablespoon; butter has 65) and saturated fat raises blood cholesterol, margarine had been considered a healthy substitute for butter. However, recent scientific evidence has shown that the trans fats in margarines affect your blood cholesterol the same way saturated fats do. In addition to raising LDL** or bad cholesterol (see Chapter 15, "To Your Health"), they are also 100% fat and fattening. One tablespoon of margarine has 90 fat calories. While still a better choice than butter, margarine should be used sparingly.

---

* Recipes in italics come from *Eater's Choice Low-Fat Cookbook* by Dr. Ron and Nancy Goor (Houghton Mifflin, 1999).

** For a fuller discussion of LDL, saturated fats, and trans fats, see *Eater's Choice: A Food Lover's Guide to Lower Cholesterol* by Dr. Ron and Nancy Goor (Houghton Mifflin, 1999).

Salad: High-Fat Choice

George concluded that salad must be good weight-loss food because he has observed so many dieters eating it. But salad is generally one of the worst choices for weight loss. First of all, the ingredient that makes salad so popular is salad dressing. In fact, for most people salad is the sociably acceptable excuse for eating salad dressing. (What people *really* want to order is a bowl of salad dressing plain, salad on the side.) Salad dressing is hardly diet food. Two tablespoons of the Italian dressing on George's small salad cost 140 fat calories. On a larger salad, half a cup (560 fat calories) is typical.

Second, even if you use lemon juice or nonfat dressing, a salad is a poor choice for someone who wants to lose weight. Salad is generally not filling and not enough to eat. Lettuce, the major ingredient, is mostly water and hardly nutritious. After a meager meal of salad greens, diet rabbits quickly turn into ravenous hogs and devour every high-fat food in sight.

The Case of the Missing Vegetable

You may have noticed that George assiduously avoids fruits and vegetables. He'll tell you he's a meat and potatoes man. (Don't tell him that potatoes are vegetables.) Perhaps his only memory of vegetables is of the soggy, overcooked vegetables of his youth. Many people have no memory of vegetables because they never had any. George is in for a treat. Vegetables and fruit provide a scrumptious variety of tastes and textures, as well as vitamins, minerals, and fiber.

Chuck the Antacids

One of the biggest surprises (and pleasures) to people following *Choose to Lose Weight-Loss Plan for Men* is that they don't have heartburn. Heartburn is not a natural result of eating. Spicy food and garlic do not give you heartburn — fatty foods do. So when you reduce the fatty foods in your diet, you eliminate heartburn.

HIGH-FAT SNACKS: ADDICTIVE AND ADDITIVE

After dinner George plays at doing work from the office. He doesn't have his heart in it. After an hour he joins his wife in front of the television. He grabs a beer, a jar of peanuts, and a bowl. Before he eases himself into his favorite chair, he thinks, "I'll measure the amount of peanuts I put into the bowl before I eat them, then I'll measure the amount left and subtract it from the original number to find out how many fat calories I consumed."

Good idea, George. He measures three-quarters of a cup into the bowl. At the end of the evening, George's bowl is empty. "Did I do that?" he asks. He almost passes out when he reads the jar label and determines that his "light" snack cost him 485 fat calories. He adds the item to his food record.

			CALORIES	
George's Evening Snack				
TIME	FOOD	AMOUNT	TOTAL	FAT
9:00–11:00 P.M.	Peanuts	¾ cup	620	**485**
	Beer	2 (12 fl oz each)	300	**0**
		Total Fat Calories:		**485**
		Accumulated Fat Calories:		**2106**
		George's Fat Budget:		416

Snack foods are guaranteed to send your Fat Budget into a tailspin. The salty, fatty taste makes it impossible not to eat "just one more." It is humanly impossible to eat one peanut or potato chip or corn chip. One leads to another and another, until finally there are none left. The snacker eats without thought. Hand to bowl to mouth to bowl to mouth. When the bottom of the bowl appears, he can't imagine where all the snacks went.

A *Choose to Lose Weight-Loss Plan for Men* tip: Keep high-fat snacks out of your home. Try air-popped popcorn instead.

THE AWFUL TRUTH

George shakes his head in disbelief. There must be a mistake. His records show that he ate 1621 fat calories from breakfast through dinner. By the time he finished his evening snack, he had eaten 2106 calories of fat.

You may think that his fat calorie intake is unusually high, but George's diet is typical of many American men.

He adds up the numbers again. He has made no mistake, in adding that is.

			CALORIES		
TIME	FOOD	AMOUNT	TOTAL	FAT
8:15 A.M.	Eggs	2	158	**100**
	Shortening	2 tsp	73	**73**
	Bacon	2 strips	72	**56**
	Toast	2 pieces	150	**20**
	Butter	1 tbsp	100	**100**
	Coffee	1 cup	0	**0**
	Table cream	1 tbsp	29	**26**
10:30 A.M.	Glazed doughnut	1 large	240	**130**
12:30 P.M.	Big Mac	1	560	**280**
	Fries	1 order	450	**200**
	Diet Coke	12 oz	0	**0**
3:30 P.M.	Snickers bar	59 g (2 oz)	280	**130**
8:00 P.M.	Sirloin steak	6 oz	474	**276**
	Baked potato	1 large	100	**0**
	Margarine	1 tbsp	90	**90**
	Lettuce salad	1 cup	5	**0**
	Italian salad dressing	2 tbsp	140	**140**
9:00–11:00 P.M.	Peanuts, dry-roasted	¾ cup	620	**485**
	Beer	2 (12 fl oz each)	300	**0**

George's Baseline Food Record

Total Calories: 3841

Accumulated Fat Calories: 2106

George's Fat Budget: 416

Before You Know It . . .

Even if your diet is not as poor as George's, fat calories have a sneaky habit of accumulating. It is like your monthly credit card bill. "A thousand dollars?" you cry in disbelief. "There must be a mistake. I didn't spend that much money." You take out your calculator. A $45 shirt, a $30 gasoline charge, a $59 TV repair bill, and on and on. Nothing big, but it all adds up to a whopping $1000. Fat calories work the same way. A glass of 2% milk (45 fat calories), 3 crackers (30 fat calories), a slice of bologna (59 fat calories). They all add up until you've wildly overspent your Fat Budget.

Food Records = Insight

Reviewing his day's food intake gives George insight. He can see exactly why he is overweight (he is 1690 fat calories over his Fat Budget of 416) and why he is always hungry: lots of fat and not much food. Looking over his baseline food record, he can easily find the sources of fat in his diet, so he can choose to eliminate them, eat them in smaller amounts, or eat them less often. With his newly acquired insight, he won't regard eggs or margarine as benign. He'll save doughnuts, candy bars, and peanuts for special treats instead of gobbling them up with no thought. He'll choose snacks that are healthier and lower in fat. He'll make fast-food restaurants his last choice rather than his first. He'll read labels *before* eating a food so he can decide if it's worth the cost.

Getting to the Minimums

George is amazed to see how little food he consumes and how little of it is nutritious. Look at George's food record. Do you see any fruit? What is the only vegetable? (French fries don't count because they have too much fat to be considered nutritious.) George can already think of many places where he could have enjoyed nutritious food instead of his high-fat choices. (Look on page 37 to see how George turned his meal plan around.)

Eating a well-balanced diet is essential for long-term as well as current health. Vegetables and fruit contain fiber, vitamins, and minerals, add color and texture to your meal, and taste wonderful. They fill you up, improve your bowel function, and help reduce your risk of prostate and colon cancer. What's more, vegetables and fruit can be eaten with abandon because they contain little or no fat.

If you avoid vegetables because you think you don't like them, give them another chance. Try steaming vegetables until they are crisp but tender. Try vegetables you've never eaten, like butternut squash, spaghetti squash, or cauliflower. Have 2 carrots with lunch. Your world will open up.

Whole grains are also vital for your health. Choose whole-wheat bread over white. Cereal makes a great breakfast and snack. Try to find low-fat cereals with dietary fiber higher than 3 or 4 grams per serving.

Include nonfat or low-fat dairy such as flavored nonfat or low-fat yogurts, skim milk or 1% milk, and 1% cottage cheese. These foods provide the calcium you need for strong bones and teeth.

Don't think that just because you are older you don't need as many vitamins, minerals, and fiber. You never outgrow your need for these nutrients.

In Chapter 6, "A Celebration of Food," we will delve more into the Food Guide Pyramid and you.

Making Changes: Easier Than You Think

Hard as it is to believe, changing from George's skimpy, sky-high-fat diet to an abundant, low-fat, delicious, nutritious diet is very easy. It just takes a little thought and planning. For some, the changes will need to be made gradually. If you are used to dumping 2 tablespoons of butter into your baked potato, eating it plain may jar your taste buds. You may need to move from 2 tablespoons to 1 tablespoon to 1 teaspoon to eventually eating it plain. After all, diet habits were not developed in a day. For others, change can be made swiftly with no turning back. "Throw away that greasy fried shrimp," you cry. "Give me steamed shrimp dipped in cocktail sauce instead." Whether your style is to make gradual changes or to cut the fat all at once, you'll love your new style of eating.

GEORGE GOES COLD TURKEY

On page 37, you can see how George has modified his original meal plan. He is plunging headlong into *Choose to Lose Weight-Loss Plan for Men*. No intermediate measures for George. (You may want to make a slower transition.) He didn't poach his eggs rather than fry them. He eliminated eggs and chose oatmeal. He chose *Grainy Mustard Chicken* served over steamed rice rather than a smaller piece of high-fat beef. He packed a turkey sandwich for lunch instead of choosing fast food. Instead of causing terminal damage to his Fat Budget with his peanut snack, he enjoyed 8 cups of air-popped popcorn.

ORIGINAL MEAL PLAN			REPLACEMENT MEAL PLAN		
	CALORIES			**CALORIES**	
FOOD	**TOTAL**	**FAT**	**FOOD**	**TOTAL**	**FAT**
Breakfast			**Breakfast**		
2 fried eggs	158	100	2 cups Wheaties	220	20
2 tsp shortening	73	73	12 fl oz skim milk	120	0
2 strips bacon	72	56	1 banana, sliced	105	5
2 slices white toast	150	20	2 slices whole-wheat	160	20
1 tbsp butter	100	100	toast		
8 fl oz coffee	0	0	1 tbsp jelly	55	0
1 tbsp cream	29	26	8 fl oz nonfat fruit	200	0
			yogurt		
Snack			8 fl oz coffee	0	0
1 large doughnut	240	130	8 fl oz orange juice	110	0
Lunch			**Lunch**		
1 Big Mac	560	280	2 turkey sandwiches		
1 large order fries	450	200	4 slices whole-wheat	320	40
12 oz Diet Coke	0	0	toast		
_____			4 oz turkey breast	124	8
_____			4 slices tomato	24	0
_____			2 tbsp mustard	30	0
_____			2 tbsp hot peppers	10	0
_____			2 carrots	60	0
			1 orange	60	0
Snack			**Snack**		
1 Snickers bar (59 g)	280	130	1 toasted onion bagel	230	10
_____			1 apple	81	0
Dinner			**Dinner**		
6 oz sirloin steak	474	276	2 cups *Carrot Soup*	138	0
1 large baked potato	100	0	*Grainy Mustard Chicken*	193	13
1 tbsp margarine	90	90	1 cup white rice	264	0
1 cup lettuce salad	5	0	1 cup broccoli, steamed	0	0
2 tbsp Italian dressing	140	140	1 tsp balsamic vinegar	0	0
_____			1 baked sweet potato	118	0
			2 fat-free Fig Newtons	100	0
Snack			**Snack**		
¾ cup peanuts	620	485	8 cups air-popped	240	0
2 beers (12 fl oz each)	300	0	popcorn		
TOTAL	3841	2106	**TOTAL**	2962	116

Food weight: 5 lbs 11 oz
Fruit = 0; Vegetables = 1½; Dairy = 0;
  Grains = 0

Food weight: 7 lbs 10 oz
Fruit = 4; Vegetables = 4; Dairy = 2½;
  Grains = 11

You will notice that George is eating much more really delicious and satisfying food in his modified plan than in the original, and yet the fat and total calories are significantly lower.

How About YOU?

To learn the skills that will further empower you to take control, read on.

5. Keeping Track

GEORGE GAINED AMAZING INSIGHT from keeping track of every food that he devoured. In this chapter, you will acquire the specific skills you need to evaluate your diet and make changes. You will learn how to use the Food Tables to find the "cost" of foods and how to keep track of the foods you eat.

In Chapter 8, you will master reading a nutrition label. In Chapters 9, 11, and 12, you will learn how to cope in any eating situation. You will soon have all the tools you need to make significant and lasting changes. The world will be yours.

KEEPING TRACK GIVES YOU INSIGHT

Establishing a Baseline

Before you can analyze and change your eating habits, you need to know what they are. Consider the following strategy:

1. Keep a baseline food record for 3 days — two weekdays and one weekend day — as George did. See Appendix A, page 405, for a detailed explanation of how to keep a food record using George's example.
2. Analyze your food records for:

   • Fat: Where's it coming from?
   • Total calories: Are you eating enough?
   • A balanced diet: Are you eating 2 to 4 servings of fruit, 3 to 5 servings of vegetables, 2 to 3 servings of dairy, and 6 to 11 servings of grain? (See the Minimum Basic Nutritional Requirements table in Chapter 6, "A Celebration of Food," for definitions of serving sizes.)

3. Begin making changes.

Food Records Are the Ticket

People who keep track of the foods they eat are much more likely to lose weight. Or you could say the reverse. People who do not keep track are much less likely to lose weight. After all, how do you know how much fat you are consuming unless you look it up and write it down? How can you make choices if you don't know the cost? Keeping accurate food records will give you insight into your eating habits and empower you to take control.

Some Men Love Keeping Track

You may actually *enjoy* keeping food records. Choosers to Lose have told us they actually *liked* keeping track of their fat calories. Mike Pierce, from South Dakota, said, "Keeping food records is like a game. You can see at any time how you are doing. It's a challenge to get where you want to be at the end of the week."

Keeping Track Made Easy

You can jot down your food record on a small notepad that you keep in your pocket. But to make keeping track easier, we recommend purchasing an inexpensive *Choose to Lose* Passbook and Balance Book Refills, which have everything organized for you. (See order form on the last page of this book.)

Don't Panic

Even if you aren't wildly ecstatic about keeping food records, you won't have to do it forever. After a short while, it won't even take much time. You don't eat that many different foods. And sooner than you think, you will learn the combinations of foods you like to eat that fit within your Fat Budget and you won't have to write everything down. You will have developed a new low-fat style of eating that will be as natural to you as your current eating pattern.

Of course, when a new food crops up, you will want to refer to the Food Tables or to nutrition labels to determine the cost and decide if or how it can fit into your Fat Budget. If you find your weight is creeping back up, you will want to start keeping track again to make sure you have complete control of your diet.

DETERMINING FAT CALORIES IN FOODS

Many people are overweight because they don't realize how much fat they are eating. To make informed choices, you need to know the exact amount of fat lurking in the foods you eat. You will use several sources to determine this amount. *Choose to Lose Weight-Loss Plan for Men* Food Tables list fat calories, sat-fat calories, and total calories for over 6000 foods. As we just mentioned, you will learn in Chapter 8 how to read nutrition labels so you can figure out the fat in commercial products.

Sound simple? It is.

THE FOOD TABLES

First, the Food Tables. Turn to page 183 and flip through the Food Tables. These extensive tables will give you invaluable information about the foods you eat. Not only can you use them to look up the fat calories of foods you eat, ate, or plan to eat, you can browse through them to find low-fat alternatives for high-fat foods.

Organization

The Food Tables are organized alphabetically into major food groups such as **BEVERAGES, DAIRY AND EGGS, FAST FOODS.** You will find a list of these groups in the Food Tables contents on page 185. You may want to stick tabs at the beginning of each section so you can find them quickly.

Within each major food group, food categories are listed alphabetically. For example, the first subheading in the **FATS AND OILS** group is *Animal Fats,* and the next subheading is *Butter Substitutes.* Likewise, within these secondary categories, foods are also listed alphabetically. Listed under *Animal Fats* is Beef tallow, then Butter.

Food Tables Index

If you have trouble finding a food in the Food Tables, check the Food Tables Index on pages 391–401 where foods are listed alphabetically rather than grouped by type.

Is the Food Tables Amount Your Amount?

Always check the amount column before you record the fat calories for a food. The amount listed may or may not be the amount you plan to eat. For example, 70 fat calories are listed for beef bologna, but for what amount? Look closely. The amount is 28 grams (1 oz) or 1 slice. How many slices did you pack into your sandwich yesterday? Two (2 x 70 = 140 fat calories) or three (3 x 70 = 210 fat calories)? Or was it more likely four (4 x 70 = 280 fat calories)? The amount you actually eat clearly makes a difference.

Comparison Value. To make it easier to compare the fat in foods, data for many foods are given in similar amounts. For instance, soups are given in 1-cup amounts, and ice creams are given in half-cup amounts. Cheeses and meats are given in 1-ounce (28 g) amounts. You can easily compare the fat in half-cup of Häagen-Dazs strawberry ice cream with the fat in half a cup of Breyers strawberry ice cream or the fat in 1 ounce of flank steak versus 1 ounce of sirloin steak. Of course, you probably eat more than half a cup of either ice cream, and be assured that no one eats only 1 ounce of either flank or sirloin steak. So you must always adjust the fat calories to the amount you actually eat.

Amounts in the Food Tables are often listed in grams.
28 grams = 1 ounce*

Finding Better Choices

Not only can you use the Food Tables to determine the cost of the foods you might eat, you can also use them to find better choices. Here's a true life example. At the Au Bon Pain kiosk at the Boston train station, we each ordered a turkey sandwich on a 4-grain roll for our trip home. When we arrived home, we checked the RESTAURANT FOODS section of the Food Tables under *Au Bon Pain* (we should have been carrying our *Choose to Lose* Passbook with abbreviated food tables!) and found to our dismay that the 4-grain roll costs 99 fat calories. Ninety-nine fat calories! We would have been just as happy had we chosen a baguette (French bread) for only 18 fat calories. We could have averted this disaster had we looked at our choices in the Food Tables first.

---

* Actually, 1 ounce equals 28.35 grams.

GETTING SERIOUS

Approach #1: One Fell Swoop

If you know you can slash your fat to fit your Fat Budget in one fell swoop and not shed a tear, go for it. Each to his own approach.

Approach #2: Easy Does It

You have been eating a high-fat diet for years. You are accustomed to bacon and eggs and big fat greasy hamburgers. You are ready to change your eating habits, but whoa, not all at once. If this is your style, take a few weeks to work up to total *Choose to Lose Weight-Loss Plan for Men* immersion. Reduce your fat intake gradually. For many, changes made gradually are more permanent.

Go for the Worst First and Make Changes in Stages

If "easy does it" is your style, start by targeting the worst culprits first. You don't have to wipe them off your plate completely. You can moderate your intake of high-fat foods by doing one of the following:

1. Consume smaller amounts.
2. Eat them less often.
3. Replace them with low-fat substitutes.
4. Eliminate them entirely.

Choose Smaller Amounts. Reviewing your food records, you find that margarine is a major high-fat offender. Margarine is a prime candidate for downsizing for two reasons. Not only is margarine full of fat (90 fat calories per tablespoon), it contains trans fats that act like saturated fat in the body and raise blood cholesterol. You can easily reduce the 2 tablespoons you inflict on your bagel to 1 tablespoon. Next try 2 teaspoons. How about 1 teaspoon? You might surprise yourself and enjoy your bagel plain or with jelly.

Choose Less Often. Your food records show that you ate cheese and crackers every evening before dinner during this three-day period. Instead of consuming 10 crackers (about 70 fat calories) + 10 slices of cheese (about 160 fat calories), why not skip your daily cheese and cracker fix and move directly to dinner? Save that cheese and cracker splurge for one Friday evening a month. You'll really appreciate the taste, and you'll be doing your arteries a favor.

Choose Low-Fat Alternatives. You find that whole milk represents a major contributor to your fat calorie bank. At 75 fat calories per 8-fluid-ounce glass (4 glasses = 300 fat calories), milk can give your Fat Budget a nervous breakdown. Try drinking 2% milk (45 fat calories per cup) instead. It tastes almost the same because it *is* almost the same. Get used to 2% and try the tip on page 68 to move to 1% (14 fat calories per cup) or skim (0 fat calories per cup).

Use the Food Tables to find alternatives for other high-fat foods as well. For example, if you normally fry up a rasher of bacon for breakfast, check the MEAT (*Pork*) section in the Food Tables for a lower-fat substitute. For about one-third fewer fat calories, you'll get four times more Canadian bacon.

Choose Not at All. Are there high-fat foods you used to eat that are just not worth the bite they take out of your Fat Budget? Did you really enjoy that bag of potato chips 270-fat-calories-worth? Did you eat them because they were there and you were bored? If so, make potato chips a no-no and eliminate them entirely. Are there foods that cry, "Just say yes," but if you aren't subjected to them, you don't miss them? For example, can you live very well without chocolate candy unless it is stuck under your nose? Eliminate those high-fat foods you can live without.

Your Turn

The information in this chapter may seem pretty abstract now, but once you start following *Choose to Lose Weight-Loss Plan for Men,* you will see how to evaluate your food choices and make constructive changes.

For the nitty-gritty on keeping food records, check out Appendix A, pages 405–408. Try keeping your own. It will be an insightful and rewarding experience.

Skimming the Fat Is Not Enough

So far our focus has been on fat. You know how to find it, and you have learned strategies to keep it in check. But as we have also emphasized, reducing fat is not enough. You also need to eat a lot of nutritious food. You need to make sure you are getting enough vitamins, minerals, and fiber for good health and so you are NOT HUNGRY. The next chapter will show you what a full, magnificent diet you will be enjoying.

6. A Celebration of Food

Choose to Lose Weight-Loss Plan for Men is not just about what you can't eat or what you should limit. It's about what you *can* eat. It's about eating delicious, nutrient-dense, fiber-rich foods. *Choose to Lose Weight-Loss Plan for Men* is a celebration of food.

In the first few chapters, we have given you the tools to reduce fat in your diet. But reducing fat is not enough. You must replace some of the fat you eliminate with foods rich in complex carbohydrates — whole grains, vegetables — and fruits. You need to eat low-fat or nonfat dairy products. You need to change your focus from high-fat to low-fat meats such as chicken, turkey, fish, and seafood.

Enjoying some of these foods — like fruits and vegetables — may be a new experience for you. According to numerous population studies, one-third of Americans eat no fruits and vegetables. If this means you, you have a real treat in store. Fruits and vegetables are delicious, and they contain vitamins, minerals, and fiber, which are vital for keeping you healthy.

Health Benefits

Here are a few examples of the benefits of eating fruits, vegetables, and whole grains: Eating foods such as sweet potatoes, carrots, cooked spinach, and cantaloupe — rich sources of beta carotene — may help prevent cancer, heart disease, and cataracts. On the other hand, *not* eating foods such as whole-grain cereals, cooked lentils, spinach, and asparagus — foods high in folic acid (a B vitamin) — may increase your risk for stroke, heart disease, or colon cancer. Eating bananas, chicken, and rice — good sources of vitamin B_6 — and oranges, strawberries, broccoli, and red peppers — good sources of vitamin C — can give your immune system a boost.

A Pill Is Not Food. If you're thinking, "Hey, I'll just buy vitamin and mineral supplements and avoid the food," you're jumping to the wrong solution. Scientists know that people who eat a low-fat diet and lots of vegetables, fruits, and whole grains have reduced risks of cancer and heart disease, but they cannot say if just eating the isolated nutrients in foods will help improve long-term health. So taking megadoses of vitamins or other supplements is not the answer. Moreover, when taken in too great amounts (and the optimum amount is often unknown), vitamin and mineral supplements can be harmful.

Eating nutrient-dense, fiber-rich foods has added benefits beyond supplying essential vitamins, minerals, and fiber. It keeps up your metabolism and keeps you from being hungry. Besides, it is extremely enjoyable.

Nutrient-Dense, Fiber-Rich Foods Are Self-limiting

Choose to Lose Weight-Loss Plan for Men allows you to eat lots of carbohydrates, but not just any kind of carbohydrates. Be sure the carbohydrates you choose are nutrient-dense and fiber-rich. If you are eating nutrient-dense, fiber-rich carbohydrates, it is almost impossible to overeat them. They are so bulky and filling they will limit themselves. Imagine eating 15 carrots (450 total calories). You'd have trouble doing it. On the contrary, inhaling two-fifths of an Entemann's Fat-and-Cholesterol-Free Butter Crunch Cake (440 total calories) leaves you ready for more. It is almost impossible *not* to overeat fiber-free, nutrient-free foods.

For guidance in choosing foods to reach your goal to be healthy and lean, follow the recommendations of the lower half of the Food Guide Pyramid. If you fulfill those requirements, you will be too full to even think of overdosing on high-fat or empty calories.

USING THE FOOD GUIDE PYRAMID

The Department of Agriculture developed the Food Guide Pyramid to help people make wise food choices. The pyramid shape clearly shows the relative nutritional value of basic foods and the importance of eating more of some foods than others.

Start at the base. The base gives you a healthy foundation. You should consume whole-grain breads and cereals, rice, and pasta. (Note: Pastas,

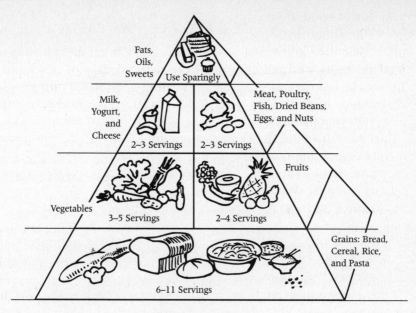

Fats,
Oils,
Sweets   Use Sparingly

Milk,
Yogurt,
and
Cheese

2–3 Servings

Meat, Poultry,
Fish, Dried Beans,
Eggs, and Nuts

2–3 Servings

Fruits

Vegetables

3–5 Servings

2–4 Servings

Grains: Bread,
Cereal, Rice,
and Pasta

6–11 Servings

Food Guide Pyramid

white breads, and white rice are grains that should be consumed in moderation, as they are highly processed and relatively low in fiber or fiber-free. Pastas topped with high-fat sauces and bread slathered with butter are to be considered fats, not grains.) Add lots of vegetables and fruits. Milk products and meat (preferably low-fat) come next and may be eaten in smaller amounts, and fats, oils, and sweets at the tip should be eaten sparingly. In general, Americans have turned this pyramid on its head and have, as a result, been totally out of balance for years.

A Tip for Meeting the Recommendations

Nancy Ochsner of Woodland Park, Colorado, thought of a great idea to ensure that you meet the Food Guide Pyramid recommendations: Each morning, place your fruit, vegetable, grain, and dairy requirements for the day on a plastic tray in the refrigerator and make sure you have emptied it by the time you go to sleep.

WHOLE-GRAIN BREADS, CEREALS, RICE, AND PASTA (at least 6–11 servings)

Eating starches used to be considered a no-no for weight loss. Now we know that carbohydrates are great diet food. You should eat bread. You should eat rice. You should eat spaghetti, and you should eat cereals. In fact, you should eat lots of whole-grain breads, cereals, rice, and pasta. But that does not mean bread slathered with peanut butter, rice mixed with gravy, or spaghetti floating in tomato-cream sauce. That also does not mean 10 slices of bread or 4 cups of pasta. Use sense. Don't push the system.

Not every grain that you eat has to be whole-grain. You may happily eat a plain bagel. But the best grains to eat are the whole grains because they are the most nutritious. Whole-grain breads are rich in fiber, protein, thiamin, riboflavin, niacin, folic acid, vitamin E, iron, phosphorus, magnesium, zinc, and other trace minerals. Check labels. The first ingredient should be whole-wheat flour. Some breads labeled "wheat bread" may contain no whole wheat. Almost all bagels labeled whole-wheat are made from white flour.

Grains: Eat at Least 6–11 Servings

Choose first from:

brown rice	oatmeal	whole-wheat cereals
buckwheat groats	pumpernickel bread	whole-wheat pastas
bulgur	whole-grain breads	

Whole grains contain loads of minerals and vitamins and fiber.

Choose less often from:

bagels	noodles	white breads
low-fiber cereals	pasta	white rice

FRUITS AND VEGETABLES (at least 2–4 servings of fruit and at least 3–5 servings of vegetables)

Because fruits and vegetables are healthy and almost fat-free (except avocado), you can eat them to your heart's content. They taste great! You

---

Make It Count

Warning: Before counting a food toward fulfilling your Food Guide Pyramid recommendations, be sure it meets the criterion for good health. Ask these questions. Is it a grain or is it a fat? Is it a dairy or is it a sweet? Is it a fruit or is it a candy? For example, don't count a croissant as a grain. A croissant is made of flour (grain) and lots of butter (fat — about 110 calories of fat). Croissants will do nothing to enhance your health. Don't count cookies, cake, or crackers either. They're entertainment, not nutrition. Don't count foods that have all the nutrients processed out of them, such as pretzels. (A pretzel or two make a nice snack, but since they don't really add to your health, don't count them.)

Don't count ice cream, frozen yogurt, or pudding as dairy. Some of these foods don't even contain dairy products. Remember, you want to meet the Food Guide Pyramid requirements to benefit your health, not just to reach a number on a piece of paper. You want to eat an abundance of foods that are rich in fiber, vitamins, and minerals — foods that will enhance your long-term health.

---

can even eat baked potatoes (hold the butter or sour cream) until you pop. Potatoes are no longer on the forbidden foods list.

The key to good health is eating a variety of fruits and vegetables because different ones offer different protections as well as making life more interesting. Choose vegetables with different colors and textures: orange (sweet potatoes, carrots, squash) provide an excellent source of vitamin A; leafy green (spinach, kale, bok choy) contribute vitamins A and C, riboflavin, folic acid, iron, and magnesium; and cruciferous (broccoli, cauliflower, and Brussels sprouts) help fight cancer.

Become a human fruit bowl. Eat oranges, grapefruit, apples, cantaloupe, honeydew melon, watermelon, strawberries, raspberries, peaches, pears, nectarines, plums, kiwi, and bananas, and you'll be consuming a multitude of life-enhancing vitamins and minerals. Fruit can be truly divine.

Bring a bag of fruit and carrot sticks to the office and dig in whenever hunger strikes. Try vegetables you have never tried before. Have you ever baked spaghetti squash? When you scrape out the cooked interior,

Try some of these!

Take this list with you to the grocery store:

FRUITS

- Apples
- Apricot
- Banana
- Blackberry
- Blueberries
- Boysenberries
- Cantaloupe
- Carambola
- Cherimoya
- Cherries
- Currants
- Dates
- Figs
- Grapefruit

- Grapes
- Guava
- Honeydew
- Kiwi fruit
- Kumquat
- Lychee
- Mango
- Nectarine
- Orange
- Papaya
- Passion fruit
- Peach
- Pear

- Persimmon
- Pineapple
- Plantain
- Plum
- Pomegranate
- Prickly pear
- Prune
- Quince
- Raspberries
- Rhubarb
- Strawberries
- Tangerine
- Watermelon

VEGETABLES

- Alfalfa sprouts
- Artichoke
- Arugula
- Asparagus
- Beets
- Bok choy
- Broccoli
- Celery
- Cabbage
- Carrots
- Cauliflower

- Collards
- Cucumber
- Corn
- Eggplant
- Endive
- Green Beans
- Kale
- Leeks
- Mushrooms
- Okra
- Parsnip

- Peas
- Peppers
- Pumpkin
- Potato
- Radicchio
- Rutabaga
- Squash
- Spinach
- Turnips
- Watercress
- Zucchini

List compiled by Shari Bilt, R.D.

it separates into strands, exactly like spaghetti but more nutritious and delicious. Top it with a low-fat tomato sauce or nonfat yogurt mixed with Dijon mustard. Cut carrots and zucchini into match-size strips and steam them until just tender and press garlic or grind pepper over them or sprinkle them with herbs. Bake a potato. Fill it with nonfat yogurt or salsa or eat it plain. Eat vegetables plain or with vinegar, herbs, or spices. You'll appreciate their superb taste. Mmm, this discussion is making us hungry.

Make sure you eat **at least 2 fruits and 3 vegetables a day** — *at least* 2 fruits and 3 vegetables. See the box opposite.

Ruining Fruit and Vegetables

Of course, fried zucchini sticks, French fried onion rings, French fries, cherry ice cream, and caramel apples don't count as fulfilling your vegetable or fruit requirement. Once you fry, butter, melt cheese over, or cover them with high-fat sauces, vegetables are no longer vehicles for good health. Likewise, fruit combined with candy, ice cream, sour cream, or sweet cream loses its slimming properties. (Substitute nonfat yogurt or nonfat frozen yogurt with fruit for a similar taste but non-fattening effect.)

When you add up your vegetable intake, disregard lettuce. Lettuce has very little to recommend it nutrition-wise.

When you are calculating the number of fruits you ate for the day, count only real sources of fruit. Froot Loops and fruit roll-ups are not fruit. Apple pie is a sweet, not a fruit. A blueberry muffin is a sweet, not a fruit. A fruit drink that is mostly water is not a fruit. Eat the real thing. Your body knows.

FIBER

In addition to just plain gustatory pleasure, fruits, vegetables, and whole grains add fiber to your diet. And you need it. Fiber is *the* missing ingredient in the American diet (which, along with a high-fat diet, may explain why we have such high rates of colon cancer). Fiber is essential for good health. A high-fiber diet reduces the risk of colon cancer and may reduce the risk of breast cancer. It helps prevent diverticulosis and hemorrhoids as well as constipation. It can even lower blood glucose levels.

Dietary Fiber in Foods

FOOD	AMOUNT	DIETARY FIBER (g)	FOOD	AMOUNT	DIETARY FIBER (g)
Vegetables, cooked			**Legumes, cooked**		
Broccoli	½ cup	2.0	Baked beans, canned	½ cup	9.8
Brussels sprouts	½ cup	3.4	Kidney beans	½ cup	7.3
Potato (with skin)	1 medium	3.6	Lentils, cooked	½ cup	3.7
Spinach	½ cup	2.0	**Breakfast cereals**		
Sweet potato	½ medium	1.7	All-Bran	⅓ cup	8.5
Zucchini	½ cup	1.3	Bran Chex	⅔ cup	4.6
Vegetables, raw			Bran flakes	¾ cup	5.3
Carrots	1 medium	2.3	Cheerios	1 cup	3.0
Celery	1 stalk	0.6	Cornflakes	1¼ cup	0.6
Cucumber, sliced	½ cup	0.5	Granola	¼ cup	3.2
Lettuce, romaine	1 cup	1.0	Oat bran, raw	⅓ cup	4.9
Mushrooms	½ cup	0.5	Oatmeal, cooked	¾ cup	1.6
Spinach	1 cup	1.5	Raisin bran	¾ cup	4.8
Tomato	1 medium	1.6	Wheaties	1 cup	3.0
Fruits			**Breads, grains, and pasta**		
Apple (with skin)	1 medium	3.0	Bagel	1	1.2
Banana	1 medium	1.8	French bread	1 slice	0.8
Blueberries	½ cup	1.7	Pumpernickel bread	1 slice	1.9
Cantaloupe	¼	1.1	Rice, brown, cooked	½ cup	1.7
Figs, dried	2	3.5	Spaghetti, cooked	½ cup	1.1
Orange	1 medium	3.1	Whole-wheat bread	1 slice	1.9
Peach (with skin)	1	1.4	**Snack foods**		
Pear (with skin)	1 medium	4.3	Popcorn, air-popped	1 cup	0.9
Prunes, dried	3	1.8			
Raisins, seedless	¼ cup	1.9			
Strawberries	1 cup	3.9			

J.A.T. Pennington, *Bowes and Church's Food Values of Portions Commonly Used,* 15th ed. (Philadelphia: J.B. Lippincott Co., 1989).

The Food and Drug Administration recommends eating 25* grams of fiber a day. Most Americans eat less than 10. The chart opposite shows you the amount of fiber found in a variety of foods.

Keep fiber in mind when you are choosing food. Don't just drink orange juice; eat an orange. Eat the potato and the skin. Compare cereal labels and choose the ones with higher fiber content.** (Of course, you have to like the taste too.) Eating the *Choose to Lose Weight-Loss Plan for Men* way ensures you will be eating enough fiber.

DAIRY
(at least 2–3 servings)

Dairy products are excellent sources of calcium and some vitamins, but many are high in fat. You don't have to give up dairy, just choose low- or nonfat substitutes for your high-fat favorites. Work your way down to skim milk; try nonfat yogurts. Even if you don't think you like yogurt, try fruit-flavored varieties. Many people find they *like* strawberry or peach or blueberry yogurt when they actually try them. Find nonfat yogurts without artificial sweeteners. Small amounts of sugar won't harm you, but artificial sweeteners may.

Do take care in your dairy choices. An 8-fluid ounce glass of whole milk contains 75 fat calories. An ounce of cheddar cheese contains 85 fat calories. (Count whole-milk dairy products as fats, not as dairy.) Choose low-fat dairy products such as low-fat or nonfat yogurt, low-fat cottage cheese, and skim milk. Fit cheeses into your budget sparingly, and you will really enjoy them.

Eat at Least 2–3 Servings of Dairy

When you are determining if you met your daily dairy requirement, don't count nonfat frozen yogurt. It may not even contain dairy. Count nonfat frozen yogurt and ice cream as sweets. Don't consider butter and margarine dairy. They are fats.

---

* But don't overdo a good thing — eating more than 50 to 60 grams of fiber a day may decrease your body's ability to absorb vitamins and minerals.

** Nutrition labels of commercial foods list dietaryfi ber (see page 95).

MEATS

Meats, poultry, fish, and eggs are good sources of protein, phosphorus, niacin, iron, zinc, and vitamins B_6 and B_{12}. Eating too little meat is not a problem for most Americans. In fact, Americans probably eat more meat than is necessary for good health.

For your health, limit greatly or eliminate red meat (beef, lamb, pork). Red meat is filled with fat and saturated fat and has been shown to increase risk for heart disease and a variety of cancers.

There are no meat minimums, only maximums. **Limit your meat consumption to no more than 4 to 6 ounces a day.**

Your best bets are the following:

White-meat chicken with no skin   White-meat turkey with no skin
Fish   Shellfish

Take note:

- Frying or breading and frying these recommended meats turns them into nonrecommended meats.
- Lean red meats are acceptable on occasion, but be sure to check out the amount of saturated fat in the meat you choose. Save high-fat red meats for a splurge.
- Organ meats such as liver, pancreas, and brain are loaded with cholesterol. Pancreas and brain are also high in fat. Limit your consumption of organ meats.
- Egg yolks are high in fat (50 fat calories) and cholesterol, so they should be chosen with thought. Don't eat eggs raw. They may contain unhealthy bacteria.

MEAT SUBSTITUTES

Beans

Cooked dried beans or peas may be substituted for meat as a source of protein. However, as these plant foods lack vitamin B_{12}, this vitamin must be supplied by other foods. All beans are very low in fat except for soybeans.

Soy Products

Soy, usually in the form of tofu, may be substituted for meat as a source of protein. Soy is low in saturated fat but may be quite high in total fat. Choose low-fat soy products.

THE TIP OF THE PYRAMID: FOODS TO LIMIT

The tip of the Food Guide Pyramid contains foods you need to limit — fats, oils, and sweets.

SUGAR

Sugar: Nothing Added (Nutritionally), Nothing Gained (in Fat)

You should not overdose on sugar. Sugar does nothing for your health. It is nutrition-free, it makes holes in your teeth, and in large quantities it is burned in preference to fat. However, it is the fat — not the sugar — in the cheesecake that settles snugly in your fat stores. It is the fat — not the sugar — in the candy bar that makes your arteries shudder.

You may eat a little bit of sugar without feeling any guilt. In fact, it may give you a psychological lift. You can use *real jelly* or jam on your bagel without a twinge of conscience. (Jelly is a far superior choice over margarine or butter.) You can pour maple syrup (try the real stuff) and forget the margarine or butter for your pancakes. You can suck an occasional peppermint, jelly bean, or hard candy (not butterscotch, which is called *butter*scotch for a reason) without guilt.

Sweet Warning. Lest you think we are urging you to eat sugar, we are not. We will say it again. Sugar provides a lot of empty calories and contains no vitamins, minerals, or fiber. Eating too much simple sugar can push out nutritious foods you should be eating instead. If you are diabetic or have high triglycerides, you should limit sugar. If you eat too many high-sugar, low-fat treats, you won't gain weight, but you won't lose weight either. Save high-sugar desserts — even fat-free sugar desserts — for a splurge.

FATS AND OILS

You know how we feel about fats and oils.

FAT-FREE FOOD

There is a new category of foods that should be added to the tip of the Food Guide Pyramid: fat-free processed foods.

Fat-Free Food Abuse

The food industry is having a ball. Every week a new fat-free or nonfat product pops up in your grocery store. People gobble up crates of fat-free crackers, nonfat cakes and cookies, nonfat frozen yogurt, and olestra*-filled chips and wait to see the weight drop off. It's going to be a long wait.

"But," you say, *Choose to Lose Weight-Loss Plan for Men* promotes eating lots of food." Right. But not any food. You need to eat lots of nutritious, fiber-rich food like fruits, vegetables, whole grains, and also nonfat dairy, low-fat poultry, fish, and seafood. A few fat-free treats are okay. But if you think a diet of nonfat processed foods will make you thin, think again.

The problem is that these foods have so many calories — so many empty calories in the form of simple sugars and starches — that your body burns them first in preference to your stored fat. The result is either that you don't lose weight or your weight loss is stalled.

In addition, stuffing yourself with empty calories will deprive you of vitamins, minerals, and fiber that you need for good health.

Can You Trust a Fat-Free Label?

There is also the problem of whether food labeled fat-free is truly fat-free. A few years ago, *New York* magazine had the fat contents of a variety of low- and nonfat foods sold in New York City food shops evaluated by a laboratory. The results serve as a warning. A "fat-free" tofu cheesecake contained 221 fat calories per slice. Tofu is a high-fat food, so how could tofu cheesecake be fat-free? A diet corn muffin billed as fat-free and sugar-free had 204 fat calories. Tasti D-lite Frozen Dessert (peanut butter**) claimed to have less than 9 fat calories per small serving when it actually contained 58 fat calories. You need to be a critical — spell that "suspicious" — consumer. Ask to see a list of the ingredients. If all you get is a blank stare, take your business elsewhere.

Keeping up the High-Fat Taste

Because the food industry knows that Americans have a fat tooth but still want to be thin, it has produced a multitude of nonfat high-fat-tast-

---

* For more information on olestra, see page 171, Chapter 16, "Frequently Asked Questions."

** Beware of peanut butter nonfat yogurt. Although the basic yogurt may contain little or no fat, the peanut oil added for flavor is not required to be fat-free.

ing foods. Nonfat cheeses, nonfat cream cheeses, nonfat salad dressings, nonfat sour creams, nonfat margarines, and nonfat mayonnaises allow us to continue indulging our high-fat taste without adding the fat calories. But can you really have your nonfat cheese and eat it too?

An occasional tablespoon of nonfat cream cheese on a bagel or a few tablespoons of nonfat dressing on your salad won't greatly hinder your progress. However, if you slip a few slices of cheese into every turkey sandwich, melt fat-free cheese over your broccoli, or mix half a cup of fat-free mayonnaise into your tuna salad, then you will have a difficult time ever giving up your craving for fatty foods.

The most successful men who follow *Choose to Lose Weight-Loss Plan for Men* are those who wean themselves from fatty foods or fatty-, cheesy-, creamy-tasting foods and replace them with high-fiber, tasty, nutritious foods. You can learn to love a potato plain. Mustard tastes great on a turkey sandwich. A sprinkling of balsamic vinegar enhances steamed broccoli. If you are a nonfat fat junky, ask yourself, when you are no longer keeping track of what you eat, will you slip back to your old high-fat ways because you never really let go of your taste for fat?

Giving up Your Fat Tooth

Scientific experiments have shown that it takes about 12 weeks to change from a high-fat to a low-fat taste *if* you don't keep subjecting yourself to your old high-fat tastes. Give yourself a chance to let the change take place.

NONFOOD: ALCOHOL

You may think that since alcohol contains no fat, you can guzzle it to your heart's content. Sorry. Although alcohol is fat-free, its consumption should be limited for other reasons. First, alcohol can wreak havoc on your health. If you drive drunk, you can also wreak havoc on the health of others. Alcohol calories are empty calories and provide no nutritional benefits.

You may also find that alcohol disconnects your self-control button and causes you to eat more fat than a sober you would allow. In addition, alcohol may have a more direct relationship to fat loss. Scientific research has shown that alcohol consumption affects fat metabolism. The body can't store alcohol so it must burn it right away. Consequently alcohol is burned in preference to fat stored in your fat stores. So when you drink that 6-pack of beer in one sitting, your body will burn the alcohol instead of burning fat from the fat stores. Those proverbial beer bellies are a result of nachos, nuts, and the beer! The bottom line: Limit alcoholic beverages to a maximum of 1–2 drinks a day.

MAKING WISE CHOICES

The following chart will give you a guide to suggested serving sizes for meeting the recommendations of the Food Guide Pyramid. You need not limit your intake of whole grains, fruits, vegetables, and nonfat dairy to these amounts. Except for meat, these recommendations are minimums. Use this table and chapter as a reference to guide your choice of foods. Remember, your goal is to eat healthfully. Choose foods that are chock-full of nutrients and fiber. Eat broccoli rather than lettuce. Eat whole-wheat rather than white bread. Eat higher-fiber cereals rather than no-fiber or scant-fiber cereals. Eat whole fruit rather than just drinking fruit juices.

Enjoy yourself. If you don't cook, get someone else to and incorporate fruits and vegetables into dishes such as chilis and chicken stir-fries, soups and rices. Eat delicious dishes you prepare from scratch (such as the easy, healthy, low-low-fat, scrumptious recipes from *Eater's Choice Low-Fat Cookbook*), and following *Choose to Lose Weight-Loss Plan for Men* will be a joy. When you start changing your eating habits and eat tasty low-fat foods, your whole attitude toward life will change. Not only will your fat melt away, your psyche will be at peace. You will be content and full. Just wait and see.

Use Sense

Choose to Lose Weight-Loss Plan for Men is about eating lots of nutritious food, but lots of nutritious food within reason. Eight cups of rice is not within reason. Four cups of cereal is not within reason. You need to use sense. You can't eat too much of fiber-rich foods such as potatoes because you get too full before you overeat them, but if you eat huge portions of pretty healthy foods that are not fiber-rich, you are faced with two problems. One, the total carbohydrate calories add up to gigantic amounts. Instead of burning fat from the fat stores, your body is burning those carbohydrates. Two, some nutritious foods have some fat, which while negligible in small servings, in large portions can add up to a lot of fat. For example, an adequate portion of oatmeal — ⅔ cup dry (1½ cups cooked) — contains 33 fat calories. An overdose of oatmeal — 2 cups

	Minimum Basic Nutritional Requirements		
FOOD GROUP	MINIMUM RECOMMENDED DAILY SERVINGS	EXAMPLES	ONE SERVING
Grain	6–11	Whole-grain cereal Bagel Rice Pasta	$\frac{1}{2}$–1 cup $\frac{1}{2}$ $\frac{1}{2}$ cup 1 cup
Fruit*	2–4	Apple Grapefruit pieces	1 fruit $\frac{1}{2}$ to 1 cup
Vegetables	3–5	2 carrots Spinach	1 $\frac{1}{2}$ to 1 cup
Dairy	2–3	Skim milk Nonfat yogurt** 1% cottage cheese	8 fl oz 1 cup $\frac{1}{2}$ cup

Meat
  Poultry
  Turkey
  Fish
 	
Meat Alternatives
	No minimum
	Maximum 6 oz
		Chicken breast without
		  skin
		Turkey breast without
		  skin
		All fin fish
		Shellfish
		Dried beans, peas, lentils
			2–3 oz
			
			2–3 oz
			3–4 oz
			3–4 oz
			$\frac{1}{2}$ cup

Note: When a food is high-fat, it is not counted as satisfying a nutritional requirement. For example, a croissant is not counted as a grain serving, nor is ice cream counted as a dairy serving.
* except avocado
** not frozen

dry ($4\frac{1}{2}$ cups cooked) — contains 100 fat calories. You don't need $4\frac{1}{2}$ cups of oatmeal.

If you are not sure how many servings you have been eating, try this experiment: If you are having pasta, fill your bowl as you would normally. Then use measuring cups to measure the amount. Figure out the calories you are consuming. You may be surprised. Try the same experiment with cereal, rice, and bagels.

Choose to Lose Weight-Loss Plan for Men is the only weight-loss plan that does not limit total calories except for fat calories and empty calories. However, that doesn't mean that you should push the system. You always need to pay attention and use sense.

And in the Next Chapter . . .

Where to find the fat so you can control it.

7. Fat City

FAT IS EVERYWHERE. It is difficult to avoid. Turn on your television set and watch the melted cheese gently enfold a thick, juicy hamburger, or sweet, creamy chocolate swirl smoothly around a gooey nougat center, or cheese joyfully bubble atop a pizza crust. Drive through your town and count the fast-food restaurants as you whiz by. Take a good look at the dishes displayed behind the glass showcase in your office cafeteria. Fat! Fat! Fat!

And because fat is so available and convenient, Americans are getting fatter and fatter. Statistics show that more than 54 percent of Americans — 97 million people — are overweight. Of those, 39 million are obese.

It's easy to do. Americans are eating out (much of it fast-food), carrying in, or popping high-fat convenience foods into the microwave. They are eating high-fat snacks and avoiding fruits and vegetables. Americans are driving more and walking less.

But this doesn't have to be you. Now that you know your Fat Budget, you have the power to take control of the high-fat world around you. Once you know that fat is the culprit and where you can find it, you can root it out. You have the power. You can make educated choices. You can make lifestyle choices to reduce your exposure. You won't suffer. You can even splurge once in a while — you know the cost.

In this chapter, we will briefly discuss fat-filled land mines and their lower-fat alternatives. But this generalized information is not enough. It is essential to look up fat calories in the Food Tables or on nutrition labels for every food you eat because fat content is not always obvious. Some is visible, like the strip of fat on a sirloin steak. But much is hidden, like the fat marbled throughout the steak and the fat added to processed frozen dinners.

Stay Cool

It may distress you to discover that fat lurks in so many of the foods you love, but don't feel hopeless. You won't have to eliminate anything. You will just have to decide how often and in what amounts you can comfortably fit it into your Fat Budget. Okay, you won't be eating an ice cream sundae after every meal, but when you decide you can afford to fit one in, you'll *really* taste it. You will also learn to love foods you once considered "health food" — vegetables, fruits, and grains. You won't feel deprived. You're going to love being lean, eating healthfully, and feeling full and satisfied.

RED MEATS   (pages 284–89, Food Tables)

Steer Away

Most of us were raised with the notion that you need to eat lots of protein to be healthy and fit. And what is usually considered the best source of protein? Red meat — beef, lamb, veal, and pork. Not true. Just as good sources are chicken, turkey, fish, seafood, and beans — and they are low in fat. As you read on page 12, almost everyone gets enough protein no matter what their diet, and overeating protein can be dangerous to your health. And more than being a good source of protein, red meat is a super source of fat. Instead of building bulging biceps and triceps, eating lots of red meat builds bulging bellies, hips, and thighs. A lot of the fat is the worst kind — saturated fat. It's the kind that clogs your arteries and leads to heart attacks.

Even athletes no longer bulk up on steaks and eggs. Now they eat carbohydrates for energy.

Turn to the **MEAT** category of the Food Tables for some surprises. The numbers won't seem so bad because they are listed in **1 ounce** portion sizes for easy comparison. Of course, no one eats just 1 ounce of meat. Be sure to multiply the fat calories by the number of ounces you eat. For instance, sirloin steak, broiled, has 46 fat calories per ounce. If you eat 8 ounces, multiply 8 x 46 for a total of 368 fat calories. How does 368 fat calories fit into your Fat Budget?

Don't just stop at beef. Look at lamb, pork, and veal too. If you thought that veal was a low-fat, heart-healthy choice, look again. Does veal breast, braised, at 54 fat calories an ounce (6 oz = 324 fat calories) fit your low-fat criteria? Check out pork. The pork lobby's definition of pork as "the other white meat" is a whitewash. At 296 fat calories for a loin chop, pork is not even a distant relation to the real white meat — 13 fat calories for an entire chicken breast without skin.

You Can Fit It In

For those of you who cannot envision life without a daily red meat fix, you can fit it into your diet. Obviously you can't afford a 10-ounce porterhouse steak (540 fat calories) or two 3½-ounce lamb chops (530 fat calories) or 8 ounces of spare ribs (616 fat calories) as daily fare, but if you plan for it and save up fat calories, an occasional red meat splurge can be budgeted in.

Be sure to check the **MEATS, FAST FOODS, FROZEN, MICROWAVE, AND REFRIGERATED FOODS,** and **SAUSAGES AND LUNCHEON MEATS** sections of the Food Tables to familiarize yourself with the fat in meats and meat products not mentioned in this chapter.

Losing the Taste for Beef

You may not believe it now, but if you limit your consumption of high-fat meats, you may even lose your taste for them after a while. A lineman from Virginia who had been following *Choose to Lose Weight-Loss Plan for Men* for about 6 months, totally avoiding fast food, told us that he decided to give himself a birthday treat — a McDonald's quarter-pounder. He bought the sandwich and found it so greasy he couldn't eat it. Scientific studies have shown that it takes about 12 weeks to change from a high-fat to a low-fat taste.

Better Choices: Fish

If you want a steak, occasionally fit in a swordfish, tuna, or salmon steak. Although higher in fat than many fish, most of these big chunks of fish are lower in fat than cuts of beef, and in addition to being delicious, contain omega-3 polyunsaturated fats, which reduce the risks of heart disease and stroke by lowering high blood triglycerides and reducing blood clotting. At 10 fat calories per ounce for swordfish, 12 for tuna, and 9 to 27 for salmon depending on the type, these fish steaks are not as low-fat as many fish (cod is 2 fat calories per ounce, snapper 3 fat calories per ounce, and sole 3 fat calories per ounce), but the fat is a healthy fat. However, don't go overboard — even healthy fats are fattening.

Better Choices: Poultry

Chicken is a great substitute for beef and pork. It is also more versatile than beef. You can prepare chicken in a million tasty ways.* At only 13 fat calories for a boneless, skinless chicken breast, chicken is a buy — fat-calorie-wise.

Even lower in fat at 2 fat calories per ounce, white-meat turkey can be turned into a multitude of scrumptious dishes. It is even delicious eaten plain.

POULTRY   (pages 293–99, Food Tables)

I Eat Only Chicken, Turkey, and Fish . . . Why Am I Overweight?

Although chicken has the potential to be a healthy choice, don't automatically equate chicken with low-fat. White-meat chicken prepared without skin and little added fat is a low-fat food, but chicken *with* the skin has a fat content approaching or even surpassing that of many cuts of beef. When fried, breaded and deep-fried, or smothered in high-fat sauces, chicken joins the high-fat food brigade. Look at the chart below to see how easy it is to fatten up a chicken.

PREPARATION OF CHICKEN BREAST	FAT CALORIES
Roasted without skin	13
Roasted with skin, then skin removed	28
Roasted and eaten *with* skin	69
Fried *with* skin, flour coated	78
Fried *with* skin, batter dipped	166
KFC Extra Crispy	216
Chicken pot pie (Marie Callendar's)	880

Turkey: Throw away the Wrapping

Eat the turkey (white-meat turkey without the skin has 2 fat calories per ounce; dark meat without the skin has 9) but unless you have been

---

* *Eater's Choice Low-Fat Cookbook* contains scrumptious chicken recipes such as *Orange Chicken Chinoise, Barbecue Chicken,* and *Indonesian Chicken with Green Beans,* as well as turkey recipes such as *Turkey Mexique* and *Turkey with Capers.*

banking fat calories for a Thanksgiving Day blowout, toss the skin. At 100 fat calories per ounce, even a little skin contains more fat than you need.

Chicken and Turkey Burgers

When you see chicken burger or turkey burger on a menu, don't automatically jump to order one. They may be lower in fat than a hamburger, but once the chef grinds in skin and fat, molds it into a burger, and fries it in oil, your poultry burger becomes a fat patty.

You also need to take care if you buy ground turkey at the grocery store. Ground turkey can be a good substitute for ground beef, but not if it is loaded with turkey skin and fat. Ground turkey can contain as much as 33 fat calories an ounce. Read the nutrition label if there is one; don't buy if there isn't.

Your best bet is to buy boneless chicken breasts without skin and grind your own meat in your food processor. Mix in some chopped carrots, celery, green pepper, onion, and some herbs, form patties, broil them, and you have a truly low-fat treat.*

Redi-Serve Fat

The food industry is always up-to-the-minute in creating foods that will save us time, but at what expense? A new category of ready-made, prepared meats has cropped up in the market. But be sure to pick and choose carefully. For example, you can buy Redi-Serve breaded and cooked chicken patties (white meat) at a mind-boggling cost of 150 fat calories per patty. What did you say your Fat Budget was? These patties have even more fat than the veal patties made by Redi-Serve.

Tyson makes roasted chicken that you just heat up. At first glance it looks pretty low in fat — 25 fat calories for a chicken breast. That's only 12 more fat calories than if you roasted it yourself. Look again. With the skin, the chicken contains 120 fat calories a breast. Make sure you read every label carefully.

Duck: Super Splurge   (page 296, Food Tables)

A duck needs all that fat to keep it warm and afloat while it frolics in freezing water, but you don't. Half a duck with skin contains 975 fat cal-

---

* For more specific directions, see *Suzanne's Chickenburgers* in *Eater's Choice Low-Fat Cookbook*.

ories — and that's without a sauce. However, if duck à l'orange is one of your absolute favorites in all the world, save up fat calories for a very, very, very special occasion and enjoy the treat.

Be sure to check the **POULTRY, FAST FOODS, FROZEN, MICROWAVE, AND REFRIGERATED FOODS,** and **SAUSAGES AND LUNCHEON MEATS** sections of the Food Tables to familiarize yourself with the fat in poultry and poultry products not mentioned in this chapter.

SEAFOOD (pages 231–39, Food Tables)

Snapper, shrimp, lobster, and sole — most plain, unadulterated fish or seafood contains 2–4 fat calories an ounce and can be a great low-fat choice.* Once they start swimming around in the deep-fryer or butter or cream sauces, they need to be considered weight-gain and artery-clogging food.

Choose fish that has been baked, broiled, poached, or grilled with little or no fat for a delectable, guilt-free entrée.

A *Choose to Lose Weight-Loss Plan for Men* tip: Oil-packed tuna has ten times as much fat as water-packed. A whole can of *undrained* tuna packed in water has 30 calories of fat or 4.5 fat calories per ounce. A whole can of undrained tuna packed in oil (soy oil, not even fish oil) has 297 calories of fat or 45 fat calories per ounce.

You will find the fat calories of fish listed in the **FISH AND SHELLFISH, FAST FOODS,** and **FROZEN, MICROWAVE, AND REFRIGERATED FOODS** sections of the Food Tables.

| | FAT CALORIES | |
FISH	1 OUNCE	4 OUNCES
Butterfish, orange roughy, Pacific mackerel	20	80
Sockeye salmon	22	88
Atlantic herring	23	92
Chinook salmon	27	108
Swordfish	10	40
Tuna	12	48

* Some fish are high in fat (a good fat: omega-3 polyunsaturated). Look at the chart above. You don't have to eliminate any of these wonderful fish from your diet — just keep track of their fat calories and fit them in.

SAUSAGES AND LUNCHEON MEATS

Eat Sausage and Look Like a Sausage   (pages 323–28, Food Tables)

Sausages, frankfurters, and luncheon meats need to be regarded with suspicion. They can blow away your Fat Budget. Most are crammed with fat (in addition to being filled with dangerous additives and excessive amounts of sodium).

Don't Throw Your Kids to the Dogs

It is tempting to throw hot dogs into a pot of boiling water when your kids are crying for food — it's so quick and easy — but these cancer-risky packets of fat are poor choices for both you and your children. The poor eating habits established at these tender years as well as future dire health effects are not worth the convenience. In almost the same amount of time, you can coat skinless, boneless chicken breasts with barbecue sauce and broil them, steam some vegetables, and cook up some basmati rice (10 minutes) for a full, delicious, healthy, low-fat dinner.

SAUSAGES AND LUNCHEON MEATS	AMOUNT	FAT CALORIES
Pork bratwurst	1 wurst (84 g)	198
Smoked link pork sausage	1 link (85 g)	230
Polska kielbasa	1 inch (28 g)	75
Frankfurter		
Turkey	1 frank (57 g)	70
Chicken	1 frank (56 g)	100
Beef	1 frank (57 g)	150
Cheese dog	1 frank (45 g)	120
Beef knockwurst	1 link (85 g)	210
Pepperoni	15 slices (28g)	120

Turkey and Chicken Franks: More Expensive Than You Think

Knowing that the American public associates chicken and turkey with low-fat, food manufacturers have created turkey and chicken hot dogs and sausage. Before you rush to buy, look at the labels. At 100 fat calories, a chicken hot dog is no buy. Turkey sausage may have 81 fat calories for a 3-ounce link.

Low-Fat Cold Cuts: Still a Poor Choice

If you use the cold cuts that have less fat (read the labels*) and make your sandwiches less thick, you can fit cold cuts into your Fat Budget. But eat them with care. Although a hefty amount of fat has been removed, the excessive sodium, unhealthy preservatives, and high-fat taste remain.

This is true for low-fat and nonfat hot dogs too.

Keeping up Your Fat Tooth

Before you make a low-fat or nonfat hot dog your daily fare, remember that if you continue to subject yourself to a high-fat taste, albeit from a low-fat food, you will never lose your craving for high-fat foods.

Sliced Turkey Breast: A Good Choice

At 2–8 fat calories per ounce, white-meat turkey that you buy at the deli counter is a good lunch choice. However, if you are buying packaged turkey breast, read the label. "Turkey" is *not* always synonymous with "low-fat."

MILK AND MILK PRODUCTS

Whole Milk: Not Wholesome   (pages 189–94, Food Tables)

Most of us have grown up with the notion that whole milk is wholesome and pure and good for us. It's not. At 75 fat calories a glass (8 fl oz), whole milk is high-fat (and high-sat-fat, for that matter) and thus an unhealthy, fattening food. Drink 3 glasses a day (225 fat calories) and you have shot more than half of your Fat Budget. Don't give up milk — just choose lower-fat varieties.

2% Milk: High-Fat Milk

If moving directly from whole milk to skim makes you shudder, make the move slowly. First switch to 2% reduced fat milk. It tastes almost the same as whole. Whole milk contains about 3% fat.

---

* Cold-cut packages claiming "⅓ fewer calories, 50% less fat" may still have 35 fat calories a slice. Four slices and you have 140 fat calories.

Although labeled "reduced-fat," 2% is not a low-fat food. The "2%" refers to the fact that 2% of the *weight* of the milk is fat; the rest is water. At 45 fat calories per 8-ounce glass, 2% milk is far from low-fat. Get used to 2% milk, then switch to 1%. It tastes almost the same but has 20 fat calories per glass. A painless way to work your way down from whole milk or 2% milk can be found in the box below.

Milk Drinker's Tip

If you are drinking whole milk, when half the milk in the container is gone, fill it up with 2% milk (45 fat calories per cup). You'll never notice the difference. When half the combination milk has been consumed, refill the container with 2% milk. Keep filling the container with 2% milk. Soon the bottle will be entirely 2% milk and you won't miss whole milk at all. After drinking 2% milk for a while, apply this trick to working your way to 1% milk (25 fat calories per cup) and then skim (0 fat calories per cup).

Skim Milk: Work Your Way Down

Skim milk should be your goal. It has 0 fat calories per glass. Don't worry about calcium content. Skim milk has just as much, or even a bit more calcium than whole milk. Follow the tip in the box above for an effortless way to become a skim-milk lover.

Cream in Your Coffee   (page 191, Food Tables)

Keep a watchful eye on cream, for it is an insidious Fat Budget destroyer. Even innocent cream in your coffee can add up to large amounts of fat. One tablespoon of light table cream has 26 calories of fat. Four cups of coffee a day adds up to 104 fat calories, and for what? At 15 fat calories a tablespoon, half-and-half is better, but four cups of coffee quickly adds up to 60 fat calories.

If you are a dyed-in-the-wool creamaholic, cut the fat by drinking fewer cups of coffee. Better yet, be flexible, be adventuresome — try whole milk at 5 fat calories per tablespoon, 2% at 3, or skim milk at 0. Best yet, enjoy your coffee black.

Cream in Soups and Sauces

When you see the word *cream,* pay careful attention. Cream added to soups adds hundreds of fat calories. A cup of cream of mushroom soup has about 155 calories of fat; vichyssoise (creamed potato soup) has 210. When eating out, be sure to ask if the soup contains cream, and if it does, you may want to choose something else. You can budget it in, but if after a spoonful you find it is not worth the expense, push it away. Better choice: order broth or tomato-based soups. Best choice: prepare any of the 47 delicious soups from your *Eater's Choice Low-Fat Cookbook* and eat them at home.

Be wary of cream sauces. The creamy Alfredo sauce drowning your fettucine may cost you 873 fat calories. Even a half-cup of creamed chipped beef can cost you 100 fat calories. If every choice on the menu is covered with a cream sauce, ask that the sauce be served on the side. Try the dish sauceless. It may taste great without the sauce. If not, don't pour on the sauce. Use it sparingly. Measure out a tablespoon, spread it on, and taste the dish. Enough? More? Keep track of the amount you use. Spoonfuls quickly add up to cupfuls.

Whipped Cream: A Pricey Choice

Whipped cream adds a festive touch to ice cream sundaes, waffles, and hot chocolate. Enjoy a look, and then remove it. The perky dollop that floats on your cafe latte costs you 60 fat calories. The little cloud that nestles atop your ice cream sundae may cost more than 350 fat calories. Whipped cream splurges should be saved for extremely special occasions.

Cheese: Another Expensive Choice   (pages 189–91, Food Tables)

The piece of cheese fits so nicely on the little cracker and tastes so good as it slides into your mouth. But it is rarely one little cracker and one slice of cheese. As you repeat this ritual over and over, talking, sipping a glass of wine, barely paying attention, you are consuming hundreds of fat calories. At 70–85 fat calories per ounce of cheese (of course the crackers contribute a stack of fat too), you have soon spent your Fat Budget for a day or two. Pay attention! You don't have to give cheese up completely, but you do need to watch the amount you eat. Buy a small quantity of your favorite as a rare treat. Eat it slowly. You will taste every bite.

Eggs: A Fat Packet   (page 194, Food Tables)

Eggs pack a lot of fat — 50 fat calories in the yolk. Just the eggs in a four-egg omelet contain 200 fat calories. That's without the 100 plus fat calories added to cook them. To reduce the fat, ask for an omelet that has one egg and three egg whites. It won't be low-fat, but it will be a better choice. Egg substitutes are also an option. Ask that your fat-free omelet be cooked in a Teflon pan. If that isn't possible, find out the amount and what kind of fat is being used so you can figure out how much the cooking fat is costing you. If the price is too high, order something else.

FATS   (pages 189, 226–27 Food Tables)

Butter and Margarine: Spreads That Cause Spread

Of course everyone knows that butter is fattening. But how fattening? A tablespoon contains 100 fat calories. Think about that each time you prepare to slather butter over a piece of toast or drop it into a baked potato. Think about the assault on your Fat Budget when you eat your vegetables drowned in butter. One hundred fat calories for one little tablespoon.

Many people think margarine is lower in fat, but it isn't. It is a somewhat better choice because it is less saturated than butter (18 sat-fat calories per tablespoon versus 65). Saturated fat contributes to raising blood cholesterol and thus risk for heart disease.* However, it is now known that the trans fats in margarines (see page 72) behave like saturated fats in the body. So, although margarine has a heart-healthy reputation, it is just as fattening as butter, almost as heart-risky, and should be limited.

A *Choose to Lose Weight-Loss Plan for Men* tip: Always say, "Hold the butter!" when you order a sandwich. Sandwiches often come buttered no matter what the ingredients.

Olive Oil: The Most Heart-Healthy Fat

Olive oil contains mainly monounsaturated fat and little saturated or polyunsaturated fat. Extensive research has determined that olive oil lowers bad cholesterol (LDL) without lowering good cholesterol (HDL).

---

* See *Eater's Choice* for a discussion of everything you need to know about saturated fat, cholesterol, and heart disease.

Fat Facts

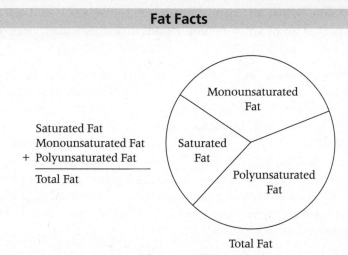

Saturated Fat
Monounsaturated Fat
+ Polyunsaturated Fat
——————————
Total Fat

Total Fat

Total fat is the sum of three types of fat: saturated, monounsaturated, and polyunsaturated fat. While all three types of fat are fattening, each has a different effect on your heart health.

Saturated fat raises your LDL-cholesterol (bad cholesterol) and your risk of heart disease. Saturated fat is found predominantly in animal fats (beef fat or beef tallow, veal fat, lamb fat, lard or pork fat, chicken fat, turkey fat, and butterfat) and the following vegetable fats: coconut oil, palm kernel oil, palm oil, cocoa butter, and hydrogenated and partially hydrogenated vegetable oil. Hydrogenated or partially hydrogenated vegetable fats are rampant in processed and convenience foods. Saturated fat is the only fat that is solid at room temperature.

Monounsaturated fat lowers your LDL-cholesterol (bad cholesterol) without lowering HDL-cholesterol (good cholesterol) and thus lowers your risk of heart disease. It further lowers your heart disease risk by preventing oxidation of LDL-cholesterol. Excellent sources of monounsaturated fat are olive oil and canola oil. We prefer olive oil because Mediterranean cultures have been using it for centuries and they have low rates of heart disease. Canola oil has been in use only for a short time, so its long-term effectiveness and safety are not yet known.

(*continued on next page*)

Warning: Before you begin guzzling the nearest bottle of olive or canola oil as an elixir of health, be advised: One tablespoon contains 119 fat calories.

Polyunsaturated fat lowers LDL-cholesterol but may also lower HDL-cholesterol. The major sources of polyunsaturated fat are vegetable oils such as soy, corn, cottonseed, and safflower. Because consumption of large quantities of polyunsaturated fats has been implicated in the development of certain cancers in animals, we recommend limiting your use of polyunsaturated oil and using olive oil instead (even in baking breads and pie crusts). In addition, when polyunsaturated vegetable oils are hydrogenated or partially hydrogenated, they become trans fats, which act like saturated fats in the body.

Trans fats are chemicals that are produced when the polyunsaturated fats and oils in foods are hydrogenated (hydrogen is added) to make them solid at room temperature and to increase their shelf life (the time before they become rancid). Trans fats are found in many processed foods, but they are not listed or included in the saturated fat calories listed on nutrition labels. They act like saturated fat in the body and raise your risk of heart disease.

In addition, by preventing the oxidation of LDL remnants, olive oil helps prevent the first step of the atherosclerotic process. Having said all this, we still urge you to use caution in eating olive oil. One tablespoon of olive oil contains 119 fat calories! So, when choosing a fat, choose olive oil, but don't use a lot.

Mayonnaise: Pure Fat   (page 229, Food Tables)

One tablespoon of regular mayonnaise has 100 calories of fat. That explains why tuna salad, chicken salad, and shrimp salad sandwiches are so high in fat — they are swimming in mayonnaise. Think twice (or maybe three or four times) before you eat a meat salad sandwich (unless you make them yourself with nonfat mayonnaise). Make sure that your bread is mayonnaise-free. Use mustard instead and save yourself 100 fat calories.

Salad Dressings (pages 227–31, Food Tables)

A little girl interviewed on television was asked what her favorite vegetable was. She answered, "Salad dressing." What refreshing honesty! Salad dressing is the number-one reason salad is so popular.

Salad dressing is a killer. One tablespoon of ranch dressing has about 85 fat calories, 1 tablespoon of creamy French about 70. But who eats 1 tablespoon? Or 2 (170 fat calories)? Or even 4 (340 fat calories)? Isn't it more like 8 (680 fat calories)? See page 124 for a way to get the taste of the dressing without the fat calories.

PASTA (page 279, Food Tables)

Not Just Any Pasta

Many people complain that they are eating pasta but not losing weight. But which pasta dish are they eating? Lasagna (475 fat calories)? Spaghetti with meatballs (351 fat calories)? The sauces atop the pasta are the problem. Even one-quarter of a cup (one-quarter cup!) of Contadina's reduced-fat (reduced-fat!) pesto sauce has 170 fat calories.

For no strain on your Fat Budget, boil up your own pasta and cover it with a low-fat sauce. Sauté some tomatoes, lots of garlic, and a generous pinch of oregano in a teaspoon of olive oil, and within minutes you'll be enjoying a feast. You can also find commercial low-fat or nonfat tomato sauces in the grocery store. But remember, use sense. Eating a 16-ounce box of pasta will not make you fat, but your body will burn those 1600 total calories instead of burning fat from your fat stores.

FROZEN MEALS (pages 239–64, Food Tables)

If you or your significant other are active members of the microwave age, we beg you to let your membership lapse. Take a few minutes and make your own food from scratch. It tastes much, much better, you can have more to eat, and it is much more nutritious. What's more, cooking is easy, fun, and creative. Express yourself.

A Box Is Not Dinner

If you want to change your ways slowly and are not quite ready to try cooking entrées, at least buy fresh vegetables to enhance your frozen dinners. Buy an inexpensive metal steamer in a kitchen store, department store, drug store, hardware store, or dime store. Place it in a saucepan with about an inch of water. Cut a vegetable — broccoli, carrots, zucchini, etc. — into bite-size pieces and put them on the steamer. Bring the water to a boil, cover the pot, and steam until tender. It only takes about 3 to 5 minutes to cook most vegetables. Bake a sweet potato or butternut squash. Boil up some rice. It's easy and well worth the effort. Remember *Choose to Lose Weight-Loss Plan for Men* is all about eating. You need to eat delicious, nutritious foods to lose weight and enhance your health.

Nutrition Labels: You Gotta Read Them

If you do buy frozen dinners, learning how to read a label is essential for survival (see Chapter 8). The package may advertise a low-fat entrée such as fish, turkey, or chicken, but that is no guarantee the dinner is low-fat. The name may imply good health, like Lean Cuisine, Weight Watchers, and Healthy Choice, but that is no guarantee that the contents are low in fat and healthy. For example, Healthy Choice's Country Breaded Chicken has 80 fat calories. This doesn't seem like such a healthy choice to us. Read the nutrition label to be safe.

Ruining a Good Thing

Hesto Presto Chango! See how the commercial food processors transform a low-fat chicken breast (13 fat calories) into a high-fat food:

CHICKEN	FAT CALORIES
Chicken breast without skin	13
Stouffer's Chicken Breast with Barbecue Sauce	210
Kid Cuisine Cosmic Chicken Nuggets	230
Banquet Fried Chicken Meal	240
Marie Callendar's Chicken Pot Pie	880

Take a look at the FROZEN, MICROWAVE, AND REFRIGERATED FOODS section of the Food Tables for a true shock.

Less Fat Means Less Food

In response to the public's desire to become thin, the food industry has reacted by creating hundreds of new low-fat products. A variety of truly low-fat dinners (fat calories ranging from 9 to 45) can be found in your grocery's freezer cases. Why aren't we applauding? The problem is that many low-fat dinners are low-fat because they contain so little meat* (many contain about ½–1 ounce of meat). As a result, eating one dinner doesn't satisfy you. That is not to say that we recommend eating he-man portions of any meat. Eating modest amounts of meat is fine (and even healthy), but if consuming one low-fat dinner (45 fat calories) leaves you hungry for another (45 + 45 = 90 fat calories) and another (45 + 45 + 45 = 135) or leads you to binge on high-fat snacks to fill up your stomach and psyche, then low-fat frozen dinners are not a healthy choice.

CONVENIENCE-STORE FOODS

High Cost of Convenience

You stop at your local 7-Eleven and pick up a beef and bean burrito for lunch. You zap it in the office microwave, and in an instant your 240 calories of fat is ready. How convenient! As a bonus, you get to consume 90 sat-fat calories too. Or try one of these microwave sandwiches if you want to blow your Fat Budget away. A set of little twin sausage sandwiches costs 210 fat calories, and a set of Chicken Chimichangas costs 200 fat calories. The Big 'Un is a humdinger at 440 fat calories. A Ham 'n Cheese Hot Pockets costs 220 fat calories; a Pepperoni Pizza Hot Pockets costs 260 fat calories.

The offerings at convenience stores are limited, but almost every one is a Fat Budget destroyer. You will notice that almost every food is packaged for an individual to pick up and eat on the run. Chips, crackers, cookies, cakes, doughnuts, hot dogs, chili dogs — the package is small but the fat content is huge.

Even the few foods that don't contain a lot of fat — breakfast cereals, for instance, such as Frosted Flakes, Cocoa Frosted Flakes, Fruit Pebbles — are the poorest choices of that type of food. These cereals are high in empty sugar calories and artificial coloring and low in fiber and nutrition.

Convenience foods can be dangerous to your health.

---

* See page 94 to find out how to determine the amount of meat in a frozen dinner.

FAST FOODS   (pages 194–226, Food Tables)

Fa(s)t Food

It's so easy to stop for breakfast, lunch, and/or dinner at a fast-food restaurant because there are so many and they are everywhere. But if you are interested in your health and physique, stay away. Don't join the thousands of Americans who will die from fat-related, or more specifically, fast-food-related diseases (heart disease, diabetes, and colon and prostate cancers).

To see the devastating effect fast food has on health, look at Japan. In the few years since we began importing fast food to Japan (a country in which both fast-food restaurants and heart disease were once virtually nonexistent), heart disease has increased fivefold and obesity has become a problem. Take a look at Hardee's Big Country Breakfast with Sausage in the FAST FOODS section of the Food Tables if you want to know why. Check out all your favorites. Here's a selection of foods whose fat content may surprise you:

FAST FOOD	FAT CALORIES
McDonald's Fish Fillet Deluxe	250
Arby's Roast Chicken Club	279
KFC Hot Wings	297
Carl's Jr. CrissCut Fries, large	306
Taco Bell Nachos Bellgrande	360
McDonald's McDLT	396
Burger King Double Whopper with Cheese	570
Jack-in-the Box Colossus Hamburger	756

If you want to be successful following *Choose to Lose Weight-Loss Plan for Men*, the best course of action is to put fast-food restaurants on your Most Unwanted List. Even if you go with the best intentions, it may be hard to resist the high-fat fare. However, if you are kidnapped at gunpoint, tied up, dragged to a fast-food restaurant, and forced to order, or if a fast-food restaurant provides the only food available for 50 miles and you haven't eaten for two days, here are some choices that won't give your Fat Budget a heart attack.

FAST FOOD	FAT CALORIES
Carl's Jr. and Roy Rogers Baked Potato, plain	0
Chick-Fil-A Chargrilled Chicken Sandwich	30*
Subway Turkey Breast on Wheat Bread	36*
KFC Tender Roast Chicken Without Skin	39
Long John Silver's Baked Shrimp	45
Hardee's Roast Beef Sub	45*
Arby's Light Roast Chicken Deluxe	54*
Carl's Jr. Barbecue Chicken Sandwich	54*
Roy Rogers Roaster White Meat without Skin	54

* without mayo, oil, or butter added

Be sure that you check the *Choose to Lose Weight-Loss Plan for Men* Food Tables for better choices. Be suspicious if the fat content for the dish seems too low, such as the Dairy Queen BBQ Beef Sandwich entry at 36 fat calories. Don't assume that chicken or fish or vegetarian means low-fat. Always check the Food Tables.

But remember — you'll become much leaner and healthier if you avoid fast-food restaurants and pack your own huge, healthy lunch.

Wrap Rap

The newest rage at some fast-food restaurants as well as other types of restaurants around the country are wraps. Wraps are made by filling a tortilla with one of a variety of stuffings — chicken, shrimp, vegetables — and rolling it up. You might think wraps would be a good choice because often many of the ingredients are quite healthy, but the glue that holds them together and gives the wrap taste is generally fat — fat in the form of cheese, mayonnaise, or oil. It is difficult to know how much injury a specific wrap will inflict on your Fat Budget, but the following examples will give you ballpark figures. At Long John Silver's the Chicken Classic Wrap has 320 fat calories. The wraps at Taco Bell range from 170 fat calories for a Veggie Fajita Wrap to 230 fat calories for a Chicken Fajita Wrap Supreme.

PIZZA   (pages 217–18, Food Tables)

Scratch "American as apple pie." The expression should be: "American as pizza." Pizza is one of the most popular foods in America. It is certainly one of the most convenient. You don't even have to go out for pizza anymore. You can order it over the phone, and within 30 minutes a steaming disk of fat can be yours. Although there are dieters who try to claim pizza as a carbohydrate, almost everyone admits that pizza is a high-fat food. A Pizza Hut Personal Pan Pepperoni Pizza has 261 fat calories; 2 slices of Domino's 12-inch Deluxe Pizza contain 207 fat calories (but who eats 2 slices?). Pizza is delicious, but treat it as you treat an expensive vacation: Fit in pizza as a major and occasional splurge.

If you are stuck in a pizza parlor with no options but to order pizza and you haven't budgeted in the splurge, you can save some fat calories by ordering the pizza without cheese. Don't spend too much time polishing your halo. You are still getting a lot of fat in the crust and tomato sauce.

RESTAURANT FOOD

Eating out at restaurants is hazardous to your Fat Budget. All restaurants are fat traps. However, you can limit the damage if you choose the right restaurant, ask the right questions, and make the right menu choices. (See Chapter 11, "Dining Out," for tips on coping with restaurant food.)

Even if you can make low-fat choices at some restaurants, we recommend limiting your restaurant excursions to seldom or very seldom. Why subject yourself to all that temptation? If you are at home eating delicious dishes, you are thinking, "Mmm, good!" but if you are at a restaurant, you're probably thinking, "I'm eating the broiled chicken on the menu, but I'd rather be eating the ribs." For many people, knowing they aren't consuming the many high-fat choices offered makes them feel sorry for themselves. "How unfair!" they cry. Soon they decide they deserve to have a high-fat choice too. Eventually all their choices are high-fat, and they fall off the low-fat wagon. If they ate scrumptious homemade meals at home, they wouldn't feel deprived and they would avoid being constantly subjected to temptation and guilt.

Any restaurant poses problems. We'll discuss a few. For more specifics, look in the RESTAURANT FOODS section of the Food Tables.

Chinese: Ultra-High-Fat Splurge   (page 304, Food Tables)

Myth: Chinese restaurant food is healthy and low in fat. Truth: The fat in one Chinese dish is enough to put your Fat Budget in hock for days.

Yes. Chinese food does contain lots of nutritious vegetables and rice, but not only do many Chinese restaurants fry and deep-fry ingredients in large amounts of oil, they often blanch them (pass meat or vegetables through hot or warm oil) first. How does a dish of kung pao beef at 1706 fat calories or moo shu pork at 1053 fat calories fit into your Fat Budget? Check out the fat calories in the box below and under *Chinese Restaurants* in the RESTAURANT FOODS section of the Food Tables and prepare your own Chinese food at home.

CHINESE RESTAURANT DISH	AMOUNT	FAT CALORIES
Egg roll	1	103
Chicken with vegetables	1 whole dish	652
Sweet and sour shrimp	1 whole dish	805
Chicken with cashews	1 whole dish	1075
Orange beef	1 whole dish	1216
Barbecued spareribs	1 whole dish	1232
Sweet and sour pork	1 whole dish	1509
Kung pao beef	1 whole dish	1706

Chinese Restaurant Syndrome. This is the real Chinese Restaurant Syndrome: When eating at a Chinese restaurant, instead of limiting ourselves to one modest portion, we take a healthy portion from each dish that is passed around. Our hunger seems to know no bounds. When Chinese food was considered the road to health, this behavior was acceptable, but now that we know the steep price paid for every bite, we have to choose with extreme care and eat with restraint.

Actually the best policy is to limit visits to Chinese restaurants severely. Make your own Chinese food at home at one-fifth the cost. If you find yourself at a Chinese restaurant, you can attempt to make your choices lower in fat by asking that the vegetables and poultry or seafood be steamed and the sauce be served on the side.* If no adjustments can

---

* However, you can never be sure your requests have been carried out.

be made in the kitchen, take a heaping portion of rice and no more than a cup of an entrée. Choose one that is heavy on vegetables. You'll still be giving your Fat Budget a hernia.

Italian: Eat It in Italy   (pages 311–12, Food Tables)

You are probably not surprised that Italian restaurant food in the United States is loaded with fat. The dishes are drowned in oil and cheese, the preparation is fattening, and the serving size of these high-fat dishes is staggering. Most Italian dishes could easily be shared by 3 people. American Italian restaurants seem to feel that if a little is good, a huge amount is much, much better. Even an innocent entrée like spaghetti with tomato sauce comes as a 3½-cup serving containing 160 fat calories. That's the low end of the offerings. Consider fettucine Alfredo at 873 fat calories for 2½ cups or lasagna at 477 fat calories for 2 cups.

Fat calories also sneak in on the garlic bread (360 fat calories for 8 ounces) and salad dressing.

Check out the fat calories of the entries under *Italian Restaurant* and under *Olive Garden* in the RESTAURANT FOODS section of the Food Tables and then make your own low-fat Italian dishes at home.

Mexican: Montezuma's True Revenge   (page 312, Food Tables)

Cheese nachos — 500 fat calories; beef burrito with beans, rice, sour cream, and guacamole — 711 fat calories; two chili rellenos with beans and rice — 864 fat calories; taco salad with sour cream and guacamole — 639 fat calories. Need we say more?

Check out the fat calories under *Mexican Restaurants* in the RESTAURANT FOODS section of the Food Tables and stay away.

Chain Restaurants*: Fat Depots   (page 303, Food Tables)

One of the reasons Americans are so fat is that we eat out so often at restaurants like these. Look at some of these statistics for chicken choices: grilled chicken — 270 fat calories; chicken fingers — 306 fat calories; Oriental chicken salad with dressing (4 cups (!) — 441 fat calories. How about an order of onion rings — 576 fat calories or a loaded baked potato — 279 fat calories?

Check out the fat calories under *Chain Restaurants* in the RESTAURANT FOODS section of the Food Tables and make your visits rare.

---

* Such as Applebee's, Bennigan's, Chili's, T.G.I. Friday's, Hard Rock Cafe, etc.

Chicken Out = Pig Out   (pages 301–2, Food Tables)

Chicken is low-fat, so chicken restaurants such as Boston Market (née Boston Chicken) or Chicken Out must be great choices. Yes? NO! Never jump to conclusions when it comes to food. Look at some of the fat calories of these chicken dishes: original chicken pot pie (300 fat calories); ¾ cup chunky chicken salad (270 fat calories); ¼ white-meat chicken with skin (150 fat calories). Consider some of the side dishes: ¾ cup baked beans (80 fat calories); ⅔ cup mashed potatoes (80 fat calories); ¾ cup coleslaw (140 fat calories). It appears that chicken restaurants are not such a great choice after all.

Check out Boston Market in the RESTAURANT FOODS section of the Food Tables and you'll be convinced to make delicious low-fat chicken dishes at home.

Fish Restaurants: Here's the Catch   (pages 315–16, Food Tables)

You might also assume that a fish restaurant would be a healthy, low-fat choice because fish can be so low in fat and healthy. Again, don't be an assumption jumper. The fish offered at fish restaurants is rarely plain broiled fish. The typical fare is breaded and deep-fried. The fried seafood combo contains 450 fat calories; the fried clams 423. Even items such as broiled salmon may contain 189 fat calories a serving.

For the lowest-fat and healthiest fish dinner, have your fish broiled, baked, or blackened with no fat added. If you feel your fish needs a butter coating (34 fat calories a teaspoon), have the waiter bring some on the side so *you* can determine the amount used.

Although it is expensive, a great low-low-low-fat choice is the shrimp cocktail. Both the boiled or steamed shrimp and the cocktail sauce contain almost no fat.

Be wary of extras such as cole slaw (81 fat calories per half-cup), tartar sauce (72 fat calories per tablespoon), and rum buns (at least 80 fat calories a bun). Ask for a plain baked potato.

Check out Red Lobster in the RESTAURANT FOODS section of the Food Tables and you'll choose scrumptious, healthy, homemade (at your home) fish dishes.

Coffee Bars: Be Alert   (pages 304–9, Food Tables)

Coffee bars have sprouted up all over the country. They have gained popularity because they offer a relaxed atmosphere for socializing. Coffee bars would seem to be safe low-fat havens, but you have to watch out for the high-fat booby traps that can blow your Fat Budget to smithereens. If you choose black coffee or caffe latte with skim milk (5 fat calories) or cappuccino with skim milk (0 fat calories), you're at no risk. If you choose other fancy coffee drinks, hold steady for the blast. At Starbucks, a short caffe mocha (8 fl oz) with whole milk and whipping cream contains 150 fat calories; with 2% milk it contains 120. Even a short caffe mocha with skim milk has 100 fat calories. A 12-ounce cappuccino made with whole milk at the Coffee Beanery contains 81 fat calories; made with 2% milk, it has 54. Check out the fat calories under *Coffee Bar Coffees* in the RESTAURANT FOODS section of the Food Tables.

Watch out for the coffee bar sweets. The scones and muffins look innocent but are riddled with fat. A maple oat nut scone contains 250 fat calories; a "very blueberry" scone contains 210. The no-cholesterol scones are no buy either. A blueberry no-cholesterol scone contains 100 fat calories.

Starbucks muffins are killers: a cranberry orange muffin weighs in at 5 ounces and contains 300 fat calories; a 5-ounce chocolate chunk muffin contains 280 fat calories. Starbucks baked goods vary from store to store, but it's probably safe to assume the choices will make deep cuts in your Fat Budget.

DESSERTS

It should come as no surprise that desserts can cause your Fat Budget to self-destruct. But what's the point of being alive if you can never have a dessert? The virtue of *Choose to Lose Weight-Loss Plan for Men* is that it allows you to eat an occasional high-fat dessert. You know the cost. Just save up for the splurge by undereating your Fat Budget for a few days. Before you indulge yourself, set limits so you won't overdo. For example, plan to eat one slice of cherry cheesecake and you won't find you have eaten half the cake. But use caution. Too many splurges and you are off *Choose to Lose Weight-Loss Plan for Men* and on Choose to Gain.

For fat calories in specific desserts, check out the SWEETS section of the Food Tables.

Candy: Small but Deadly   (pages 356–60, Food Tables)

Perhaps it is because candy bars are often so small, perhaps it is wishful thinking — whatever the reason, people often are shocked at the megafat calories packed into a candy bar. It should not be a surprise because candy contains all the highest-fat and highest-sat-fat ingredients — butterfat, cocoa butter, and nuts (and sometimes coconut).

Grab a small bag of M&Ms and you'll be getting 90 fat calories. A Baby Ruth contains 110 fat calories, a Payday 120, a Snickers 130, and a Butterfinger 100.

Candy can be an expensive treat. Save it for rare occasions.

Power Bars: Candy Bar in a Healthy Wrapper

If you pop a power bar for quick energy, you are throwing your money away. Most power bars are extremely expensive packages of empty calories. Some are also high in fat. They look like candy bars because they are candy bars. A 1¾-ounce Balance Bar will cost you 50 fat calories. Even when it contains some fiber, vitamins, and minerals, a power bar is no substitute for a full, satisfying meal or even a piece of fruit.

Cookies Add Up   (pages 360–67, Food Tables)

Cookie consumption is a miraculous occurrence. Somehow, when you are not even looking, scores of cookies jump from the plate or package into your mouth. Cookie monsters — pay attention. Even one little cookie can be a fat whammy. One small Fudge-Covered Oreo has 50 fat calories, and one Pecan Sandie has 45. The only person in the world who ate just one cookie is listed in the *Guinness Book of World Records.* Most people intend to eat just one cookie but end up eating many. The last one always turns out to be the next-to-last one. And those fat calories add up. If you know that you are a cookie monster, keep your home and office cookie jars filled with fruit.

Nonfat Cookies: Not Free. The above advice applies to nonfat cookies too. Eating one or two for dessert is just fine, but eating half a box will do nothing for your weight-loss goals. Eating all those hundreds and hundreds of empty calories pushes out nutritious calories and stalls your weight loss. For a discussion of nonfat food abuse, see Chapter 6, page 00.

Frozen Desserts   (pages 370–76, Food Tables)

Ice Cream: An Expensive Treat. Rich ice creams such as Ben & Jerry's or Häagen-Dazs can cost 160–210 fat calories for half a cup. (That's 320–420 fat calories a cup, and who eats just a cup?) Even ordinary vanilla ice cream has about 144 fat calories a cup. Some ice creams advertised as "light" are light only in the minds of the manufacturers. Edy's Grand Light French Silk Ice Cream has 90 fat calories per cup. Read the label. Don't keep ice cream in the freezer. Save your ice cream treats for a much less convenient visit to ye olde ice cream shoppe.

Keep Ice Cream Novelty Bars a Novelty. If you are eating Ben & Jerry's Cookie Dough Peace Pops to save the rain forests, think about saving your arteries first. This little ice cream bar contains 230 fat calories — 126 of these are saturated (that's more than half the Sat-Fat Budget for a man wanting to weigh 170 pounds). The fat calories of the following ice cream novelties should make you think carefully before you indulge. A Häagen-Dazs Vanilla and Almond Bar contains 240 fat calories; a Dove Milk Chocolate/Vanilla Ice Cream Bar has 200 fat calories; even a little Snicker's Ice Cream Bar weighing less than 2 ounces costs 110 fat calories.

Frozen Yogurt: Get the Scoop. Just because it's frozen yogurt doesn't mean it's low in fat. You need to ask the server to look for nutrition information on the container. If he can't supply the fat calorie facts, move on.

Nonfat Frozen Yogurt: The Best Buy. The greatest treat is nonfat frozen yogurt, which has 0 calories of fat and is truly delectable. But here are 3 cautions: First, the claim of nonfat may not be true, so don't overdo. Second, although the basic frozen yogurt may be almost fat-free, the almonds, Oreo cookie pieces, peanuts, M&Ms, and coconut you load on top are not. Eat your frozen yogurt plain or with fruit toppings. Third, don't make frozen yogurt a breakfast, lunch, dinner, and bedtime treat. While frozen yogurt may have little or no fat, eaten in excess the empty calories can add up to great amounts and slow down or even stop your weight loss.

Doughnuts   (pages 368–69, Food Tables)

Doughnuts should be added to the old favorite "Old MacDonald Had a Farm" — "Here a doughnut, there a doughnut, everywhere a dough-nut-doughnut." This delectable sweet can be found everywhere: in every office, at every conference, at every PTA, church, or choir meeting. It is difficult to resist, but resist you must. (Of course you may save a doughnut for a special splurge.) Each doughnut costs between 90 and 160 fat calories. The omnipresent glazed doughnut costs 130 fat calories.

Your best bet is to urge your compatriots to stop thinking doughnuts and start thinking bagels (0–15 fat calories each).

Cakes and Pies   (pages 349–55, 379–80, Food Tables)

You need not avoid cakes and pies completely, but they should be saved for splurges. Even fat-free cakes and pies should be considered special treats.

Always check the fat calories AND the serving size on the food label. On first glance, the fat calories for the package of 2 small chocolate cupcakes doesn't look too, too high — 50 fat calories. Look again — carefully. The serving size is 1 cupcake. Who eats half a package? The whole package of 2 cupcakes is 100 fat calories.

HIGH-FAT SNACKS   (pages 329–44, Food Tables)

Caution advised. Unless you are capable of eating one potato chip or one nacho or one peanut, then leave snacks out of your house. Just look under SNACK FOODS in the Food Tables for an eye-opener. An ounce of potato chips has 90 fat calories; an ounce of potato sticks, 90; an ounce of corn chips, 80. Do you know how small an ounce is? About 18 chips. A tiny can (2.8 oz) of French's French Fried Onions contains 330 fat calories. A small deli bag of Fritos may contain 270 fat calories. Are they really worth all that salt and fat?

Chips — High Stakes   (pages 329–31, Food Tables)

If you are like most human beings, you will find it impossible to refrain from eating potato chips if they are in your house. Potato chips are truly addictive. The last one always invites another. Since 1 ounce (about 14 chips) has 80 to 100 fat calories and the ounces go down so easily, in very little time you can consume enough chips to do severe damage to your Fat Budget.

Any chips — Fritos, Chee-tos, nachos — should be eaten with considerable thought. Chips are basically fat stiffened with a bit of vegetable and the fat calories show it. Our strong recommendation is to leave temptation out of the house by not bringing chips in. No one needs them.

If this information is making you sad because chips are your greatest joy in life, then budget them in for a rare treat. However, we bet their absence will make your heart grow less fond of them.

The Truth About Popcorn

Hot-Air-Popped Popcorn: A Real Buy. Let's start with the good news. Plain, unadulterated popcorn is one of the healthiest snacks known to mankind. It's almost fat-free and it's chock-full of fiber — half insoluble (important for effective bowel function and reducing risk of colon cancer) and half soluble (helps a little bit to lower blood cholesterol and risk of heart disease). It satisfies your hand-to-mouth needs and tastes delicious. We admit that plain air-popped popcorn may at first taste like Styrofoam, because with no fat coating it won't hold salt. However, we guarantee that in no time you will love it madly. Hot-air-poppers are the dream machine. They are inexpensive (about $20), and you never have to clean them.

Microwave Popcorn: Questionable Buy. Don't buy microwave popcorn for the speed and convenience. With microwave popcorn you're getting neither speed (microwave popcorn takes 4½ minutes to pop; air-popped takes only 3) nor more convenience (air-poppers need no cleaning), but you may be getting a lot of fat. Microwave popcorn ranges from 6 to 40 fat calories per cup (versus almost no fat for plain air-popped popcorn). That could amount to 320 fat calories for 8 cups.

Movie Popcorn: Risky Business. Usually popped in coconut oil (the most heart-risky fat) and drowned in butter, movie popcorn can torpedo your Fat Budget out of the water. The cost can get as high as 1134 fat calories for a 20-cup tub popped in coconut oil with "butter." Check movie popcorn under SNACK FOODS in the Food Tables and then hot-air-pop and bring your own. If the usher questions you, tell him you are following doctor's orders.

Fat in a Nutshell   (pages 290–93, Food Tables)

Before you stick your hand into the bowl of nuts or sweet talk the stewardess into giving you a few extra bags of peanuts, take a look at the NUTS AND SEEDS section of the Food Tables. The half-ounce bag of airplane peanuts will cost you 65 fat calories. One ounce of cashews will cost you 118 fat calories, macadamia nuts 196 fat calories, walnuts 158 fat calories. Considering that 1 ounce of nuts isn't many, it turns out to be a lot of fat calories. This is also true of seeds and trail mixes that contain nuts.

Don't be conned into thinking that nuts are healthy because they are

	Popped in:	Coconut oil		Coconut oil with butter		Canola shortening*	
		CALORIES		CALORIES		CALORIES	
AMOUNT	SIZE	TOTAL	FAT	TOTAL	FAT	TOTAL	FAT
5 cups	Small (A);	300	180	472	333		
	Kids (C)	300	180	472	333		
7 cups	Small (C, U)	398	243	632	450		
	Small (A)					361	198
11 cups	Medium (A)	647	387	910	639	627	342
16 cups	Medium (C, U)	901	540	1221	873		
	Large (A)					850	468
20 cups	Large (all)	1161	693	1642	1134		

Movie Popcorn

A = AMC; C = Cineplex Odeon; U = United Artists
*Some AMC theaters use canola oil.
Sources: Nutrition Action Healthletter; Center for Science in the Public Interest; SGS Control Services, Inc.

high in protein and vitamin E. Their ultra-high-fat content negates any positive benefits you may derive from eating them.

When you see that nuts or seeds have been added to a food, such as cereal or muffins, you know that food is going to be much higher in fat. If you are nuts about nuts, save them for a rare treat. By cutting them out, you may be saving thousands of fat calories.

Crackers: Always the Last One   (pages 331–35, Food Tables)

Like most snack food, crackers are addictive. If you could eat just one (sometimes only 10 fat calories), you would be in good shape. But before you take a second sip of soda, you've eaten 10 (100 fat calories). And then there's the cheese you *have* to put on each one. If you are tempted at a party and can stop at one or two, then do. Otherwise, don't get started.

This advice also holds for fat-free crackers. Too many crackers means too many empty calories, and your body will burn them instead of the fat you want to lose.

Pretzels

Most pretzels are nonfat or low-fat — but not all. Be sure to read the labels because some pretzels, such as Snyder's of Hanover Honey Mustard and Onion pretzel pieces (60 fat calories per ounce), or Cheddar Cheese Pretzel Combos (45 fat calories per ⅓ cup) are pretty pricey, fat-calorie-wise.

In moderation fat-free pretzels are a lovely treat. They are crunchy and satisfying. We often eat a few for dessert. However, keep your passion for pretzels in tow. One or two large ones a day should be a ceiling. They are highly processed, often oversalted (sodium raises blood pressure in some people), and when eaten in abundance are burned in preference to fat.

Go Slow on Pork Rinds

Pork rinds or cracklins make a poor snack, health- and fat-wise. Half an ounce — half an ounce! — of Utz Pork Cracklins has 90 fat calories (70 sat-fat calories). One ounce of Smithfield pork rinds has 90 fat calories (36 sat-fat calories). For the sake of your heart and weight-loss goals, think long and hard before budgeting in pork rinds.

"Healthy" Snacks

Even snack food that appears to be low in fat or "healthy" is subject to suspicion. For example, you might pick up SmartFood Reduced Fat Air-Popped Popcorn because the package implies it is a smart, healthy, low-fat food. Its ingredients are, after all, *"all natural"* and the popcorn is *"air-popped."* Check out the nutrition label: fat calories per serving — 50; 1 serving — 3 cups. Who eats 3 cups? Try 100 fat calories for 6 cups. Is that smart food?

Snack Sense

Even low-fat snacks should be eaten with restraint. Of course it is better to chomp on nonfat baked chips than nachos and peanuts while watching the Super Bowl, but try to convince yourself that you don't need to have a constant stream of food flowing into your mouth. You could just watch the game without eating or eat air-popped popcorn you make yourself in your own hot-air-popper. If you do eat high-fat snacks, measure a limited amount into a bowl and consume only that amount. Eat a big lunch or dinner before the game begins so you are too full to have a high-fat snack breakdown.

DRY YOUR TEARS

If you have been reading this chapter with a lump in your throat and tears billowing down your cheeks because so many of your favorites turn out to be fat bombshells, cheer up. You have a Fat Budget, and with a little planning you can occasionally fit some of these fat-laden foods into your diet. The advantage of learning the fat in foods is that you won't inhale foods without thinking about the cost. You won't waste fat calories on foods you hardly like. Is that little greasy cheese dog worth 120 fat calories? Do you want to spend 100 fat calories on mayonnaise for your turkey sandwich when mustard (0 fat calories) tastes just as good? Refer to this chapter and to the Food Tables in the back of the book to make educated choices that will produce a lean, fit you.

Give yourself a chance to change your palate to a low-fat taste that will shrink your belly and enlarge your world.

Nutrition Label Know-how

Knowing the fat calories in foods is the key to making choices. The Food Tables in the back of the book list thousands of foods and their fat calories. You also need to judge the fat cost of packaged food that you buy. In the next chapter, you will learn everything you need to know about deciphering nutrition labels. They look complicated, but after reading Chapter 8, we guarantee you will be able to analyze a nutrition label in 5 seconds flat.

8. Decoding Nutrition Labels

IN THE PAST you may have grabbed packages from the supermarket shelf with nary a glance at the nutrition label. When you did look at the package, you might have been impressed by a "40% less fat" or an "all natural" claim, but you had no way of interpreting if the product was healthy or low-fat. You may not have even cared. Now you *must* care!

All the hype — "50% fewer calories!" "⅓ less fat!" "Cholesterol-free!" "Healthy Choice!" — is designed to win over people like you who are interested in eating a healthier diet or losing weight. In this chapter, you will learn everything you need to know about nutrition labels so you will be able to ignore the bright letters, stars, and exclamation marks and zero in on the only information you need: fat calories per serving and serving size.

FDA Regulates for Consistency

The Food and Drug Administration has made navigating through the food claim jungle much easier by setting guidelines for nutrition labeling. (On first glance, nutrition labels look impossible, but they don't have to be.)

By reading the nutrition label, you will know what you need to know — how many fat calories are in the amount of food you want to eat. You will know which foods are good choices for you. It's a snap.

INGREDIENT LIST

What's Inside?

Get your own can or package so that you can examine the label.

First, find the list of ingredients on the package you chose. It is often grouped with the Nutrition Facts label, but you may have to search for it elsewhere. The ingredient list does not give you quantitative information, but it does give you useful information. Ingredients are always listed in descending order by weight. Would you choose a food with coconut oil as its first ingredient?

BAR-B-Q FLAVORED POTATO CHIPS

INGREDIENTS: POTATOES, VEGETABLE OIL (CONTAINS ONE OF THE FOLLOWING: CANOLA, CORN, COTTONSEED, OR PARTIALLY HYDROGENATED SOYBEAN OIL), SALT, SPICES, DEXTROSE, SUGAR, HYDROLYZED SOY PROTEIN, MSG, ONION, TOMATO, CITRIC ACID, ARTIFICIAL AND NATURAL FLAVORS, AND GARLIC.

First Ingredient: Potatoes. Reading this label tells you that potatoes account for more weight than any other ingredient. Unfortunately, since neither the actual weights of the ingredients nor each ingredient's percentage of the total weight are provided, you have no way of knowing if the chips are mostly potatoes or half potatoes and half the next ingredient — oil!

Second Ingredient: Oil. Vegetable oil is listed second, which probably means there is lots of it. The type of oil may be canola, corn, cottonseed, or partially hydrogenated soybean oil. Manufacturers typically list a variety of oils so they can use whichever is cheapest at the time. You have no idea if they are using canola oil — low in saturated fat and thus heart-healthy — or cottonseed oil — high in saturated fat and thus heart-risky and possibly full of pesticides.* They may be using partially hydrogenated soybean oil, which is also heart-risky — the more hydrogenated an oil, the more heart-risky. All of the oils are 100% fat and fattening, but the type of oil determines the impact on your arteries. (See pages 71–72 for a discussion of the health effects of saturated, monounsaturated, and polyunsaturated fats.)

---

* Because cotton is not regulated as a food, pesticide levels in cottonseed oil may be higher than is considered healthy for consumption.

Salt. Next comes salt. So basically, this food is potatoes, oil, and salt.

Just reading this ingredient list would give you a big clue that it is not a nutritious food. If this general information is not enough to spoil the chips for you, you will next learn how to decipher the Nutrition Facts box for the rest of the awful truth.

Before you read the next section, look at the ingredient list on the package you chose. What does it tell you?

NUTRITION FACTS BOX

A much more specific and thus much more helpful item on a package is the Nutrition Facts box. Congress has legislated that the format be standardized so that every product includes the same nutrition information.

The Nutrition Facts box has the essential information you need to make wise decisions — calories from fat and serving size. Saturated fat is also listed (albeit in grams, not calories). Fiber is an important category.

You may also find a lot of information on the labels that seems confusing. You really don't need to look at anything other than calories from fat and serving size, but we will explain the rest so you can understand it.

One Serving

First, you should know that all the numbers listed — calories, calories from fat, total fat, and cholesterol, even the amounts of vitamin A and vitamin C — are for one serving of the food. The package may hold more than one serving, but the nutrition information is for only one serving.

Be warned: The serving on the nutrition label may not be what you consider a serving — one-fourth of a candy bar, half a 5" chicken pot pie, one cookie — so you must *always* determine what one serving means before you determine how much fat you are consuming.

Calories from Fat

Find Calories from Fat on the corn chips label. One serving of corn chips has 90 fat calories. But don't stop there. You need to know the size of a serving.

Corn Chips

Nutrition Facts	
Serving Size 1oz. (28g/About 32 chips)	
Servings Per Container About 3	
Amount Per Serving	
Calories 160 Calories from Fat 90	
	% Daily Value*
Total Fat 10g	**16%**
Saturated Fat 1.5g	**8%**
Cholesterol 0mg	**0%**
Sodium 160mg	**7%**
Total Carbohydrate 15g	**5%**
Dietary Fiber 1g	**4%**
Sugars 0g	
Protein 2g	

Serving Size

Next look under the Nutrition Facts heading for the Serving Size. The Serving Size is "1 oz (28g/About 32 chips)." If you were to eat one serving, you would be consuming 90 fat calories. But keep reading, you need to know how many servings you plan to eat.

Is the Serving Size What You Eat? In this case, a serving is 1 ounce or 32 chips, but is that what you would eat? When the serving size is smaller, the amounts of fat, saturated fat, and sodium listed on the label are also smaller, and the product looks a lot healthier. This distortion benefits the food manufacturers, but not you. If you want your belly to melt away and your cholesterol level to plummet, you need to know exactly how much fat you are consuming. Always multiply the fat calories per serving times the number of servings you are planning to eat to determine what a food will cost you in fat calories.

Servings per Container

It is natural to look at the fat calories on the label and assume they are for the entire package. For example, if you were to hold this tiny deli bag of corn chips, you would assume that it contains one serving of chips. DON'T MAKE ASSUMPTIONS! Look at the Servings Per Container. There are **3** servings in this little bag. The entire bag holds 3 x 90 fat calories per serving or 270 fat calories.

Because you would never share this bag of chips with 2 other people (we bet the food manufacturer wouldn't either), you cannot assume that the food manufacturer shares your notion of a serving or the number of servings in this bag. You must always look at the serving size and multiply it by the number of servings you are planning to eat to figure out the amount of fat you will be consuming (in this case, the entire bag).

These listings may also be of interest to you:

Saturated Fat

Find Saturated Fat on the corn chips label. Saturated fat is listed as 1.5 grams. There are 9 calories per gram of saturated fat. Thus, in one serving of the chips there are 1.5 x 9 fat calories per gram, which equals about 14 sat-fat calories or 41 sat-fat calories in the whole bag. Since saturated fat is the main culprit raising blood cholesterol levels, you want to limit your consumption of saturated fat. To help put the 41 sat-fat calories into perspective, a sedentary male who wants to weigh 160 pounds has a Sat-Fat Budget of 224.*

Cholesterol

On the chips label, Cholesterol is listed as 0 mg. This information is useful, but not in the way you might assume.

A listing of 0 mg of cholesterol tells you that the potato chips are a vegetable product. Only animal products contain cholesterol. Cholesterol content will not help you judge if a product is heart-healthy because dietary cholesterol has a very minor effect on raising blood cholesterol (saturated fat is the culprit). In fact, cholesterol-free foods such as coconut, palm, and hydrogenated plant oils are highly saturated and thus extremely heart-risky. You need to determine the calories of sat-fat to determine if the food is heart-healthy.

The cholesterol listing is useful because you can use it to determine the amount of meat in the product. All meats — beef, veal, lamb, poultry, and fish (except for shrimp at 43 mg per oz) — contain 18–28 mg of cholesterol per ounce. Say the cholesterol listed for a chicken dinner is 25 mg per serving. Since 1 ounce of chicken contains about 24 mg of cholesterol, by dividing the 25 mg cholesterol listed on the package by the 24 mg of cholesterol per ounce for chicken, you would determine that the chicken dinner contains about 1 ounce of meat (25 ÷ 24 = about 1 oz). Note: The reason that frozen dinners may leave you hungry and dissatisfied (and annoyed you paid so much for so little) is because they often contain less than 1 ounce of meat.

Dietary Fiber

The FDA did us a big favor by including dietary fiber in the nutrition label. Fiber is an essential element of a healthy diet. (See page 51 for a discussion of the benefits of consuming dietary fiber.)

By listing dietary fiber, the new nutrition labels help you choose higher-fiber foods when possible. (Caveat: Because of an unclear definition of dietary fiber, the only reliable dietary fiber listings may be those for cereals.) For example, look at the Dietary Fiber entries of the two cereal labels below. Check out which cereal would be a better choice, fiber-wise. The corn flakes have 1 gram of fiber, and the raisin bran has 8. Choose the higher-fiber cereal when you can, but if you have to hold

---

* For everything you need to know about saturated fat, read *Eater's Choice: A Food Lover's Guide to Lower Cholesterol.*

Corn Flakes

Raisin Bran

Nutrition Facts

| Serving Size | 1 Cup (28g/1.0 oz.) |
| Servings per Package | About 12 |

Amount Per Serving	Cereal	Cereal with ½ Cup Vitamins A & D Skim Milk
Calories	100	140
Calories from Fat	0	0
	% Daily Value **	
Total Fat 0g*	**0** %	**0** %
Saturated Fat 0g	**0** %	**0** %
Cholesterol 0mg	**0** %	**0** %
Sodium 300mg	**13** %	**15** %
Potassium 25mg	**1** %	**7** %
Total Carbohydrate 24g	**8** %	**10** %
Dietary Fiber 1g	**4** %	**4** %
Sugars 2g		
Other Carbohydrate 21g		
Protein 2g		

Nutrition Facts

| Serving Size | 1 Cup (61g/2.2 oz.) |
| Servings per Package | About 7 |

Amount Per Serving	Cereal	Cereal with ½ Cup Vitamins A & D Skim Milk
Calories	200	240
Calories from Fat	15	15
	% Daily Value **	
Total Fat 1.5g*	**2** %	**2** %
Saturated Fat 0g	**0** %	**0** %
Cholesterol 0mg	**0** %	**0** %
Sodium 370mg	**15** %	**18** %
Potassium 360mg	**10** %	**16** %
Total Carbohydrate 47g	**16** %	**18** %
Dietary Fiber 8g	**32** %	**32** %
Sugars 18g		
Other Carbohydrate 21g		
Protein 6g		

your nose while you choke it down, choose a lower-fiber cereal you enjoy. By following *Choose to Lose Weight-Loss Plan for Men* you will get lots of fiber in fruits, vegetables, and whole grains, so you need not suffer through a 10-gram-fiber bowl of wood chips. Like anything else, give yourself time — you might find you love the taste of wood chips.

The dietary fiber in our corn chips example is a big 1 gram. No surprise. We doubt that anyone eats corn chips to fulfill their fiber quota. Even if the fiber content were 10 grams per serving, the fat content should still discourage you from eating them.

FDA's Folly: Daily Value and % Daily Value

Here's where the FDA compromised the value of the nutrition labels. The FDA knew that the numbers on the nutrition label mean very little without a way of putting them into perspective. So it developed nutrition budgets for every American irrespective of size or activity level. It called these Daily Values (DV*) and gave Daily Values for fat, saturated fat, cholesterol, sodium, total carbohydrate, and dietary fiber. There are three problems:

1. People differ in size and energy needs. The same Daily Values do not meet the needs of everyone.
2. The Daily Value the FDA chose for fat was much too high.
3. Most people are confused and turned off by all the Daily Values, so they disregard the label completely.

You may be asking smugly, "What do these Daily Values have to do with me? I have my own personal Daily Value for Fat — my Fat Budget — tailored just for me." Right. On *Choose to Lose Weight-Loss Plan for Men* you zero in on calories from fat and serving size. You can ignore the Daily Values. However, if you are curious about the elaborate, confusing, superfluous system the FDA developed and want to understand what the other numbers mean, read on.

Chocolate Chip Cookies

Nutrition Facts	
Serving Size 1 cookie (20g)	
Servings Per Container about 26	
Amount Per Serving	
Calories 100 Calories from Fat 45	
	% Daily Value*
Total Fat 5g	**8%**
Saturated Fat 2g	**10%**
Cholesterol 2mg	**1%**
Sodium 75mg	**3%**
Total Carbohydrate 14g	**5%**
Dietary Fiber less than 1g	**2%**
Sugars 8g	
Protein 1g	
Vitamin A 0% • Vitamin C 0%	
Calcium 0% • Iron 2%	

	Calories:	2,000	2,500
Total Fat	Less than	65g	80g
Sat Fat	Less than	20g	25g
Cholesterol	Less than	300mg	300mg
Sodium	Less than	2,400mg	2,400mg
Total Carbohydrate		300g	375g
Dietary Fiber		25g	30g

*Percent Daily Values are based on a 2,000 calorie diet. Your daily values may be higher or lower depending on your calorie needs.

Total Calorie Intake

Look at the circled area at the bottom of the chocolate chip cookies label. It says "Percent Daily Values are based on a 2,000 calorie diet." This means that everyone, regardless of sex, activity, height, desirable weight, or frame size, has to be consuming a 2000-calorie diet for this system to work.

Now look at the information below that on Total Fat.

Daily Value Total Fat: Too Much

Instead of recommending that every man, woman, and child in the United States follow *Choose to Lose Weight-Loss Plan for Men* or *Choose to Lose* and determine their own personal Fat Budget based on 20% of their BMR, the FDA

---

* On smaller Nutrition Facts boxes, Daily Value is abbreviated to DV.

tried to develop a Fat Budget that would fit everyone in the country. For their Fat Budget, called Daily Value for Fat, they chose 30% of 2000 total calories. By creative multiplying, they determined that 30% of 2000 equals 585* fat calories or 65 grams. This Daily Value for total fat — 585 fat calories! — is so huge it comes with a money-back guarantee for weight gain.

The Daily Value of 585 fat calories applies to everyone, whether a 6 foot 7 inch basketball player or a 4 foot 10 inch jockey, whether your goal weight is 195 pounds or 120. How does 585 fat calories compare with your Fat Budget?

Now find Saturated Fat, which is listed below Total Fat.

Daily Value Saturated Fat: A Healthy Prescription

Although not tailored to individuals, the FDA's Sat-Fat Budget (Daily Value for saturated fat) is reasonable. At less than 20 grams (180 sat-fat calories), the Daily Value for saturated fat is actually low for most people, and that's healthy.

% Daily Value: Complicating a Simple System

To help people understand how the fat calories or sat-fat calories per serving on the label fit into their Daily Values, the FDA invented % Daily Value. Instead of clarifying nutritional needs, these percentages compound the confusion.

This is how % Daily Value works. Look at the circled section of the chocolate chip cookie label. On the left is a list of nutrients and the amount of each nutrient found in one serving of the product. On the right is a list of the percentage of the Daily Value for that nutrient contained in one serving of this product. Come again?

Maybe this will help. Look at % Daily Value for total fat. The label lists

Chocolate Chip Cookies

Nutrition Facts	
Serving Size 1 cookie (20g)	
Servings Per Container about 26	
Amount Per Serving	
Calories 100 Calories from Fat 45	
	% Daily Value*
Total Fat 5g	8%
Saturated Fat 2g	10%
Cholesterol 2mg	1%
Sodium 75mg	3%
Total Carbohydrate 14g	5%
Dietary Fiber less than 1g	2%
Sugars 8g	
Protein 1g	

---

* We have always found that 30% of 2000 is 600 fat calories or 67 fat grams. We have no idea why the FDA determined that 30% of 2000 is 585 fat calories.

Total Fat 5g* _____ 8%. This means that the total fat per serving (45 fat calories) represents 8% of the Daily Value for fat or 8% of 585 fat calories. Each time you eat a cookie — 45 fat calories — you are eating 8% of your Daily Value for Fat. Does the consumer understand that if he eats 2 cookies (90 fat calories), he will be consuming 16% of his Daily Value for fat? Is he going to add up all his % Daily Values throughout the day until he reaches 100%? Will he figure out the % Daily Value for noncommercial food that he eats and include it? Sure.

Actually, most people think that the % Daily Value means that the food contains 8% fat — not a big percentage — and gobble up half the bag (585 fat calories). (See page 102 to understand why percentage of fat in individual foods is irrelevant and misleading.)

Now that you understand % Daily Value, you can forget it. The information is irrelevant to you.

BUYER BEWARE!

Armed with your Fat Budget, you can enter a grocery store with no fear. However, you need to keep on your toes at all times to avoid being duped. Always remember that no matter what the package claims, you must find the Nutrition Facts box, look at calories from fat per serving and serving size, and determine the fat calories for the amount you plan to eat. Never make assumptions. Here are some traps to avoid.

"All Natural": So?

Just because a food is listed as "all natural" does not necessarily mean it is healthy. Cream (792 fat calories per cup), cheese (80 fat calories per ounce), and macadamia nuts (196 fat calories per ounce) may be pure and natural, but they are too fat-packed to be healthy. Arsenic is also "all natural."

Although the food manufacturer does not claim outright that 100% Natural cereal is healthy, the package has been designed so you will leap to this conclusion on your own. Just calling it 100% Natural conjures up visions of ruddy-cheeked campers merrily digging into their bowl of 100% natural oats, honey, and raisins. Stop. Never make assumptions. The label tells the true story.

---

* The fat calories are converted to grams here. There are 9 calories per gram of fat. By dividing 70 fat calories by 9 you get 7.777 or 8 grams. Ignore this number. Calories of fat are a more accurate measure.

Find Calories from Fat: 80. 80! Eighty fat calories is a heap of fat. Find Serving Size: ½ cup. Is ½ cup what you eat? Or is it more like 1 cup, or 160 fat calories? The ingredients listed include dried coconut and partially hydrogenated cottonseed and soybean oils. Coconut is what scientists feed rats, an animal naturally resistant to heart disease, to give them heart attacks. Being 100% natural certainly doesn't guarantee that this is a healthy product.

Cholesterol-Free: So?

Not only does the label boast "100% Natural," it also shouts "CHOLESTEROL FREE FOOD." "Must be heart-healthy" is what the food manufacturers want you to assume. But "cholesterol-free" only tells us that 100% Natural Granola is a vegetable product. We know it is not heart-healthy because it contains heart-risky coconut and partially hydrogenated oils, which are among the most heart-risky foods available.

Chicken: Low-Fat?

Chicken frankfurters! You lick your lips in anticipation. You know that chicken is a low-fat meat. It is certainly lower in fat than beef or pork. The package even says "40% less fat." Must be a good thing. Stop. Look. Read the label.

Granola

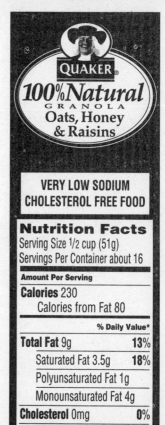

Be Suspicious of All Claims

Since the FDA does not have enough inspectors to keep on top of all the health claims, YOU have to be your own inspector and check out the truth and/or relevance of the health claims you encounter. Always read the Nutrition Facts box to get the facts, man, just the facts.

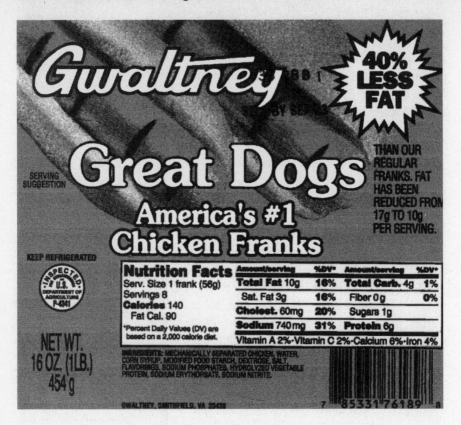

Calories from Fat: 90; Serving Size: 1 frank (56g). Although white-meat turkey and chicken without skin may be low in fat in their virgin state, when they are packed with fat and skin in processed poultry products, they turn into high-fat fare. This hot dog may contain less fat than an all-beef frankfurter (150 fat calories), but 90 fat calories for 2 ounces of meat is far from a low-fat and healthy food.

A Name Is Just a Name

You reach for this frozen dinner because you *think* it is a healthy choice. It says "Weight Watchers," so you *assume* it's low in fat. It says, "Smart Ones," so you must be smart to choose it.* It is pasta, which you

---

* Smart Ones was the brand name given to a line of Weight Watchers frozen dinners that contained 1 gram of fat (9 fat calories). The number of grams is no longer limited to one but the name is still used.

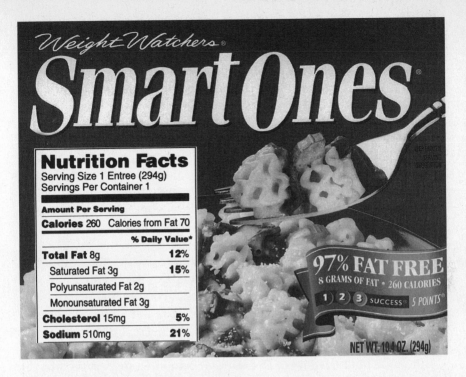

think is a good, low-fat choice. And it is also "97% fat free." Wow! What a great choice! Really? Read the label.

This package may say Weight Watchers and Smart Ones, but these are just brand names. Weight Watchers, Lean Cuisine, and Healthy Choice are not required to be true to their names and produce healthy or low-fat products, and some of their products are neither. If you were to consume this tiny box of pasta at a cost of 70 fat calories, you would neither be acting smart nor watching your weight (unless you are watching it grow).

% Fat-Free: So?

When packages brag that their contents are "97% fat-free" (3% fat), they are only telling you that fat accounts for 3% of the weight of the product. You have no idea if the product is low-fat. You only know that the *weight* of the fat in the product is a lot less than the *weight* of the product as a whole. In this case, the weight of the fat is 8 grams and the weight of the pasta dish is 294 grams. Divide 8 grams by 294 grams and you have 3% fat. So? All you need to know is that the fat content is 70 fat calories for a little bit of food.

% Fat in Individual Foods

While we're talking about "percent fat-free" and % Daily Value, we want to discuss another percentage that is often misunderstood — % fat in individual foods.

Most health agencies recommend that your daily fat consumption be less than 30% (we recommend less than 20%) of your total caloric intake for the *whole day*. In an effort to simplify this recommendation into an action plan, some health writers recommend that *each* food you eat should be less than 30% fat. Not only would this recommendation be very restrictive — you could never eat any oil, cheese, beef, etc. — it would be misleading, as the following example shows.

A malted milk that contains 1060 total calories, 225 coming from fat, is 21% fat — not a high percentage. Two malted milks (450 fat calories) are still 21% fat. Three malted milks (675 fat calories!) are still 21% fat. The percent fat — 21% — doesn't give you a clue that the malted milks are loaded with fat. On the other hand, a food that contains 10 total calories, 8 coming from fat, is 80% fat. But you would never avoid a food that contains a mere 8 fat calories. The percentage of fat in an *individual* food is irrelevant and tells you nothing about how low-fat the food is. You need to know the number of fat calories to make choices.

CLAIMS AND THEIR TRUE MEANING

1. CLAIM: Reduced-Fat

   TRUTH: A food can sport a "reduced-fat" label if it contains at least 25% less fat than the normal product. However, "reduced-fat" does not necessarily mean low-fat. Consider these two "reduced-fat" examples. Nabisco Better Cheddar Crackers are normally 70 fat calories an ounce. Their reduced-fat version is a heaping 50 fat calories an ounce. Utz Ripple Cut Potato Chips normally cost you 90 fat calories an ounce. The reduced-fat version at 60 fat calories an ounce is still a high-fat choice.

2. CLAIM: 2% Reduced-Fat Milk

   TRUTH: 2% milk is now called "reduced-fat." While better than the old "low-fat" label, "reduced-fat" also implies a low-fat food. At 45 fat calories a cup, it is hardly low-fat. The 2% is misleading. If, as most people think, the percentage referred to the percent of calories that come from fat (which is irrelevant — see box above), it would be called 35% milk. Somehow, we doubt if 35% milk would be a great seller. Actually, the 2% refers to the fact that fat accounts for 2% of the *weight* of the milk. Milk is mostly water, so the percentage contributed by fat to the total weight is small. The percentages are totally irrelevant. The important fact is that one 8-ounce glass of 2% milk has 45 fat calories, 2 have 90, and 3 have 135. Work your way down to 1% milk, ½%, and then skim. (See page 68 for a painless way to move from whole to skim milk.)

3. CLAIM: % Fat-Free

   TRUTH: "% fat-free" used to be a very popular form of deception, particularly in cold cuts. Since the FDA issued its new guidelines, it is not as prevalent. The "percent fat-free" information was and is never inaccurate. It is just irrelevant and misleading. (See the Smart Ones pasta discussion, page 101.)

4. CLAIM: Fat-Free, Nonfat

   TRUTH: In the last few years there has been an explosion of fat-free and nonfat products. "Nonfat" foods produced by large companies are probably nonfat. The most fat the product may contain is less than 4.5 fat calories per serving. Of course, if the serving is ¼ teaspoon and you want to eat 1 tablespoon, the fat calories add up.

   Be careful of foods billed as fat-free or nonfat when they have no labeling (such as in bakeries or candy stores). They may only be fat-free in the imagination of the provider.

   When a high-fat food is added to a nonfat food, it is no longer nonfat. The nonfat frozen yogurt with Oreo pieces may be called nonfat, but Oreo cookies remain fat-laden goodies, even when they cohabit with nonfat frozen yogurt.

5. CLAIM: Sugar-Free

   TRUTH: The sugar-free label is a red herring. First of all, a product may not have sugar but may be loaded with fat. Sugar contains empty calories, causes tooth decay, and can force out nutritious foods, but in reasonable quantities does not make you fat (see Chapter 2). To produce sugar-free products, un-healthy sugar substitutes replace sugar. Aspartame (Nutra-sweet) may have harmful side effects. Since it is not neces-sary to eliminate all sugar consumption to lose weight, why take a chance? Avoid sugar-free products unless you are a diabetic. And of course, don't overdose on empty sugar calories.

6. CLAIM: Lite or Light
   TRUTH: Food manufacturers can claim that a product is "light" or "lite" even if the product contains loads of fat. Lite is often used as a relative term. The Boston Lite popcorn has less fat than regular Boston popcorn, but nonetheless it contains 50 fat calories for a mere 4 cups.

7. CLAIM: Lean
   TRUTH: The FDA definition of a "lean" meat is hardly lean at 90 fat calories per $3\frac{1}{2}$ ounces.

8. CLAIM: Extra-Lean
   TRUTH: The FDA defines an "extra-lean" meat as containing less than 45 fat calories per 100 grams ($3\frac{1}{2}$ oz). We would define an extra-lean meat as containing 7 fat calories (turkey breast or cod) or 10 fat calories (chicken or flounder) per 100 grams ($3\frac{1}{2}$ oz).

The Bottom Line

Ignore the claims. Never make assumptions. Go directly to the Nutri-tion Facts box for all the information you need. With your Fat Budget in mind, look at the calories from fat and the serving size, figure out how many fat calories you plan to eat, and how that amount fits into your Fat Budget. Take a look at the ingredient list to make sure you still want to eat the product. If you want to be a healthy person, you need to be a wise consumer.

Coming next . . . better breakfast, lunch, and dinner.

9. Eating In: Best Choice

No More Eating on the Run

Does the following describe you? You pop a frozen dinner into the microwave, order pizza over the phone, or dump lettuce and croutons into a Styrofoam container at a supermarket salad bar and call it dinner. The only vegetables you eat are French fries and ketchup, and the only fruits are Froot Loops and fruit roll-ups. Well, maybe your diet is not this bad, but if you don't eat three, full, well-balanced meals every day, this is the time to start.

This is a great opportunity to enhance your life. Experiment. Cook or encourage a loved one to cook for you. Cooking doesn't have to be difficult. Try new foods, new preparations, new dishes. Do you think you hate squash? Try it. You might love it. Is your diet boring and bland? Add spices. Use *Choose to Lose Weight-Loss Plan for Men* as an excuse to lift yourself out of your rut. Who knows where it will lead?!

SETTING UP FOR SUCCESS

Wipe the Slate Clean

First you need to de-fat your kitchen. Pizza in the freezer, potato chips in the cupboard, cold cuts in the refrigerator — out they go. Otherwise, they may cry, "Eat me! Eat me!" and weaken your resolve. Forget what they cost you in dollars. You will pay a heavier toll in weight gain and poor health by eating them than by pitching them. Don't use the excuse that you're keeping them for the children, your spouse, your mother, Uncle Fred, the dog, the baby-sitter, the Fuller Brush man. They don't need those foods either. You might find it gratifying to tally up the fat calories as you drop them into the garbage rather than into you.

Fill the Larder

Next step is to stock your kitchen with delicious, nutritious, low-fat food. Create a shopping list and go wild at the supermarket. Make sure your fruit bowl is filled, a jar of popcorn kernels awaits air-popping, and a variety of vegetables are at the ready for lunch and dinner.

EATING IN: BREAKFAST

Do NOT Skip Breakfast!

Skipping breakfast does not help you lose weight. People who skip breakfast are so hungry they lose control and pig out on a high-fat lunch. Not eating breakfast (and/or lunch) slows your metabolism. Remember, you need to eat enough calories to keep up your metabolism and to keep from being hungry.

Are you one of those people who claim you can't stomach food or even the thought of food in the morning? This is why. If you don't eat breakfast (and sometimes no lunch), by the time dinner comes around, you are famished. As a result, you gorge yourself until bedtime. No wonder you can't think about food in the morning. You are stuffed from the night before.

You *can* break the cycle. Start tomorrow with a light breakfast, and then eat a normal lunch and dinner. Eat fruit or air-popped popcorn for a nighttime snack. Soon you will be so hungry at breakfast time you will eagerly eat a hearty low-fat breakfast.

Eat at Home

Now that you know the importance of eating breakfast — eat it at home. There is really no reason to eat breakfast out unless you are traveling in a different city. Breakfast out can be one of the most fattening of meals. A low-fat breakfast at home can be nourishing and delicious and quick and easy. Here's a list of some quick and easy low-fat breakfast choices:

- Whole-grain toast (whole-wheat bread has more fiber and nutrients), English muffins, or bagels instead of sweet rolls, biscuits, muffins, Danish pastries, doughnuts, or croissants.
- Spreads such as jelly, honey, apple butter, or nonfat cream cheese instead of butter, margarine, or cream cheese.

- Hot cereals such as oatmeal, Wheatena, cream of wheat, farina, or oat bran (check the label for fat calories), plain or with skim milk (*not* 2% or whole).
- Cold cereals (check the nutrition label for fat and dietary fiber), with 1% or skim milk (*not* 2% or whole). Find cereals you like with at least 4 or 5 grams of dietary fiber.
- Half a cantaloupe filled with 1% cottage cheese.
- Fruit-flavored nonfat yogurt or vanilla nonfat yogurt + cut-up fruit.
- An omelet made with egg whites and one egg yolk or egg substitutes instead of whole eggs. Remember — an egg yolk contains 50 fat calories.
- Ron's favorite: whole-wheat bread with 1% cottage spread on top twice toasted. If commercial bread, put toaster on low so it won't burn.
- Nancy's favorite: whole-wheat toast covered with banana slices, topped with 1% cottage cheese.
- Fruit: banana, orange, a bowl of strawberries, blueberries, raspberries, half a cantaloupe, melon slices.
- A weekend treat: waffles or pancakes made with buttermilk and skim milk, nonfat yogurt and skim milk, or orange juice and skim milk instead of whole milk, sour cream, or sweet cream. Substitute a small amount of olive oil in the batter for butter or margarine. Spray a nonstick waffle iron with canola or olive oil spray before you plug it in. Use a cast-iron grill with a light application of margarine or olive oil for the pancakes. For superior taste, use real maple syrup, not cane or maple-flavored syrup. Ron eats maple syrup with waffles on the side.

Here are some breakfast foods that are more expensive than you might think:

- Convenience foods such as Great Starts breakfasts ranging from French Toast Sticks (90 fat calories a serving) to Sausage, Egg, and Cheese on a Biscuit (250 fat calories a serving).
- Pop Tarts and Granola Bars. Some are candy bars in disguise. A brown-sugar cinnamon Pop Tart has 60 fat calories.
- Egg dishes (made with whole eggs), sausage, bacon, and home fries.

EATING IN: LUNCH

Do not skip lunch. **Do NOT skip meals!** Treat yourself as well as you treat your car. Would you expect your car to perform well on an empty tank? Your car (and you too) need energy to get going and keep going. Skipping meals just slows your metabolism and makes you exhausted, irritable, and HUNGRY. What do hungry people do? They gobble up dinner like there is no tomorrow. They use no restraint and eat three times their Fat Budget. Be sensible and satisfied. Eat a large low-fat breakfast and a large low-fat lunch and low-fat snacks in between and you'll be cool and collected when you dig into your delicious, low-fat dinner.

- The best advice is to bring lunch from home. To save time in the morning, make lunch and refrigerate it the night before. Invite your co-workers to bring their lunch and join you. Have picnics if the weather permits.
- Make a sandwich of last night's *Bar-B-Que Chicken*. Fill a whole-wheat pita with *Indonesian Chicken with Green Beans* and heat it in your office microwave.
- Cook up a large batch of *Pawtucket Chili* or *Chili Non Carne,* and prepare one to two cups of rice. Keep them in the refrigerator and bring a bowl of chili over rice to work and heat it in a microwave. You can also put it in a whole-wheat pita pocket, heat it up, and add lettuce, tomatoes, and onion.
- Spruce up your turkey breast sandwich with tomato slices, mustard, and hot peppers. Avoid mayonnaise, butter, or margarine.
- Use poultry, fish, or lean meat in place of processed meats, such as salami, bologna, or frankfurters.
- Be wary of any processed meats — even, or especially, innocent-looking franks made with chicken or turkey. Read labels for fat content and be sure to adjust fat calories for amount eaten.
- Beware of low-fat cheeses or meats. How much do you eat? Fat calories add up quickly.
- Eat nonfat cheeses with care. Eating fatty-tasting (although nonfat) food prevents you from losing your high-fat taste.
- Make your tuna salad sandwich with low-fat or nonfat mayonnaise mixed with nonfat yogurt. Again, don't overdo the high-fat tasting mayonnaise if you want to lose your high-fat tooth.
- Have plenty of fruit available.
- Pack carrot or celery sticks.
- Pack a nonfat flavored yogurt.
- Bring air-popped popcorn (take it with you to the movies too). Or better still, keep a hot-air-popper in your office and make a fresh batch each day.

EATING IN: DINNER

Three Cheers for Eating Home-Cooked Meals at Home

We realize that some of you are single, so the following plea doesn't apply, and some of you are on the road seven days a week, so you can't take our advice, but for the rest of you, eating at home with your family is a goal well worth attaining.

Don't just pencil in "dinner at home" on your daily calendar — use indelible ink. Arrange your schedule, job, hobbies, and activities — and have your family do the same — so that you dine together almost every night. It's a MUST. The emotional benefits of sitting together at a table every evening and sharing a meal and conversation with spouse and children are immeasurable. For your own mental health, sitting down to a meal, taking time to eat, to digest, to think, to talk, to unwind can have long-term psychological rewards.

The physical benefits are also substantial. When you eat food prepared at home you can include an abundance of vegetables, fruit, dairy, and grain. You know that you and your family will be consuming lots of vitamins, minerals, and fiber. You know that the meat you buy is low-fat because you have purchased it. You know the preparation is low-fat, because you prepared it. You are not tempted by high-fat no-no's because you don't have them in the house. Dinner can always taste divine, because you are in control of the cooking.

Spice up the Main Course

Low-fat doesn't have to mean boiled chicken. It can be *Blackened Chicken* or *Lemon Chicken* or *Alex's Chinese Chicken with Onions, Mushrooms, and Zucchini*. It can be *Turkey with Capers* or *Spicy Shrimp Louisiana*. In other words, it can be delicious. As Dan King, a Chooser to Lose who has lost 100 pounds, put it, "We found that our low-fat food selection has much more variety than we had in the old days with burgers or steak every other night."

Rethink your preferences and retrain your palate. Throw out cream, butter, margarine, and cheese. Bland, fiber-free food is unsatisfying. You keep eating and eating, trying to fulfill your need to crunch. You need some bulk to feel full. Replace cheesy, bland food with spices and vegetables for taste and texture. Don't be frightened by spices. "Spicy" doesn't necessarily mean "hot." Spicy means tasty. And despite what the ads claim on TV, spices don't give you heartburn. Greasy and fatty foods give you heartburn.

Modify favorite recipes by reducing the fat. Make "cream" sauces with skim milk, nonfat yogurt, or nonfat buttermilk. Don't eat meat in a slab — cut it up and mix it with masses of vegetables. Serve entrées on a bed of rice or pasta. Not only will it enhance the flavor, you will be eating less meat.

To achieve the most success with the least sacrifice, prepare low-fat, delicious meals at home so you eat well and know exactly what you are eating. If you haven't ever cooked, try it. You may turn out to be great chef material. Encourage your significant other to cook low-fat. Cook together. Even if you are a bachelor and don't like cooking for one, you can invite people over to eat with you and/or cook in large quantities and freeze it for future meals.

Be creative. Try different low-fat recipes. You may find that cooking is your hidden calling. See Chapter 10 for loads of low-fat cooking tips. And for those times you have to eat out, see Chapter 11 for advice on taking control at restaurants.

10. Cooking Up a Low-Fat Storm

TO OUR SURPRISE (since Ron has always been a superb eater, but never a cook), many men cook. This certainly makes sense. The greatest chefs are men. Cooking is fun, so why should cooking be limited to women? For many men, cooking is a form of relaxation.

If you don't cook already, you may want to join the legions of men who do and become a cook yourself. Because if you want to lose weight and stay healthy, the easiest way to be successful is to eat healthy, low-fat food prepared at home. Preparing food from scratch ensures you have nutritious, tasty meals.

Is Cooking from Scratch More Expensive?

No way. The foods that are a drain on your finances are convenience foods and high-fat snacks. Compare the cost of a pound of potatoes (33¢) with a pound of potato chips ($3.42). Frozen dinners are about five times as expensive as the raw ingredients used to prepare them.

In contrast, a variety of fruits, vegetables, rice, or pasta with small amounts of chicken, seafood, or lean beef keep both budget and body trim. Even if low-fat eating were more expensive — which it is not — the health and psychological benefits would be worth every cent.

MEAL-MAKING MADE EASY

Cooking need not be time-consuming or tedious. Here are some hints to make preparing dinner as quick and easy as possible:

Approach #1: Wing It

If just *thinking* about planning the whole week's entrées gives you a headache, try this approach.

First, be sure your cupboards are stocked with the basics, such as canned chicken broth, canned tomatoes, Dijon mustard, unbleached white flour, and a variety of spices.* Then, each week go to the grocery store and buy a variety of food you can use for recipes. Buy boneless, skinless chicken breasts (you can freeze them), turkey cutlets, and lots of vegetables and fruits. If you want to make seafood, you should buy it on the day you plan to cook it. Then, during the week, choose recipes in *Eater's Choice Low-Fat Cookbook*** (or other low-fat cookbooks) that strike your fancy and that use some of the ingredients you bought. *Turkey Mexique* might catch your eye, and you can make it because you have a supply of green peppers and mushrooms in your refrigerator and a jar of green olives on your shelves. As you become familiar with the recipes, you will shop for specific vegetables for specific recipes you want to make. For example, you will add asparagus to your shopping list because you want to make *Asparagus Soup*.

Approach #2: Plan Ahead

At the beginning of the week, glance through *Eater's Choice Low-Fat Cookbook* (or other low-fat cookbooks) and choose recipes for the week. Look at the ingredient lists and jot down the foods you will need to buy so you won't waste time when you shop. Be sure to add foods such as fruits, vegetables, and bread to have on hand for snacks, side dishes, and desserts.

Both Approaches: Be Well Stocked

Buy lots of fresh produce so you always have food on hand for entrées, vegetable side dishes, breakfasts, lunches, and snacks. Make sure you have a variety of vegetables so you always have two or more vegetables with dinner.

Be adventuresome. Try a new fruit and vegetable each week. Copy the list of fruits and vegetables on page 50 and take it with you when you shop.

Keep your larder (excuse the expression) well stocked with basics so you always have the ingredients you need on hand. This will prevent

---

* If you have never cooked, look at the ingredients for recipes you might want to prepare. Buy the ingredients that are not perishable and store them so you will have them on hand.

** *Eater's Choice Low-Fat Cookbook* contains more than 300 easy, tasty, low-low-fat recipes that you will love.

frustration such as when a yen for pasta with tomato sauce overcomes you and you find no canned tomatoes or spaghetti on your shelves.

When you go to the supermarket, buy from your shopping list, but be open to other possibilities. For example, if the swordfish looks firm and fresh, you might scratch your dinner plan for that night and prepare *Oriental Fish Kebabs* instead. If fresh pineapple suddenly appears in the produce section, take it home and treat yourself to a sumptuous dessert.

Time-Saving Tips

• Prepare large batches of soup (double or triple the recipe). Refrigerate some and freeze the rest (except soups with rice or beans) so you have soup to eat in the future.
• Double or triple an entrée recipe so you can eat it for more than one day. Make enough so you can also freeze some to reheat for later.
• Bake up a batch of boneless, skinless chicken breasts to refrigerate or freeze for future use (see "Cut the Fat" below).
• Marinate chicken in the refrigerator before you go to work so it will be ready for you to prepare when you arrive home.
• Make enough rice for several days. Each day put the amount of rice you need into a saucepan, add a little water, and heat it up.
• Try basmati rice. It cooks in 10 minutes and has a delicious flavor.
• To de-fat canned chicken broth, store it in the refrigerator. The cold hardens the fat for easy removal.

COOKING LOW-FAT

We pause for a short advertisement. In case you hadn't noticed (how could you miss it?), we often refer to the recipes in *Eater's Choice Low-Fat Cookbook*. That is because these recipes are low, low in fat, delicious, and easy to make. In fact, our biased opinion is that *Eater's Choice Low-Fat Cookbook* is the best low-fat cookbook around and that everyone who wants to eat healthfully and lose weight should get it. We love to eat and the only cookbook we use is . . . can you guess? *Eater's Choice Low-Fat Cookbook!*

MODIFYING RECIPES

You can also modify your own favorite recipes or recipes that you find in cookbooks that are too high-fat to keep your Fat Budget in the black. A few substitutions and modifications may be all that is needed to include them in your new low-fat eating plan.

Cut the Fat

A simple, painless way to modify a recipe is to reduce the amount of fat you use.

- Cut the fat in half, then in half again. For example, if the recipe calls for sautéing in ¼ cup oil or butter, use 2 tablespoons of olive oil instead. If the reduced amount works, try one tablespoon. If you are sautéing vegetables, you can probably cut the amount to as little as one teaspoon. Add a splash of water to help steam the vegetables. Try sautéing them in de-fatted chicken broth with no added fat.
- DON'T add the extra tablespoon of butter to the sauce or dot the top of your fish or pie with margarine or butter. The dish probably doesn't need the extra fat.
- Instead of sautéing chicken breasts in a few tablespoons of olive oil, dredge them in a mixture of flour, salt, and pepper, and then bake them in a single layer in a shallow baking pan. Add no fat. When the breasts are fully cooked, either refrigerate or freeze them for future use or cut them up and add them to the sauce you have just prepared.
- Try substituting applesauce for margarine in cake recipes. In most recipes, the results are superb.

Silent Substitutions

In most cases, the following low-fat or nonfat substitutions will greatly reduce the fat content of your recipes without diminishing the taste or texture.

WHEN THE RECIPE CALLS FOR:	SUBSTITUTE:
Cream	Nonfat yogurt, nonfat buttermilk, skim milk, evaporated skim milk
Whole milk	Skim milk
Sour cream	Nonfat yogurt, nonfat buttermilk
Veal cutlets	Turkey cutlets
Pork	White-meat chicken
Ground beef	Ground chicken or ground turkey (without skin and fat) that you grind yourself
3 egg yolks	1 egg yolk
2 whole eggs	3 egg whites or 1 egg + 1 egg white
Margarine	Applesauce

You may wonder why we don't list fake cheeses as a substitute for cheese. We urge you to move away from cheesy-tasting food even if it is nonfat. If all your recipes continue to taste cheesy or creamy or fatty, even though they are made with nonfat substitutes, you will never lose your taste for fat. Try moving toward tasty recipes instead, and your weight-loss goals will be achieved sooner and last longer.

A Recipe Modified

We easily modified the high-fat recipe for Spinach Soup into a tasty low-fat treat. (You may find it hard to believe, but this is a real recipe. Yes, the original recipe calls for *one cup* of butter.)

	Spinach Soup		
HIGH-FAT VERSION		**LOW-FAT VERSION**	
INGREDIENTS	FAT CALORIES	INGREDIENTS	FAT CALORIES
1 cup butter	1600	1 tsp olive oil	40
2 large onions		2 large onions	
4 garlic cloves		4 garlic cloves	
10 cups spinach leaves		10 cups spinach leaves	
4 cups chicken broth	90	4 cups de-fatted chicken broth	0
¾ cup chopped parsley		¾ cup chopped parsley	
1 cup sour cream	400	1 cup nonfat yogurt	0
Total Fat Calories	2090	Total Fat Calories	40
Makes 6 servings		*Makes 6 servings*	
Fat Calories per Serving	348	Fat Calories per Serving	7

This is how we made the changes:

- Sixteen tablespoons of butter was much, much, much more fat than necessary to sauté the onions and garlic. In addition, butter is a heart-risky fat. We reduced the fat to 1 teaspoon of olive oil and a splash of water and saved 1560 fat calories. (We chose olive oil because it is a heart-healthy oil.)
- Straining the fat from the chicken broth saved 90 fat calories.
- Replacing the sour cream with nonfat yogurt saved 400 fat calories.

Instead of consuming almost your whole Fat Budget in one bowl of soup as well as adding to your fat stores and plaque stores, by making the above modifications you can reduce the fat in the original soup to 7 fat calories. The soup will still taste great but will be much more nutritious.

Determining Fat Calories per Serving. To determine the fat calories per serving for a recipe, add up the fat calories of all the fat-containing ingredients and then divide by the number of servings. For example, in the high-fat recipe above, the fat calories for all the fat-containing ingredients total 2090. To determine the fat calories per serving, you divide 2090 by the number of servings, which is six. $2090 \div 6 = 348$ fat calories per serving.

FAT-CUTTING COOKING TIPS

The following cooking tips will help you stay within your Fat Budget:

- Always remove skin from the chicken breast. A chicken breast *with* skin contains 69 fat calories. A chicken breast cooked without the skin contains 13 fat calories.
- Always remove skin *before* cooking chicken to keep the chicken from absorbing fat from the skin. A chicken breast that is cooked with the skin has 28 fat calories *after* removal of the skin. A chicken breast cooked without the skin has only 13 fat calories.
- Think twice before flouring, breading, and frying fish, seafood, chicken, or vegetables — any food. Since breading absorbs fat like a sponge, you greatly increase the fat calories by preparing food this way.
- Bake, broil, grill, or poach chicken or fish. Limit the amount of fat you use. Use low-fat sauces for added taste.
- If you cook beef, lamb, pork, or veal, trim off all visible fat. Broil or bake on a rack to drain the fat. Wrap cooked meat in paper towels to remove more fat. Avoid pan-frying. Keep consumption of red meat to a minimum and your arteries will thank you.
- Cook vegetables in an inexpensive metal steamer. Put the steamer in a saucepan filled with about an inch of water. Place cut-up fresh vegetables on the open "leaves." Cover the saucepan and steam the vegetables until they are tender. This usually takes 3 to 5 minutes, depending on the vegetable. Cauliflower takes a bit longer. For added flavor, mix in some pressed garlic or herbs (thyme, basil, etc.), sprinkle cooked vegetables with vinegar (try balsamic), or top with a dollop of nonfat yogurt mixed with Dijon mustard.

- Sauté vegetables in 1 teaspoon of olive oil and add splashes of water to steam-cook them.
- Sauté vegetables in de-fatted broth.
- Always steam or bake eggplant. When it is sautéed, it absorbs gobs of oil.
- In any recipe that calls for canned chicken broth, either strain the broth or, if the fat is hardened, lift it off the soup with a spoon or use a gravy skimmer. Keep cans of broth in the refrigerator so the fat will be hardened and easy to remove.

TIPS FOR SUPERIOR TASTE

- Always use fresh garlic instead of garlic powder or garlic salt. Fresh garlic not only gives you a superior, fresher taste, it is more nutritious. Garlic stays fresh for weeks in the refrigerator. We store it in the empty butter container on the refrigerator door.
- Use ginger root (first slice off the outer covering) with superior results in recipes that call for ginger. Fresh ginger root is available at most grocery stores. To keep it fresh for many months, store it in the refrigerator in a jar filled with sherry.
- Grind your own black pepper. The superior, lively, peppery taste of freshly ground pepper will enhance your recipes. Buy yourself a peppermill (usually not expensive) and whole peppercorns (available in the spice section of your local grocery store).
- For a fresher, nuttier taste, buy whole nutmegs (available in the spice section of your local grocery store) and grate the amount called for in your recipe.

FAT-CUTTING COOKING EQUIPMENT

- Steamer: See "Fat-Cutting Cooking Tips" above.
- Cast-iron: Cut out the fat by using cast-iron griddles. Cast-iron is an effective nontoxic, nonstick cooking surface. Cast-iron griddles that fit over two stove burners quickly cook chicken breasts, turkey cutlets, French toast, and pancakes with little or no added fat. Small cast-iron griddles that fit over one stove burner are also available.
- Clay cooker: Cooking in a clay cooker keeps chicken moist and tender without added fat.
- Gravy skimmer: Gravy skimmers provide an inexpensive, simple method to remove fat from canned chicken broth or gravies.

Useful Cooking Gadgets

- Defrosting tray: If you are a last-minute-type person like Nancy Goor, the defrosting tray (one brand is called Miracle Thaw) is a life-saver. If you have neglected to thaw chicken breasts for dinner, just run the black metal sheet under hot water until it becomes very hot, place the frozen breasts across it, and 15 minutes later you will have either almost or completely thawed meat. If the meat is not completely thawed, remove the breasts and repeat the process. Replace the breasts so the more frozen side faces down.
- The best vegetable peeler in the world: Good Grips makes a vegetable peeler that works like a dream.
- Lemon zester: To get the most intense lemon taste, a lemon zester is just what the chef ordered. Press as you pull the zester down a lemon to create fragrant strips of lemon zest.
- Garlic press: The easiest way to mince garlic for most recipes is to squeeze it through a garlic press.
- Mini-chopper: You may have noticed how many of our recipes use garlic and ginger. A mini-chopper makes mincing cloves of garlic and ginger root effortless. If you have no lemon zester, you can chop strips of lemon peel (just the yellow) and create grated lemon zest.

And Coming Next . . .

We realize that you cannot make *every* meal at home from scratch — you *may* have to eat out once in a while. Check out Chapter 11 for tips on making eating out as low-fat as possible.

11. Dining Out

IF YOU *REALLY* want to be successful at turning your spare tire into a washboard, you need to limit eating out. This is why: When you eat out, no matter how careful you are, no matter how many questions you ask and how many requests you make, you never *really* know how much fat is in the food you are served. Rest assured, it will always be more than the amount you consume at home.

Whereas you could be loving every bite of your home-cooked meal, when you eat out, you are painfully aware of the multitude of high-fat choices that you are *not* enjoying. You snarl while you eat your broiled fish, plain, because you really wanted lobster swimming in butter. If you feel sorry for yourself often enough, you're off of *Choose to Lose Weight-Loss Plan for Men* and onto Fat for Life.

Of course, you can always save up fat calories for an occasional restaurant meal and really splurge. But if you are dining out 2 to 21 times a week,* you are handicapping your fat-loss progress.

Okay. Sometimes you have to eat out and you haven't saved up for it. You have dinner with a client, you're on a business trip, you work away from home. Here's some advice to reduce the damage as much as possible.

DINING AT A RESTAURANT

You are the master of your fate. You can be in control of your choices in almost all situations, beginning with your choice of a restaurant.

---

*We discourage eating out often, but you may have no other options. Read this chapter to make your choices as healthy and low-fat as possible.

Sizing up the Restaurant

The first step is to find out if a restaurant has low-fat options. Don't make assumptions. A steak house may have low-fat chicken offerings. A vegetarian restaurant may be fat heaven.

Call First. Call the restaurant and ask if they have chicken, fish, or seafood and how it is prepared. Call *before* you get there so you are not forced to eat poorly.

Review the Menu. If you can't call before you arrive, look at the menu before you sit down. If every item looks like a Fat Budget-buster, find another restaurant.

Be Choosy. Unless you have planned for a splurge, avoid Chinese, Thai, Mexican, Italian, German, chicken, and fast-food restaurants. One meal at these fat factories may sink your Fat Budget for a month.

Take Control at the Restaurant

Ask Questions. Don't be afraid to ask questions and make requests to ensure your meal is low-fat. Ask if the soup is made with cream, whole milk, or beef. Ask if the chicken is grilled with fat, and if it can be grilled without fat or skin. Ask for the salad dressing on the side so you can determine how much you want to use.

You're the Boss. Ask as many questions as you need to. Remember that you, not the waiter, are in charge. They are your arteries, not his; your love handles, not hers.

Send It Back. If your order is not prepared as desired, send it back. If you ordered your English muffin plain and it comes dripping with butter, send it back. If your potato looks like sour cream in a potato skin, send it back. You wouldn't accept a hard-topped car from the dealer if you ordered a convertible.

Look a Gift Horse in the Mouth. If the portion served is more than you should eat, get rid of the surplus immediately. Put it on a small plate and have the waiter remove it from your sight.

A Penny Saved May Cost You a Lot. Don't feel guilty about leaving half the pasta or steak unfinished on your plate. If you eat it you'll pay for it twice: once with money, once with your health. If you have a serious case of frugality, don't ever go to a buffet or smorgasbord.

If These Are Friends . . .

If your friends give you a hard time because you are trying to make changes — they rib you when you request your potato plain or roll their eyes when you request chicken without the skin — don't ignore their behavior. Let them know that you are trying to lose weight and eat healthfully. If they don't let up, you could ask why they feel so threatened by your behavior. Could it be that they know that what you are doing is exactly what they should be doing?

Don't let them derail your new lifestyle. Why should you be overweight or get diabetes or have a heart attack and die just to keep your "friends" quiet? If they can't get used to the New You, choose more caring dining partners.

DINING OUT: DINNER

Confronting the Menu

First, scan the menu to find foods that you can eat as described or that have potential to be modified. You can easily eliminate the foods that are irredeemable. For example, there is no way (save discarding the meat and eating the bones) that ribs can be modified to be low-fat. Find meats that are naturally low-fat, such as chicken without the skin, turkey, fish, and seafood. How are they prepared? Can they be prepared in low-fat ways?

If you don't cook, you might find some terms on menus confusing. What does sautéing mean? What is béarnaise sauce? See the glossary below for definitions of terms and preparation methods. If you don't find it in our glossary, or you can't remember a definition when you're at the restaurant, ask the waiter.

In the next section, we will review the typical menu offerings from appetizer to dessert and offer suggestions on how to reduce their fat impact.

Glossary of Restaurant Terms	
Amandine	Prepared or garnished with almonds
À la mode	With ice cream on the side
Au gratin	Covered with cheese or bread crumbs and then baked or broiled

Glossary of Restaurant Terms (continued)

Béarnaise sauce	High-fat sauce composed primarily of butter, egg yolks, and wine, usually served over steak
Beef Wellington	Beef tenderloin covered by layer of paté and sautéed mushrooms and baked in a crust of puff pastry
Blackened	Meat that is covered with spicy seasonings and seared, sometimes turning it black
Braised	Food that is browned, then cooked slowly in a small amount of liquid in a covered pot in the oven
Bruschetta	Bread brushed with olive oil, rubbed with garlic, and grilled
Caesar salad	Large salad made with romaine lettuce, croutons, parmesan cheese and a dressing consisting of raw egg, olive oil, and anchovies
Capers	Pickled flower buds the size of small peas that add a distinct taste to food
Chili	Highly spiced dish made of red peppers, meat, tomatoes, and beans (prepared without meat, the dish is called vegetarian chili)
Clam chowder	
Manhattan	Thick clam/potato soup with a tomato base
New England	Thick clam/potato soup with a cream base
Club sandwich	Sandwich made with 3 slices of bread, mayonnaise, bacon, and turkey or chicken
Creole	Dish usually made of tomatoes, peppers, and rice
Cumberland sauce	A fat-free sauce made of mainly red currant jelly, port, mustard, orange juice, and lemon juice
Deep-fat frying	Frying food in a basket submerged in a heavy saucepan filled with boiling fat. The fat is reused over and over, making it more and more saturated (heart-risky)
Eggs Benedict	An open-faced English muffin topped with Canadian bacon, poached eggs, and hollandaise sauce
En papillote	Food cooked and served in paper or parchment
Flambé	Food doused with alcohol and set on fire
Fondue	Swiss dish in which you dip skewered pieces of bread into a fondue pot or chafing dish of hot melted cheese flavored with wine or you dip (and cook) raw pieces of skewered meat in hot oil
French onion soup	Onion soup topped with a round of toast covered with melted Swiss or Gruyère cheese

Frittata	Italian omelet consisting of beaten eggs cooked until set; like a French omelet but firmer and not folded over
Gratinée	Having a crust of buttered crumbs or melted cheese
Gravlax	Raw salmon cured with salt, sugar, and spices
Guacamole	Mexican dip made from avocado, mayonnaise, cumin, garlic, and tomatoes
Hollandaise sauce	Sauce composed primarily of butter, egg yolks, and wine; served over poached eggs in eggs Benedict
Hungarian goulash	Beef stew with paprika
Julienne	Cut into thin strips
Louis sauce	Sauce made from mayonnaise, cream, and chili sauce usually served over crab or shrimp
Omelet	Dish consisting of beaten eggs cooked, set, and folded over a filling
Pico de gallo	Relish made from tomatoes, jalapeño peppers, onions, cilantro leaves, and lemon juice
Poached	Covered completely with liquid while cooking
Quesadilla	Tortilla filled with cheese, green chiles, jalapeño peppers, and salsa
Remoulade	Sauce composed of mayonnaise with cooked egg yolks, gherkins (little pickles), capers, and herbs
Risotto	Rice dish made with butter, cheese, and chicken stock
Roasting	Baking food uncovered in the oven
Salsa	A relish made with fresh tomatoes, onions, and hot peppers
verte Sauce	A sauce made of mayonaise with watercress and spinach leaves
Sautéed	Pan-fried quickly with butter or oil
Seared	Cooked quickly at high heat
Shish kebab	Lamb cubes marinated and cooked on a skewer
Shrimp cocktail sauce	Fat-free dipping sauce for seafood made from chili sauce, horseradish, Worcestershire, lemon juice, and hot sauce
Stir-fried	Small pieces of food quickly pan-fried in oil
Tartar sauce	Fish sauce composed mainly of mayonnaise, cream, lemon juice, and pickles
Thousand Island dressing	Salad dressing made primarily of mayonnaise with a little ketchup
Tuna melt	Tuna fish with cheese melted over it
Vinaigrette	Oil and vinegar dressing (often a ratio of 3 parts oil to 1 part vinegar)
Waldorf salad	Salad composed of apples, celery, walnuts, and mayonnaise

Appetizers

Most appetizers are fat-packed, but you can make some choices with no guilt: Try shrimp cocktail with cocktail sauce or melon in season.

Ask what is in the appetizer. Does the soup contain whole milk, cream, cheese, butter, oil, beef?

Appetizers may contain more fat than your Fat Budget can bear: pâtés, any dish wrapped in puff pastry, potato skins, taco chips, chicken wings, and other fried foods, cream, and other high-fat soups. *Remember, you don't have to have an appetizer!*

Salad Bar

Salad bars are a great temptation — unlimited food at no additional cost. But beware. Salad bars are a healthy eater's undoing. The offerings are a fat lover's delight: mayonnaise with tuna, egg, or chicken; oil mixed with a green bean or two; sour cream with apples and raisins; and great bins of salad dressing. A little bit of this and a little bit of that add up to triple your Fat Budget for the day. (See SALAD BAR FOODS in the Food Tables.)

To control fat intake, choose fresh vegetables and fruit and use the fork method (see below).

A *Choose to Lose Weight-Loss Plan for Men* tip: Choosing the salad bar as your main meal selection leaves you high and dry: Either you gorge on great heaps of fat or starve on salad greens.

The Fork Method

Want to eat real salad dressing without suffering Fat Budget annihilation? Try the fork method. Instead of having your salad served drowning in dressing, ask for the dressing served on the side. Dip your fork into the dressing and then spear a biteful of salad. You will get a taste of dressing without a lot of fat.

Entrées

High-Fat Choices. Here are dishes that will devour your Fat Budget whole.

- Casseroles and potpies. Fat is always a major ingredient.
- Dishes with cream sauces (have the sauce served on the side so you can regulate the amount you use).
- Dishes made with cheese (unless it can be removed or you can order the dish without it).
- Ultra-fatty foods such as ribs and dishes made with ground meat or sausage.
- High-fat meats such as beef, lamb, veal, pork, duck, and goose.
- Fried foods.
- The "Dieter's Plate" is invariably high in fat. Normally it consists of a hamburger without a bun and high-fat cottage cheese with a canned peach.

Turning High-Fat Choices into Low-Fat Choices. Choose foods that are naturally low in fat, such as chicken or turkey without skin or seafood so the basic meat doesn't contribute much fat. Ask the waiter questions to find out if these low-fat meats are prepared with lots of fat or covered by high-fat sauces.

Try these tricks to keep your meal low-fat:

- Have high-fat sauces, gravies, dressings, butter, or sour cream served on the side so you can regulate the amount you use, if any. First taste the dish with no sauce, gravy, etc. It may taste fine plain.
- If the low-fat foods are prepared in high-fat ways, ask if they can be prepared differently — i.e., fried chicken or fish that can be baked or roasted or broiled, with no fat, etc.
- See if you can apply the spices or low-fat sauces from high-fat foods on the menu to a low-fat food. For example, Cajun steak and fried chicken are on the menu. Ask if the chicken (skin removed) can be roasted or broiled with the Cajun sauce.
- If you cannot modify the available dishes, ask the waiter if the kitchen can prepare a low-fat dish that you like and describe it in as much detail as possible.

Important Message:

If the food does not come as you ordered — SEND IT BACK!

Vegetables

The vegetables that are served with an entrée are not always indicated on the menu. When you order, always ask which vegetables come with the dish and how they are prepared so you can be assured they are prepared in a low-fat way. If necessary, make the following requests:

- Ask for vegetables steamed with no butter added. They will still taste delicious.
- Order a baked potato, plain, with toppings on the side so you can determine how much, if any, you want to use. Ask to substitute a baked potato, plain, for French fries or other high-fat potatoes.
- If the vegetable is a salad, have salad dressing served on the side so you can determine how much you use. Use the fork method (see above).

Bread and Rolls

Bread can enhance your meal, but you need to make choices so it doesn't enhance your fat stores too.

- Ask if the bread has been buttered. If so, request an unbuttered loaf instead.
- Not all rolls or breads are low in fat. The pumpkin bread tastes like cake because it has as much fat as cake. Most muffins and biscuits are chock-full of fat. Give rolls the shadow test (see box below).

Testing for Fat: The Shadow Test

Place the suspect food on a paper napkin, leave it for a few seconds, remove the food, and see if a fat print is left.

Dessert

Most restaurant desserts would eat up a whole day's Fat Budget. Instead of ordering a dessert you will regret:

- Ask for a fruit platter or a piece of fruit (even if it isn't on the menu).
- Share a dessert with a few people so you get a taste but much less fat.
- If you know him/her well enough, ask for a small taste of your dining partner's dessert.
- Find a frozen yogurt parlor. Nonfat frozen yogurt makes an excellent

snack and/or dessert. Beware of the toppings such as M&Ms, Heath Crunch, granola, shredded coconut, etc. By the time you add these high-fat crunchies, you might as well have had ice cream. Be wary of low-fat (as opposed to nonfat) frozen yogurts. Ask the server for the *number* of fat calories (or grams of fat) per ounce and the number of ounces in a serving. Remember, percentage fat-free (e.g., 95% fat-free or 5% fat) is based on weight and does not give you enough information to make a judgment. When in doubt, don't eat the frozen yogurt.

Budget in Your High-Fat Favorites . . .

Before you cry out in despair, "Can't I ever order a hot dog again?," remember that *Choose to Lose Weight-Loss Plan for Men* is a flexible system that allows, even encourages, an occasional high-fat splurge. The reason you have a Fat Budget is so that you can save up for a thick steak or a piece of Black Forest cake. If you feel that you are a martyr, suffering the slings and arrows of an outrageous diet, you won't be a Chooser to Lose for long. The big surprise is that after you have followed *Choose to Lose Weight-Loss Plan for Men* for a while, your tastes will change and what you now consider divine you may find greasy and disgusting in a couple of months.

. . . But Not at Every Meal

You can plan ahead for a splurge (better than paying back for an overindulgence), but if you splurge too often you will be off *Choose to Lose Weight-Loss Plan for Men*. By eating high-fat or high-fat-tasting foods too often, you deny your taste buds a chance to change. A man who lost 35 pounds told us that he once considered McDonald's French fries ambrosia from the gods. After following *Choose to Lose Weight-Loss Plan for Men* for several months, just looking at those greasy yellow sticks made him queasy. If he had included French fries in his daily meal plan, *really* making permanent changes would have been impossible.

Truths!

- You don't have to finish everything on your plate.
- Re: appetizers or dessert. Take a bite. If it isn't to die for, don't finish it.

DINING AT A PRIVATE HOME

This can be tricky. Even if you know the people well, you may feel hesitant about making special requests. However, *you* can control what you eat. If you are offered a food that compromises your weight-loss goals, just eat a small amount. Eat more bread (low-fat, of course) to fill up. If the vegetables are not loaded with fat, pile them high. Eat more rice than sauce. The next time you are invited, prepare by eating some low-fat food before you leave home. Then, at the dinner, you will be able to eat enough food to be polite but not so much that you pay dearly for it the next week. You may also want to save fat calories by eating extra-low-fat for several days before. Then you will have fat calories in the bank to pay for the splurge.

   A Family Affair. If every trip to visit Mom and Pop involves a fight to keep your Fat Budget solvent, read page 147, in Chapter 14, "Obstacles and Overcoming Them."

DINING OUT: LUNCH

Here are some tricks for saving fat calories:

At a Sandwich Shop

- Make your first request: "Hold the butter or mayo on the bread." In many sandwich shops and fast-food restaurants, bread is automatically slathered with high-fat spreads — whether or not you ask for them.
- Avoid meat salad sandwiches — tuna salad, chicken salad, egg salad, shrimp salad. Mayonnaise is often the first and most plentiful ingredient.
- Use mustard on sandwiches (like turkey subs) instead of mayonnaise or oil. To jazz up sandwiches, experiment with different mustards and hot peppers.
- Ask for no chips and no fries with your sandwich. If possible, order a baked potato, plain, instead.
- Order whole-wheat bread or toast (it's healthier). Avoid croissants (110+ fat calories each) and biscuits (63–162 fat calories each).

At a Pizzeria

- Ask for vegetarian pizza with tomato sauce but no cheese or oil. Request as many vegetables as possible. The crust still contains fat, but without cheese, sausage, ground beef, and other high-fat toppings, the pizza contains much less fat.

At a Real Restaurant

- See advice on page 121 for "Dining Out: Dinner."

DINING OUT: BREAKFAST

Breakfast is so easy to whip up at home and so high-fat in restaurants, you should eat breakfast out only if you have no other choice.

- Order hot cereals plain or with skim milk and no butter. If only 2% or whole milk is available, ask for it on the side so you can control how much, if any, you use.
- Cold cereal may be an option at some restaurants. Read the nutrition label and make sure the milk you add is 1% or less.
- Don't order muffins, except English. Blueberry, corn, walnut-cranberry, etc., muffins taste like they are made with lots of fat because they are.
- Order toast (preferably whole-wheat), bagels, or English muffins plain. Eat them with jelly or jam instead of butter, margarine, or cream cheese. Butter or margarine may be ordered on the side so you can control how much you use, but you will soon find you don't need it. Two tablespoons of cream cheese have 45 fat calories.
- If your toast comes buttered, send it back.
- Avoid Danish pastries, doughnuts, or croissants.
- Pancakes (3 weighing 7.5 oz contain 108 fat calories) and waffles (plain: 133 fat calories; Belgian: 177 fat calories) are high-fat choices. If you order them, be sure to specify, "Serve with no butter or whipped cream." Use real maple syrup instead. Eat with moderation. You don't have to leave your plate clean.
- Avoid bacon and sausage. They are filled with fat, sat-fat, and cancer-causing nitrites.
- Ask if omelets can be made with egg substitutes or egg whites + one yolk. Ask that the fat be margarine (or olive oil) and minimal.

- Order half a cantaloupe filled just to the top with cottage cheese. You can ask for low-fat, but you probably will get 4% at 43 fat calories per half cup. Ask if the cottage cheese is 1%, 2%, or regular (4%) fat so you can determine the number of fat calories you are consuming.

THREE CHEERS FOR DINING AT HOME

Here's our refrain. Cook meals at home with your family. Preparing food at home from scratch gives you the ultimate power over your food choices. Take time to sit down and eat. Relax. Enjoy yourself. Eating as a family builds good relationships.

Even if you are not planning to cook every meal, you do need to shop for food. Be sure that you have a kitchen full of fruit, vegetables, low-fat and nonfat dairy, and whole-grain cereals and breads for snacks, lunches, and breakfast. Viva la food!

12. Man About Town

THE THOUGHT OF STEPPING OUT into the high-fat world where every event offers a temptation to annihilate your Fat Budget may turn you into a recluse. Don't worry! In this chapter, you will learn the skills to choose delicious, low-fat food in every social situation — at parties, at work, and while traveling. You will have the power to control every new situation and meet every challenge.

SOCIAL OCCASIONS

If you have been true to the *Choose to Lose Weight-Loss Plan for Men* principles — that is, not making it a "diet" (a four-letter word) and yourself a martyr — then you will have no trouble resisting high-fat temptation. Parties and other social events will not rattle your resolve. Conquering social events will be a piece of cake (pardon the expression).

Plan Ahead
That's really all you have to do.

- Don't starve yourself all day to "save calories" for the event. You may be so hungry you go berserk and lose control over your choices. If you eat a lot of delicious, low-fat, nutrient-dense, fiber-rich food all day, you'll be able to enjoy the party without overindulging.
- Eat something before you go — a fruit-flavored nonfat yogurt, a bagel, a bowl of cereal — so you will be full enough to regard high-fat goodies with cool contempt.
- Budget in a splurge. If high-fat desserts are your weakness and you know they will be available, allow yourself one slice of your favorite.

Do you love high-fat dips? Spoon 2 tablespoons (or 1) onto a plate and then move away to dip and enjoy. Just plan ahead for the splurge.

At the Event

- Check out the food situation. What's available? Any low-fat items?
- Choose your splurge and after that limit yourself to low-fat choices.
- Don't be an eating automaton. Think as you eat. Take a bite. Does it really taste *that* good? If so, continue and enjoy your splurge. If not, don't finish it. Don't eat a food just because it is there.
- Take your food and move to a food-free room so you won't hear plaintive cries of "Eat me! Eat me!"
- Don't focus on the food. Focus on the conversation or entertainment.
- If you cook, ask if you can bring something to the party. Bring a low-fat dish you enjoy. It might be the only thing you can eat. If it's a cookout, bring some skinless marinated chicken breasts to barbecue.

> A truth: Most of the food at a party doesn't taste *that* good.

AT YOUR OWN PARTY

Don't use a party as an excuse to eat high-fat food. What are your motives? Ask yourself if you're grilling big, thick steaks for your guests or for yourself. Why did you buy a gallon of ice cream when your guests are allergic to dairy products? You are not obligated to provide high-fat food for your guests. In fact, by providing delicious low-fat food you will be doing them a favor. You'll show them how wonderful low-fat food can be, and you'll be doing their risk factors a favor too.

AT WORK

You have more control over what you eat at work than you might think.

Meetings

See if you can have input into the choice of refreshments. It may be possible to be part of the decision-making process.

Breakfast Meetings. Although they always appear, doughnuts, croissants, or Danish pastries are not mandated in the conference code book.
Try bagels, English muffins (with a toaster), jellies, nonfat cream cheese,
dry cereal and skim milk, and a luxuriant offering of fresh fruit salad.

Lunch Meetings. When you can, intervene so that sliced turkey, tomatoes, hot peppers, pickles, and mustard are available, as well as bread
or bagels, whole or cut-up fruit, and carrot sticks (perhaps even cut-up
vegetables). Keep in mind that potato salad has about 80 fat calories per
half cup, and chips of any type have about 90 fat calories an ounce.

Office Parties

Join the planning committee and make sure that the party fare includes some low-fat dishes, dips, and desserts.

If you drink alcohol, use restraint. If you drink too much, you will lose
your inhibitions and overeat your Fat Budget. In addition, your body
will be busy burning all those alcohol calories and leave your fat calories
to wallow happily in your fat stores.

Coffee Breaks

Most people run to the vending machine — a great place to self-destruct — when they are bored or hungry. A better solution is to BYO.
Bring a bag of fruit (the greatest fast food) — bananas, oranges, pears,
whatever is in season — and a bagel or pretzel or two. Refrigerate a
nonfat yogurt with fruit. But don't overdo. This is a snack, not a feast.

If feasible, keep a hot-air-popper in your office with a supply of popcorn kernels so you can pop your snack hot and fresh when hunger
strikes.

Business Lunches or Dinners

See Chapter 11, "Dining Out." We would bet that your new eating
habits will impress your dining partner.

ON THE ROAD

Air Travel

Airplane meals are getting smaller and smaller, but they are still
packed with fat. Why waste your fat calories on mediocre food?

- Call at least 24 hours in advance and order a special meal. You might ask what their "low-fat" meal is. You can try being very specific and ask for chicken without skin or a bagel instead of a muffin, an egg-substitute omelet, etc.
- Eat beforehand. Grab a turkey sandwich at the airport before your flight. You are paying twice for lunch, but it's a small price to pay to avoid consuming fat you don't need.
- Bring some fruit and a bagel or two so you won't starve if the meal is impossible.
- If you have done none of the above and it's a long flight, don't eat everything on your tray just because it's there. Pick and choose.

Car Travel

Planning is the key.

- Pack a bag of fruit for snacks. Keep a cooler in the car and refrigerate fruit juices and nonfat yogurt with fruit. Pack a sandwich if your lunch options are nil. (These days real restaurants are hard to find.)
- If you are away from home and have use of a car, find a grocery store and stock up on fruit and bagels, buy food to make lunch, or have the grocery deli prepare you a sandwich or two.

Train Travel

Train food is notoriously fat-laden. Don't get caught unprepared.

- If you are traveling at mealtime, go to a deli or sandwich shop before you depart and buy food for the trip.
- Bring along a bag of fruit, air-popped popcorn, bagels, and pretzels for snacks.

Remember the Boy Scout Motto

As you can see from the above advice, the trick to eating low-fat in every situation is to be prepared. Think ahead. Be sure that low-fat food is available when you need it. Bring a bag of fruit and other healthy snacks so you can avoid "death by vending machine" or "death by drive-in."* Plan your splurges in advance. It takes only a little thought. But a little thought makes all the difference. Be the master of your domain no matter where you are.

---

* We thank Joseph Cejka of Exeter, California, for these apt phrases.

13. Exercise: An Essential Ingredient

YOU'RE ON YOUR WAY to becoming the new lean YOU, glowing with good health and bursting with energy. You have the first two ingredients — a low-fat diet and lots of nutritious food — down pat. Now you have to add the third — daily aerobic exercise. Daily aerobic exercise doesn't have to mean running five miles in fifteen minutes or buying an expensive treadmill programmed with 25 different terrains and speeds. Aerobic exercise can be just plain old walking.

EXERCISE

You Gotta Do It

We can't say enough good things about aerobic exercise. Exercise increases your total energy needs, thus forcing your body to remove fat from the fat depots to supply the additional energy and causing you to lose weight. It builds and preserves muscle, and since muscle burns fat, it helps you lose weight. It raises your metabolism so you burn fat at a higher rate. It keeps you limber and flexible. It makes you strong so you can continue to be independent through your old age. It helps you retain your balance so you don't fall and break bones. It makes you feel great. It helps you sleep at night. In addition to a healthy diet, it is the essential ingredient for a long, healthy, and lean life.

Because If You Don't . . .

In addition to all the positive reasons for exercising, there are disastrous consequences of not exercising.

Disastrous Consequence #1: If you don't exercise, your energy needs are minimal, and thus your fat withdrawal is minimal. This means you lose weight at a slower rate.

Disastrous Consequence #2: If you don't exercise, you lose muscle. As we explained in Chapter 2, the body uses energy stored in carbohydrates, fats, and protein (muscle) to fuel the body. Carbohydrate storage is limited, so there isn't much there to burn. Fat is not easy to dislodge because the body holds on to it for times of famine. But because muscle (protein) is constantly being broken down, it is readily available as an energy source. This means that if you don't preserve it by exercising (muscle is rebuilt only in response to use), the protein in your muscle is the number-one energy choice.

Losing muscle is disastrous if you are trying to lose weight because muscle is the tissue that burns fat. The less muscle you have, the less fat-burning capacity you have. On a positive note: The more muscle you have, the more fat-burning capacity you have.

Disastrous Consequence #3: If you don't exercise, you lose strength. Without adequate muscle mass, you can't lift or carry objects, including your own body. You have trouble walking and standing. You lose your independence.

Disastrous Consequence #4: There is a large body of evidence that not exercising — a sedentary lifestyle — increases your risks of heart disease, cancers, stroke, and diabetes. Regular aerobic exercise reduces your risks.

So get off your butt and do it!

Exercise: Better Than Sominex

Many people complain that they can't sleep at night. If they take sleeping pills, they are so drowsy the next day they doze on and off. That night they again have difficulty sleeping. Why? Because they aren't tired. In fact, they probably couldn't sleep in the first place because they weren't active enough to get tired.

The best solution for sleeping at night is to exercise during the day. Take a 30-minute walk around the neighborhood before it gets dark. Move that body. Give your body a reason to sleep.

Types of Exercise

Aerobic exercise, strength training, and stretching are all important types of exercise. We will discuss them all, but we will start with aerobic exercise because it will have the most impact on your fat loss.

AEROBIC EXERCISE

Aerobic exercise is the exercise of choice for fat loss. Aerobic exercise is repetitive and rhythmic. For maximum weight-loss benefit it must be performed nonstop for 30 or more minutes. Walking, jogging, biking, swimming, rowing, and aerobic dancing (if continuous) are examples of aerobic exercise. Tennis, bowling, golf, lifting weights, and competitive sports are not aerobic because they involve stopping and starting.

You don't need to be an athletic star or amazon to do aerobic exercise. In fact, it need not be strenuous or executed with speed. Duration is the key. Twenty, but preferably at least 30, minutes of nonstop aerobic exercise each day will maximize your weight loss.

So forget about running (unless you enjoy it) — walking for 30 minutes is more effective for fat loss than running for 10 minutes. (It is also less punishing to your body, especially your knees, shins, and feet.)

Consult your physician before you begin an exercise program if you are over 40, have heart trouble, experience pain during or after exercise, or suffer from arthritis, dizzy spells, or any condition that would lead you to believe you should consult your physician.

Why Aerobic Exercise?

Most of the carbohydrates that you eat are burned within a few hours of consumption. A small amount is stored as glycogen, a source of quick energy. When you do nonaerobic exercise, such as tennis, you use primarily glucose from the glycogen stores in your muscle. Your fat stores remain unperturbed.

When you exercise aerobically, you burn a mix of fuels. The first 20 minutes you burn mostly glucose. After that you burn more and more fat. The longer you exercise nonstop, the more fat you burn. Since this fat is supplied by the fat stores, you will lose fat and thus lose weight. The simplest way to know if you are exercising at the right intensity is that you can carry on a normal conversation without getting out of breath.

Exercise Aerobically Every Day

Fit aerobic exercise into your daily routine. If you exercise every day, you can't put it off until tomorrow. As Dan King (a Chooser to Lose who has lost 100 pounds — so far) told us: "The thing that finally worked for me was to commit a time of day that no one could take away from me with meetings or appointments or other distractions. Everyone needs to find their own time, but the commitment to doing it every single day is really important."

We concur. We have made exercise a daily part of our routine, just like brushing our teeth or taking a shower. We exercise first thing in the morning after we get up and take a walk every night before we go to bed. At these hours, the time is ours to exercise without interruption.

Tip: Get a Dog

If you have difficulty prying yourself from your armchair and pushing yourself out the door for a walk, get yourself a dog. The natural demands of your pet will force you to take several walks every day. The exercise will be good for both of you.

Tip for Dogs: *Choose to Lose*

If you already have a dog, following the strategies for *Choose to Lose Weight-Loss Plan for Men* will improve your dog's health as well. Dave Bytell, a physician from Georgia, told us that his dog is much healthier and thinner because it is rigorously following *Choose to Lose* by reducing its fat intake (scraps from the Bytells' table are now low in fat) and by joining the Bytells' new exercise program, which includes walking the dog.

TYPES OF AEROBIC EXERCISE

The most effective aerobic exercise is the one that you will continue to do. Here are a few choices.

Walking

The easiest, most convenient, safest, least expensive exercise is one you're expert at — walking. You don't need fancy equipment or special clothes. You just need a good pair of walking shoes with good support. Your walking need not be brisk, but it must be continuous. Walking 15 minutes to the bank and stopping to cash a check turns off the aerobic meter.

Normal walking gives you no upper body exercise, so you might want to enhance the aerobic and muscle-building effect. Bend your arms at the elbow and swing them back and forth so the lower arm is parallel to the ground. Walking has the advantage of being weight-bearing and thus helps strengthen your bones.

An aside: If you are very overweight, walking may be difficult. Take it easy. Start by walking for 5 minutes a day. When you feel ready, lengthen your walk to 10 minutes. Keep adding 5 minutes until you are walking continuously for 30 minutes. As you get lighter, you will find it will become easier to walk. We received e-mail from a man who told us a few years ago he was so heavy he couldn't walk at all. As he slimmed down following *Choose to Lose Weight-Loss Plan for Men*, he added more time to his walks until now, 100 pounds lighter, he walks 3 miles every morning.

Treadmill: Walking in Any Weather

If you want to be able to walk no matter what the weather, you can purchase a treadmill. Turn on the news on TV or a video and walk as you watch. Treadmills range from inexpensive, nonmotorized models to expensive super-high-tech electric models. If you are into high-tech and can afford them, treadmills are made that can be programmed to simulate different terrains at varying speeds, talk to you in French, Spanish, or Urdu, and read out your daily horoscope and stock market quotes (well, almost). Even the non-electric, self-propelled treadmills give an excellent workout.

Bicycling

Riding a bicycle outside can give you a good aerobic workout as well as lift your spirits. If the weather is accommodating and bicycle paths are convenient or your streets are safe for riding, fit in a half hour or more of riding every day.

Bicycling in All Weather

Stationary bicycle rides aren't scenic, but they sure beat riding on ice and snow. The convenience of having equipment in your own home is an added incentive to using it. Again, make sure your stationary bike is durable and well-made. Bikes with handles that move back and forth give you upper body exercise. The wheel of the Schwinn Air Dyne has a fan that cools you as you pedal.

If you love gadgets, bikes have also become high-tech. Some allow you to read your pulse as you pedal. On some you can program your terrain, either flat or hilly or a random course that includes both. One model can be hooked up to your Nintendo set so that you participate in the Tour de France and compete against the pros. Who says exercise isn't fun?

Swimming

Swimming is an effective aerobic exercise that employs muscles in both the upper and lower body. If you have trouble walking, swimming is a great choice because the water helps support your weight. The drawbacks are:

1. You need an easily accessible pool.
2. Swimming pools are often overchlorinated and overpopulated.
3. You must possess the umph to swim for 30 minutes or more nonstop.
4. Swimming is not weight-bearing so does not help prevent osteoporosis.

If swimming is possible and your choice, start slowly and work up to 30 minutes of laps 5 times a week.

Jogging

We are not fans of jogging, although we know that people think it is effective for weight loss. The injuries incurred to backs, knees, shins, and ankles do not seem worth the benefits. Jogging is not as effective for fat loss as walking because short-term joggers burn relatively more sugar and less fat than do walkers. So why not walk? Walking is more fun too. Have you ever seen a jogger smile? If you love to jog, jog on, but do it for at least 30 minutes nonstop.

Trampolining

A dyed-in-the-wool jogger will jog through snowstorms, hail, and sleet, and in the dark. If you are a less fanatical type, you can purchase a $20 mini-trampoline and take a milder jog where the weather is always good — inside. The trampoline allows you to jog in place in your family room as you watch TV. And it is less stressful to your joints.

Cross-training

To exercise different muscle groups, and to prevent boredom, combine different types of exercise. Swim in the summer and bike in the fall.

Walk on a treadmill Monday, Wednesday, and Friday. Ride your stationary bike Tuesday and Thursday. Jump on your trampoline Saturday, and walk into town on Sunday. Whichever exercise(s) you choose, do something aerobic for 30 minutes every day.

Aerobic Exercise Equipment

You do not have to purchase expensive exercise equipment to satisfy your aerobic exercise needs. You can purchase a good pair of walking shoes and walk. However, if you are interested in exercise equipment, many choices await you. We have already mentioned treadmills and stationary bikes. Cardio glides (and other glides) are also popular and give an effective aerobic workout. Ellipse machines allow you to "run" with less stress on your joints. Stationary rowing machines and cross-country skiers are also good choices.

Visit an exercise equipment store so you can try out the equipment. (If you buy secondhand exercise equipment, be sure it is in good condition.) Once you find something you like, ask if it has a money-back guarantee after a 1-month trial. Test it out every day for a month. You might find that the rowing machine is hard on your back but you can "ride" the cardio glide for hours. You need to find a machine that fits you and your needs. The most perfect exercise equipment works only if you use it.

Try It on for Size

Check out exercise equipment before buying it. Test it out. Many companies let you use the equipment for a month with the option of returning it. Make sure it is well-made. Some exercise equipment is made for the 2 weeks people with good intentions actually use it and will break down if used on a daily basis over the long term.

STRENGTH TRAINING

While aerobic exercise is vitally important for your health, spirits, and weight loss, you need to do more. Most aerobic exercises strengthen lower body muscles (rowing and swimming are exceptions) but do little or nothing for upper body muscles. Especially if your aerobic exercise is walking, jogging, or biking, you should add upper body strength training to prevent loss of muscle.

You Gotta Do It . . .

We're not talking about bulking up so you make Arnold Schwarzenegger tremble in his boots. The benefits of strength training go beyond the cosmetic. Strength training builds up your muscles and by building your muscles improves your strength. A strong body means independence. If you continue to build and preserve your muscle as you age, you will have strength to lift and carry things (including supporting your own body), walk, climb steps, be active.

In terms of weight maintenance, strength training also has benefits. Strength training builds muscles. The more muscle you have, the more fat you burn.

Because If You Don't . . .

Here's the grim truth: If you don't do strength training, your muscles will atrophy. From the age of 20 to 70 you may lose up to 40% of your muscle mass if you are sedentary. With insufficient muscle and strength, when you grow old you may lose your balance, fall, and break bones. You will be unable to lift even 10 pounds or to lift yourself out of a chair. You might have to give up living in your own home and live in a nursing home.

Look around at old people. In general they have sunken chests and spindly arms (even if they have big bellies). They are too weak to lift objects and have difficulty walking more than a few steps. Many of the people you see drooping around nursing homes wouldn't be there if they had done strength training. Is being a couch potato worth the consequences? Definitely not! It takes only a small amount of exercise to maintain your strength, your health, and your independence and is well worth the effort.

Never Too Late

If you are looking down at the flab you call muscle and feeling hopeless, don't be. It's never too late to benefit from exercise. A Tufts University study of 80- and 90-year-olds in a nursing home showed that even the aged can build muscle and regain independence. At the beginning of the study, these men and women could not even get out of bed. Following a rigorous weight-lifting program, they built sufficient muscle to walk a mile, and some could even press up to 75 pounds with their legs. No matter if you are 25 or 90, exercise improves your life.

A detailed weight-training regimen is beyond the scope of this book, but there are many good books available. One that we have found very useful and user-friendly is *Top Shape* by Joyce L. Vedral, Ph.D. (Warner Books, 1995). This book describes exercise regimens for upper and lower body using both free weights and weight machines. Photographs show the correct way to do each exercise.

Weight-Training Equipment

The best and least expensive equipment for weight training is a set of dumbbells and a bench that can be adjusted to an incline. These are relatively inexpensive and easy to store. Weight machines are safer, but they are expensive, take up a lot of room, and probably don't give you as good a workout as dumbbells and a bench. Of course, you can always join a gym and use the weights there, but having the equipment at home makes it more likely you will actually use it.

Although not really "weights," elastic bands can have the same effect on your muscles as lifting weights. These 4-inch-wide, 4-foot-long strips of rubber are inexpensive (about $10 for 3 different elasticities), portable, and easy to use. We have had positive experience with Dyna-Bands (Fitness Wholesale, 895-A Hampshire Rd., Stow, OH 44224, 800–537–5512).

Our advice is to purchase a fitness book first and read its suggestions before you invest in equipment. Or you can hire a personal trainer at your local YMCA or fitness club to teach you how to use the equipment properly and to develop a personalized regimen so you don't hurt yourself and to maximize the benefit you get from the time you invest.

Frequency

You should not exercise the same muscles two days in a row. When you stress a muscle by lifting weights, you actually tear the muscle. The muscle needs a day off to repair itself, during which time it is strengthened. Thus, you should plan to exercise the same muscles no more frequently than every other day. On alternate days exercise a different set of muscles. The only exceptions are the leg and abdominal muscles, which can be exercised every day. Thus, you can do bent-knee sit-ups every day.

A Perfect Specimen

So, go do it! Invest in your future. You'll feel so good and look so good, you'll wonder why it took you so long to get started.

STRETCHING

The third part of the exercise success strategy is stretching. Don't skip stretching because you think it is wimpy. It is extremely important. And unlike aerobic exercise and strength training, it takes almost no effort. What's more, it's easy, and doing it feels fantastic. It's essential to do stretching exercises because as you age your tendons get shorter and your muscles get tighter. You can stay limber by doing stretching exercises. You should stretch every day even if you are young. It is best to warm your muscles by using them a few minutes before stretching. This prevents damage to the tendons, which may tear if stretched while cold. Hold the stretch for a count of 20 and do NOT bounce or jerk while stretching, as this may increase the chance of injury.

As with strength training, describing a stretching regimen is beyond the scope of this book. Many good books on stretching are available. We advise either getting one or consulting with a personal trainer or an exercise physiologist before you begin to stretch to make sure you do stretches that will not cause injuries. Some of the stretching exercises recommended years ago may cause injury to your back and should be avoided.

The Bottom Line

Exercise has nothing but positives. You really gotta do it. For your mental and physical well-being, as well as to reduce your risks for all sorts of disease, you need to fit in exercise every day.

And for fat loss, there is no way around it. You can lose weight if you just reduce fat in your diet. But if you want to lose fat and not muscle and you really want to keep it off, you MUST incorporate exercise into your life every day.

14. Master of Your Domain

YOU LUCKY MAN! If you are like many men, you know you could be slimmer, but weight has never been a lifelong fixation.* You eat because you are hungry or because the food is there. You may overeat, but you don't binge because you are depressed or stressed. This lack of concern is a real advantage. You approach losing weight as a simple problem to solve, without great psychological and emotional hang-ups. We explain the system. It seems logical to you. We give you the tools and you follow through.

While your former lack of attention allows you to approach weight loss without any emotional baggage, now that you are planning to lose weight, you have to start paying attention with a vengeance. Paying attention is what *Choose to Lose Weight-Loss Plan for Men* is all about. You need to know exactly what you are eating, and you need to know why. When you know both of these, you can make significant changes and attain your goals.

WHY ARE YOU OVERWEIGHT?

Extracurricular Eating

Are you overweight but have no idea how you got that way? Think about your eating habits. Do you always eat because you are hungry? Are there other reasons? Make a list of the times you eat. Then list the reasons you are eating. Do you eat because it is there? Is it boredom? Is it the dread of facing work you don't want to do? Are the luscious food ads

---

* If weight loss *has* been a fixation, following *Choose to Lose Weight-Loss Plan for Men* will help reduce it to what it should be — a healthy goal. Knowing what you are eating, not being hungry, eating without guilt — all the *Choose to Lose* strategies — will go a long way toward making eating a joy and not an obsession.

on TV too convincing to ignore? Are you seeking comfort from food because you're lonely?

Unconscious Eating

A lot of eating is unconscious or automatic. Have you ever been so involved in a conversation you consumed an entire tray of cheese and crackers without tasting even one? At the end of a movie have you ever looked into an empty 22-cup bucket of movie popcorn and wondered who ate it? When eating is unconscious, not only do you generally eat much more than you need, you also don't get the pleasure of tasting it.

To ensure that you don't waste fat calories on food you don't need or taste, set specific consumption goals and stick to them. For example, at the office party, decide beforehand to limit yourself to 2 cheese and cracker combos (which you really enjoy because you are finally tasting them). After taking your allotted food, move away from the table. (Never have conversations within reaching distance of food.) At the movies, *bring* 10 cups of air-popped popcorn. Movie popcorn will gobble up days of your Fat Budget. Even the kiddie size (5 cups) has 180 fat calories. Turn unconscious eating into pleasurable, conscious eating.

Boredom

A major cause of mindless eating is boredom. It isn't hunger that makes you devour bowl after bowl of high-fat munchies as you stare at the tube for hours on end. You are bored. Food can't replace that empty feeling. Reject boredom. Get off of the couch and get involved. Join the men's club of your church or synagogue. Take a course in photography or woodworking. Learn how to cook or garden. Work for your local politician. Meet people, get outside of yourself — in other words, liven up your life. You'll feel better and won't have time to sit around adding fat to your fat stores.

When you find yourself in front of the television, you don't need to clog your arteries with high-fat snacks. Solution: Get a hot-air popcorn popper and pop up a big batch of fat-free air-popped popcorn. Plain, unadulterated popcorn is not only healthy, it's delicious. It satisfies your hand-to-mouth cravings and fills you up.

BYO

Another reason people eat irrationally is because they are starving. They eat a breakfast and lunch that wouldn't satisfy a small flea, so when afternoon arrives they are forced to ravage the office vending machines to soothe the wild rumblings of their empty stomachs. This hunger haunts them even after they leave the office (see "Fatigue" below). To prevent this from happening to you, make sure you eat a full breakfast and lunch so your hunger doesn't drive you to high-fat bingeing. Bring a bag of fruit, carrot sticks, nonfat yogurt, and a bagel to keep you happy and full of energy all day.

Fatigue

You come home from work pooped. You head for the kitchen and clean out the cupboards. This time you can answer the question, "Why?" with, "I'm famished." Then you have to ask, "Why am I famished?" The answer is probably that you didn't eat any or enough lunch, and you didn't take an afternoon snack. You were probably so tired you had only enough strength to tear the door off the refrigerator but not enough strength to control what you ate.

What is the solution? Easy. Eat a hearty, low-fat, fiber-rich lunch, in the afternoon eat a piece of fruit from the bag of fruit you stash in your desk, and take a nap when you arrive home. Or take a walk or run. Some people prefer exercising when they come home from work. They say it energizes them. See what works for you.

If dinner is hours off, take a snack, a healthy, low-fat snack. But as you would tell your kids, don't eat too much or you'll spoil your supper.

The Moral of the Story

Remember: If you eat a large, delicious, nutritious, low-fat breakfast, a large, delicious, nutritious, low-fat lunch, and a large, delicious, nutritious, low-fat dinner, you won't need to pig out on high-fat, low-nutrient snacks. You'll be satisfied and content.

OBSTACLES AND OVERCOMING THEM

The road to healthy, low-fat eating may not be straight and smooth. You may come up against barriers that need to be overcome. You must always remember that you are number one. Eating healthfully is the most important thing you are doing right now. You must be steadfast as a rock. It's up to you.

Undermining Your Goals

Now that you have entered into a healthy way of living, are you getting mixed messages from your loved ones? Is your wife admiring your resolve, on the one hand, but insisting she's too tired to cook "special foods," on the other? Is your obese mother telling you you're too thin and should put on some weight? Is your best buddy pushing you to eat "just one little hot dog" as he buys his third chili dog from the hot-dog vendor? Even though they really care for you, they may feel threatened by the New You. Maybe they don't want to change their own eating habits even though they know they should. Maybe they are afraid that you will look much more attractive than they. Maybe they don't want to change the way they cook. Whatever the reason, if you want to be successful, the best solution is to confront them and bring the issue out into the open. They may not even be aware of their behavior.

Speaking Out

You may find confrontations uncomfortable, but if you want to effect a change, you need to communicate.

You need to make your saboteurs aware of their behavior. They may be shocked and deny that they are trying to sabotage your success. You need to let them know that eating healthfully is extremely important to you. In fact, it's a matter of life or death. Let them know that you are not rejecting them when you choose not to eat their food; you still love them. You just don't like being out of breath and getting caught in turnstiles. You miss seeing your toes.

Enlist their help. Encourage them to join you or at least not thwart your attempt to eat healthfully. In the long run, and even the short run, everyone will benefit from a lean, healthy, energetic you.

If your plea lands on deaf ears and your wife keeps insisting that you take her out for pizza, your mother keeps stuffing cherry cheesecake down your throat, and your children cry because there's no ice cream in the freezer or cake and chips in the cupboard, you need to get tough. Repeat your argument and ask them why they want to sabotage you. That will make them think. Maybe they'll face their behavior and change it. Insist that you don't want to overwork your wife and that you adore your mom's cheesecake, but you also want to be alive to enjoy your retirement and your great-great-grandchildren.

Fight on! By your example, you may be able to turn your whole family into healthy eaters.

Self-Sabotage

Before you blame your capitulations on others, maybe you need to look at yourself. Did you eat 3 pieces of Aunt Martha's pecan pie to make her feel good, or did you want an excuse to overindulge? Did you pop into a fast-food restaurant to stop the kids from whining, the dog from barking, and your wife from nagging, or did you want a Big Mac and fries? Did you serve nachos and peanuts to the guys on Super Bowl Sunday to be a good host or to pamper yourself? Why did you bring your mother-in-law peanut brittle when you know she has no teeth? Much sabotage is self-inspired. You need to analyze your motives and stop fooling yourself. If any high-fat temptation that comes along weakens your resolve, you aren't really committed to changing your lifestyle. If you want to eat healthfully, you can. It's up to you.

Personal or Professional Crises

Let us state categorically that there is almost no situation that should make you fall off the *Choose to Lose Weight-Loss Plan for Men* wagon. Perhaps if you are in a coma, or in solitary confinement, you have a reason to stop following it. Even crises like being fired or changing your job or moving out of town or having a medical problem in your family should not affect your resolve. You have to eat, and when you eat, there is no reason not to eat a healthy diet. In fact, following *Choose to Lose Weight-Loss Plan for Men* during a crisis will give you fortitude. It will provide order in one part of your life and thus help in every other part.

When people "go off" *Choose to Lose Weight-Loss Plan for Men*, it is because they are treating it like a diet. This is *not* a starvation or exchange diet in which you eat 1200 calories of carrot sticks and celery. You go off such a diet because it is impossible to stay on it for more than a few weeks. *Choose to Lose Weight-Loss Plan for Men* is forever. You eat lots of delicious food. You lower your fat intake, but you can fit in an occasional high-fat favorite. *Choose to Lose Weight-Loss Plan for Men* should become such an integral part of your life that nothing will unhinge you.

Cheating Is Impossible

Choose to Lose Weight-Loss Plan for Men encourages you to include an occasional high-fat splurge, so you don't have to go crazy from deprivation. Why would you need to eat 3 pieces of Aunt Martha's pecan pie if you were including an occasional high-fat splurge in your diet and were eating plenty of delicious, nutritious food? You need to do the complete program. That doesn't mean just reducing fat in your diet. It doesn't mean eating a stalk of broccoli and a baked potato for dinner. It means eating nutritious foods, enjoying real meals, and fitting in an occasional splurge.

Sinning

Even if you do falter and overeat your Fat Budget for a few days, don't give up and return to your high-fat ways. Don't accuse yourself of being "bad" and then eat everything in sight. Recognize that you have gotten into sloppy habits and need to pay attention. If you eat a low-low-fat diet for several days, you can easily balance out the extra fat calories you accumulated.

Pay Attention!

The key words are PAY ATTENTION. Be aware of what you eat. Be aware of your motives and the motives of others. Be aware of the bumps in the road so you will be able to maneuver a clear course. Pay attention and enjoy yourself!

Pinpoint your problems and come up with solutions. If you don't have time to make a sandwich in the morning, make it the night before. If you get hungry every afternoon, pack a bag with fruit and a bagel and keep it in your desk. If the prospect of no desserts makes you weep, go out for dessert once a week or once a month. Remember, you can solve any problem that may arise. No obstacle is too big if you have the will and resolve to overcome it.

You are the master of your fate. You need to prioritize your needs. Eating healthfully and exercising aerobically every day should be number one. You can do it.

15. To Your Health

THE TRULY most important reason for following *Choose to Lose Weight-Loss Plan for Men* is for your health. There are compelling health reasons for eating a low-fat, high-fiber diet and exercising even if you are not overweight. You can be thin as a rail and still be at increased risk for many chronic diseases if you eat a high-fat and low-fiber diet. Both obesity and a typical American high-fat, low-fiber diet increase a person's risks for a variety of diseases and for premature death.

Here are some studies to further convince you that eating healthfully is crucial for your health:

Eat Right and Exercise to Save Your Life

Recently scientists looked at the underlying causes of all of the deaths that took place in the United States in 1990. They found that, together, lack of exercise and poor dietary habits were the second-largest underlying cause of death. (Smoking was the largest.)

Source: National Institute on Aging, National Institutes of Health.

OBESITY AND DEATH

Many scientific studies have shown a relationship between weight and total mortality (death from all causes). This research has made it clear that as weight increases, mortality increases. The lowest mortality rate occurs in people who are 10% under the average weight for people of the same age and height.

Mortality and Weight in Men

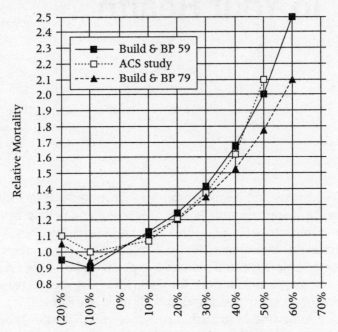

The results of three separate studies relating mortality and weight are shown in the graph above. It is evident in all three cases that mortality increases as weight increases. The American Cancer Society (ACS) study defines relative weight as the percentage above the average weight for people of the same age and height. In the graph above, a man who is 40% overweight for his age and height is 50% more likely to die at any given age than a man who is the desirable weight for his age and height. In some studies, mortality is doubled in men who are 50% overweight.

HEART DISEASE

Heart disease is the leading cause of death for both men and women, accounting for about 50% of all deaths. In the past we thought heart disease was a natural consequence of aging. We now know it is a highly preventable disease. *Choose to Lose Weight-Loss Plan for Men* will arm you with the tools to decrease your risk of death and disability from heart disease.

For those tough men who say, "I'll eat steak and just have a heart attack and drop dead," we say, "Dream on." Dying of heart disease can be a slow, agonizing process. Why would you want to sentence yourself to years of pain and disability when you can eat wonderful low-fat food and live to a ripe and healthy old age?

Heart Disease Risk Rises as Weight Rises

The relationships between diet, cholesterol, and many other risk factors, including obesity, and heart disease are well known. The graph below shows the relationship between relative weight and death from coronary heart disease (CHD) in men for all ages combined.

The graph shows that death from coronary heart disease increases steadily with increasing weight. Men who are 40% overweight (they are shown as 1.4+, which means average weight plus 40% or more on the relative weight axis) have a twofold higher death rate from coronary heart disease than men of average weight.

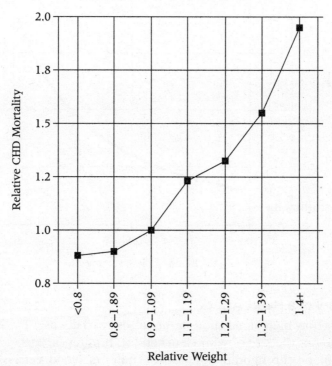

Weight and CHD Death Rates

Blood Cholesterol

One of the major risk factors for coronary heart disease is high blood cholesterol.

You can see from this curve that risk rises sharply at cholesterol levels above 200 mg/dL. Between cholesterol levels of 200 and 300 mg/dL, risk increases by 2% for every 1% increase in blood cholesterol level. The recommendation from all the health agencies is to lower your cholesterol to 200 mg/dL or less. The good news is that you can lower your cholesterol by one-third by diet alone. Even if your cholesterol is as high as 300 mg/dL (about 5% of the population have cholesterol levels this high or higher), you can lower it to 200 by eating a diet low in saturated fat. By following *Choose to Lose Weight-Loss Plan for Men*, you will be reducing both total fat and saturated fat in your diet.

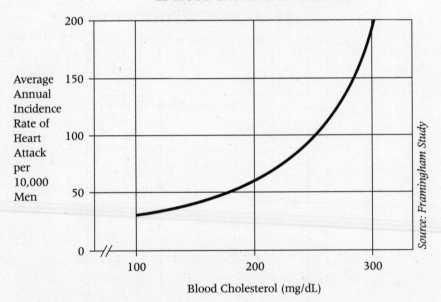

Risk of Coronary Heart Attack Rises as Blood Cholesterol Increases

Average Annual Incidence Rate of Heart Attack per 10,000 Men

Blood Cholesterol (mg/dL)

Source: Framingham Study

The Story of a Heart Attack

Here is how high blood cholesterol causes heart disease. The heart is a muscle about the size of your clenched fist. It pumps thousands of gallons of blood throughout hundreds of miles of blood vessels in your body every day. In order to do this prodigious amount of work, the heart needs an uninterrupted supply of oxygenated, nutrient-rich blood. This blood is supplied by the coronary arteries on the surface of the heart. As long as these arteries remain open, blood is supplied and the heart muscle cells are fed.

When I Was Just a Little Boy . . . But beginning in early childhood, in many people eating a high-fat diet, cholesterol-rich deposits called plaque begin to be deposited on the inner surface of the coronary arteries. Even as early as young adulthood many Americans already have significant deposits in their coronary arteries. Autopsies of young accident victims and American soldiers killed in action in Korea and Vietnam vividly reveal the extent of this accumulation in young men. Over time deposits narrow the inside diameter of the coronary arteries, especially at branch points where there is turbulent blood flow.

Blood Clot Gums up the Works. When the inside diameter of the coronary artery is reduced to 25% or less of its original diameter, a small blood clot that normally passes unhindered through the artery can get stuck in the narrowed artery. The clot blocks the blood flow and deprives the heart muscle cells downstream of oxygenated, nutrient-rich blood. The cells slowly begin to die. This is a heart attack. Once these cells die, nothing can be done to restore them. The location of the blockage determines the extent of the damage to the heart, whether the heart attack is mild, serious, or fatal, and whether the patient will survive with little or extensive permanent damage.

Solving the Problem

The key to reducing blood cholesterol levels (especially heart-risky LDL-cholesterol) and thus risk of heart disease is to eat a diet low in saturated fat. Saturated fat is the main culprit in the diet that raises blood cholesterol levels. Saturated fat is one of the three major types of fat in the diet that make up total fat (see page 71). The other two are monounsaturated fat and polyunsaturated fat. The major sources of saturated fat in the diet are animal fats, such as beef, lamb, veal, and pork, and dairy fat, cocoa butter, and tropical oils, such as coconut, palm, and palm kernel oils.

For heart health, you also need to limit your consumption of trans fats. Trans fats act like saturated fats and raise LDL-cholesterol levels and thus risk of heart disease. Trans fats are produced by the hydrogenation

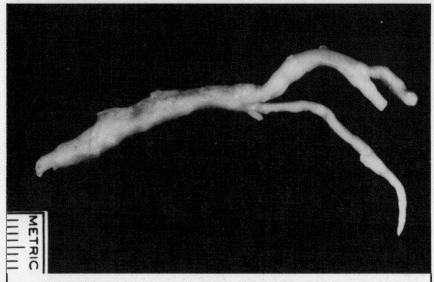

Photo by Maggie Moore, laboratory of Dr. William C. Roberts, NHLBI.

The photograph above shows the cholesterol-rich plaque that has been removed from the coronary artery of a man who died of a heart attack. The plaque is so thick it has taken the shape of the coronary artery. You probably have plaque similar to this in your coronary arteries, but not this thick or you wouldn't be reading this.

Every time you are deciding whether or not to eat a double cheeseburger or chocolate brownie whipped cream cake, conjure up the image of this coronary-artery plaque, and you won't have difficulty saying, "No thanks."

of polyunsaturated fats and are common in many processed foods. To determine if a product contains hydrogenated fats, look for the words "hydrogenated" or "partially hydrogenated."

By following *Choose to Lose Weight-Loss Plan for Men* and eating a low-fat diet, you will automatically be eating a low-saturated-fat diet, and your blood cholesterol level will come down. You can reduce your blood cholesterol level by as much as 33% by diet alone, and it takes only about 2–3 weeks with the proper dietary choices. But don't think that eating healthfully for a few weeks will lower your cholesterol for life. If you resume eating a high-fat, high-saturated fat diet, your blood cholesterol will shoot right back up, and so will your risk of heart disease. You can never be *cured* of high cholesterol. You need to eat a heart-healthy, low-fat, low-saturated-fat diet forever. How lucky! Low-fat, low-sat-fat food can be a great treat.

For More Information. The saturated-fat contents of many common and brand-name foods are listed in the Food Tables at the end of this book. A more complete discussion of diet, cholesterol, and heart disease can be found in our book *Eater's Choice: A Food Lover's Guide to Lower Cholesterol*.

Combating Heart Disease: Diet Plus Exercise

Regular aerobic exercise also reduces the risk of a fatal heart attack. This includes repetitive, rhythmic exercises such as walking, running, biking, rowing, and swimming. For maximum heart protection, you should exercise at an intensity that will maintain your heart rate within the target heart zone. Target heart zones are age-dependent. To determine your zone, first subtract your age from 220, the maximum heart rate in beats per minute. Your zone lies between 70% and 90% of this value. Thus, if you are 50 years old, subtract 50 from 220. This is 170. Your target heart zone lies between 119 beats per minute (70% of 170) and 153 (90% of 170). This is actually a higher heart rate than is optimal for weight loss. The optimal weight-loss heart rate would be between 50% and 70% of the value 220 minus your age. Exercise for fat loss need not be intense. If you are carrying on a conversation during exercise without losing your breath, you are exercising at the right intensity.

Aerobic exercise seems to be protective in at least two ways. It increases HDL-cholesterol, which acts as a scavenger to remove LDL or bad cholesterol from the bloodstream. The higher the HDL-cholesterol, the lower one's risk of heart disease. Regular aerobic exercise also strengthens the heart muscle and increases the chances of surviving a heart attack.

DIABETES

People with diabetes lack the ability to move the simple sugar glucose from the blood into the cells where it is burned for energy. There are two types of diabetes. Type 1 diabetes, also known as juvenile diabetes, is caused by the absence of the hormone insulin, which facilitates uptake of glucose by cells from the blood. This type of diabetes, which can occur at any age, is often the result of a viral infection or other disease that destroys the pancreatic cells that produce insulin. Type 1 diabetics are insulin-dependent.

Type 2 diabetes, also known as adult-onset diabetes, is much more common (95% of all diabetics) and is usually the result of obesity. In this type of diabetes the body produces insulin, but the body's cells no longer respond to the insulin and so glucose remains in the blood and the cells are starved for energy.

The graph below shows the relationship between relative weight and death from diabetes in men. There is a steep rise in death rates with increasing relative weight greater than 10% overweight. Men who are 40% overweight have a fivefold greater risk of dying from diabetes than normal-weight men.

Losing weight and maintaining a desirable and healthy weight may prevent type 2 diabetes. This is best accomplished by eating a low-fat,

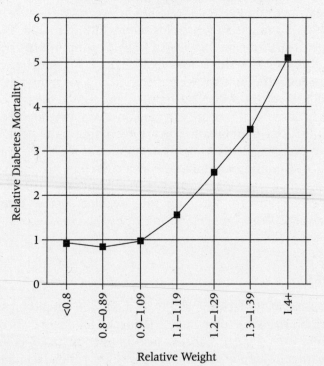

Weight and Diabetes Death Rates

high-fiber diet such as recommended in *Choose to Lose Weight-Loss Plan for Men* and doing regular aerobic exercise. For those who are glucose-intolerant — often an early stage of type 2 diabetes — losing weight may reverse this condition and normalize their glucose metabolism, thereby reducing their risk of becoming diabetic.

STROKE

Stroke is the major cause of cerebrovascular disease (CVD). A stroke is a brain attack in which the brain is deprived of oxygen-rich, nutrient-rich blood. This can be caused by either rupture of an artery or blockage of an artery by cholesterol-rich plaque. High blood pressure is a major risk factor for stroke. Obesity, in turn, is a leading cause of high blood pressure. Men who are 40% overweight have a more than twofold higher rate of dying from cerebrovascular disease (see graph below).

Losing weight and maintaining a desirable weight by eating a low-fat,

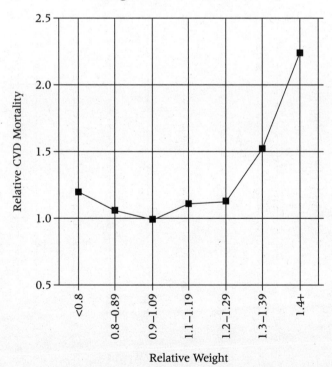

Weight and CVD Death Rates

high-fiber diet and doing regular aerobic exercise will reduce blood pressure and risk of stroke. In addition to its role in weight control, aerobic exercise has an independent action in lowering blood pressure. Reducing sodium intake will help lower blood pressure in those people who are salt-sensitive.

CANCER

The graph relating cancer death to relative weight is U-shaped. The large increase in death rates at lower than normal weights is ascribed to weight loss due to preexisting illness, probably undiagnosed cancers. From the graph below, you can see that there is a greater than 30% increase in cancer mortality in men who are 40% or more overweight. The cancers most commonly linked to obesity are prostate and colorectal, two of the three leading causes of cancer death in men. (The leading cause is lung cancer associated with smoking.)

Weight and Cancer Death Rates

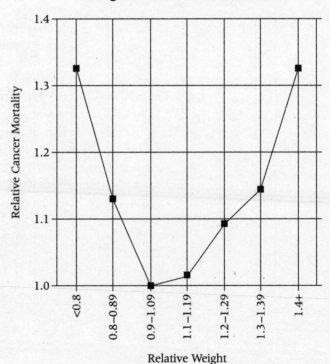

Cancer Institute Guidelines

The National Cancer Institute has issued the following dietary guidelines to reduce risk of cancers:

- Reduce fat intake to 30% or less of calories.
- Increase fiber intake to 20–30 grams per day, with an upper limit of 35 grams.
- Include a variety of vegetables and fruits in the daily diet.
- Avoid obesity.
- Consume alcoholic beverages in moderation, if at all.
- Minimize consumption of salt-cured, salt-pickled, and smoked foods.

By following *Choose to Lose Weight-Loss Plan for Men*, you will automatically be conforming to all the recommendations (except the last).

JOINT DEGENERATION

Although not a fatal condition, the degeneration of a joint, especially the knee, can have devastating effects on the quality of life. The problem occurs because the knee joint and also the hip joint and the feet are not designed to carry the excessive loads associated with obesity. Cartilage in joints breaks down with normal aging, but this process is speeded up in obese persons.

Lift a 20-pound bag. Imagine carrying this around all day. Think of your back. Think of your knees. What if the weight were 40 pounds, or 100? It is no wonder so many obese people have to use canes, crutches, walkers, or even wheelchairs. The best way to avoid the damage to your joints is to lose weight and keep it off.

The *Choose to Lose Weight-Loss Plan for Men* Refrain

The same basic dietary and exercise recommendations that help you reach and maintain your desirable and healthy weight will also help reduce your risks of heart disease, diabetes, stroke, and prostate and colorectal cancers.

What greater reason could you have to make today the first day of a long life of healthy eating and daily exercise?

16. FAQ: Frequently Asked Questions

CONTENTS
(in alphabetical order)

Alcohol

Q. Alcohol has lots of calories. Will the alcohol calories turn to fat if I drink too much?

A. Overconsuming alcohol calories is a lot like overconsuming empty carbohydrate calories. The calories don't turn to fat, but since the body can't store them, it burns them in preference to fat stored in your fat stores. Result: Your fat remains in the wine cellar and your weight loss is put on hold. In addition, drinking too much alcohol may cause your resolve to dissolve. You might find yourself ravaging the bowl of beer nuts and plate of nachos. Unlike alcohol, these high-fat snacks do turn to beer bellies and love handles.

The bottom line: Limit nonfat alcoholic beverages to a maximum of 1–2 drinks a day.

Also, beware of the company the alcohol keeps. Some mixed drinks contain high-fat ingredients. The cream of coconut in a 6-ounce piña colada makes it a 103-fat-calorie land mine. The whipped cream topping adds 99 fat calories to your Irish coffee. Look up BEVERAGES in the Food Tables and stay away from the ones with fat calories.

Football Game Passes

Q. Watching football games with friends means drinking beer and eating nuts, chips, and nachos. How do I enjoy the party without busting my Fat Budget for the week?

A. You may take several approaches. Whichever approach you take, don't go to the party hungry. Make sure that before you leave home you have eaten a sandwich, a baked potato, a bowl of cereal or air-popped popcorn — enough low-fat food so you can look at the party snacks with indifference.

- Take a small amount of whatever is offered and stop eating. If you are worried that someone will make a fuss that you aren't making a pig of yourself, don't be concerned. No one will notice. People will be too busy watching the game and eating themselves to worry about you.

- Position yourself so you are not near the food. Move the food away if it is near you. You don't *have* to have a snack to watch the game. Game snacking is generally unconscious eating.

- If you know what the host typically serves, try to match it with a nonfat substitute. For example, if the host serves popcorn, ask if you can bring your own air-popped. If he serves chips, ask if you can bring nonfat baked chips and a salsa dip.

High-Protein Diets

Q. I have friends on high-protein, low-carbohydrate diets who say they can eat lots of fat and lose weight. Why should I avoid this approach and follow *Choose to Lose Weight-Loss Plan for Men* instead?

A. High-protein, low-carbohydrate diets like the Atkins Diet, Protein

Power, and the Zone came back into vogue in the late 1990s.* These "new" diets are throwbacks to the diets of the 1950s and 1960s, which were abandoned because they were dangerous and ineffective in the long term. They are dangerous because consuming too much protein can damage the kidneys and liver and low-calorie diets slow metabolism and cause people to be deficient in vitamins, minerals, and fiber.

While these diets may work in the short term (see explanation below), their effectiveness is limited because they can't be followed for long. They are generally low-calorie and restrictive. Not eating makes people hungry, so they build up cravings and binge, and then return to their old eating patterns. People complain that these diets make them feel awful, which is an additional inducement to quit.

This is the way high-protein, low-carb diets work and why they can be very, very dangerous:

Because the carbohydrate intake on a high-protein, high-fat, low-carbohydrate diet plan is insufficient to fuel the body's physical activity and maintenance needs, the body quickly burns up its glycogen stores (not that big to begin with) for energy. (Muscle is generally not burned because the high protein intake may help reduce protein loss from the muscle.) First negative effect: Depleting the glycogen stores leaves the dieter fatigued and low on stamina.

The body next turns to the fat stores for energy. Large amounts of fat are removed from the fat stores and transported to the liver, producing a fatty liver. The breakdown of the fat in the liver occurs at a greater than normal rate.

Second negative effect: Because there is an insufficient amount of carbohydrate to metabolize the fat completely, ketone bodies are formed. When more ketone bodies are formed than the body can assimilate, the ketones build up in the blood and in the urine.

Third negative effect: Excretion of the ketones in the urine results in a loss of sodium and large quantities of fluid, leading to an imbalance of salts in the body. A tendency to nausea and consequent vomiting causes even more fluid loss.

Another negative effect: Breakdown products from the increased protein in the diet strain the kidneys and can lead to kidney failure.

Ultimate negative effects: Imbalance of salts in the body causes

---

* Hopefully protein and low-carbohydrate diets will soon be discredited and abandoned because of the numbers of people who get sick following them.

muscle cramps and difficulty in walking. Depression of the central nervous system due to fluid loss and salt imbalance can ultimately lead to profound coma.

You may be thinking that the people you know on protein diets are not in such dire straits as described above. They may be okay for the moment, but eventually they will suffer some of these serious consequences. Dietitians have told us they are seeing many high-protein dieters with serious liver problems and extremely high cholesterol levels. They are also seeing increased numbers of colon cancer associated with these diets. Many of these dieters report that they feel lousy and fatigued. In the long term a deficiency of vitamins, minerals, and fiber will result in poor health.

Fear of Insulin

Q. I have heard that you should avoid carbohydrates because eating them raises your insulin, which leads to weight gain and diabetes.

A. No way! Insulin production in response to eating carbohydrates is as normal and healthy as an increased pulse rate is to exercise. You need to produce insulin to live! When you eat carbohydrates, your body produces insulin to move the carbohydrates into the cells where they are burned (not converted into fat). The production of insulin does not cause diabetes. In fact, the inability to produce insulin is a sign of diabetes.

Goal Weight

Q. Once I reach my goal weight, can I stop following *Choose to Lose Weight-Loss Plan for Men?*

A. No! No! No! Being overweight is not like having a strep throat that you can cure by taking antibiotics. You need to follow a low-fat, nutrient-dense, fiber-rich diet with daily aerobic exercise forever or you will gain back everything you lost. You need to follow *Choose to Lose Weight-Loss Plan for Men* forever so you will be full of energy and good health. If you are truly following *Choose to Lose Weight-Loss Plan for Men* and not starving yourself, fitting in an occasional high-fat splurge, and eating lots of delicious, nutritious, low-fat food, it will be easy (and enjoyable) to maintain your weight-loss goal forever.

Q. Once I reach my goal weight, should I increase my Fat Budget?

A. No. The Fat Budget you determined is designed both to reach and maintain your goal weight.

Weight-Loss Rate

Q. How many pounds can I expect to lose each week?

A. If you expect to lose a specific number of pounds each week, you may be sorely disappointed. Weight loss depends on many things — your past history of weight loss and gain, your metabolic rate, how much exercise you do, how many changes you are making in your diet, how completely you are adhering to the three *Choose to Lose Weight-Loss Plan for Men* strategies. Besides, pounds lost is not a good indicator of fat loss and muscle gained. How your clothes fit will give you a truer picture of your progress. See "The Scale" on page 170.

Weight-Loss Standstill

Q. When I first started *Choose to Lose Weight-Loss Plan for Men,* I lost a lot of weight quickly. But now I seem to have reached a plateau. Should I give up?

A. Never! Your scale is a poor judge of how well you are doing. Check the notches in your belt and the seams in your pants for progress on your fat loss. Do not give up now. You *will* lose weight. This is only a temporary plateau. Hang on. See the next answer too.

Not Losing

Q. I have been following *Choose to Lose Weight-Loss Plan for Men* to the letter. Why am I not losing weight?

A. First, think health, not pounds. No matter what your weight loss, *Choose to Lose Weight-Loss Plan for Men* is the healthiest way to eat. You are reducing your risks for all sorts of diseases and improving your long-term health outlook. Second, people lose at different rates. You may not lose for the first few weeks, then suddenly you drop ten pounds. On the other hand, maybe you aren't being as religious at following *Choose to Lose Weight-Loss Plan for Men* as you think. The explanation for your weight-loss standstill may be found in your answers to these questions:

1. How often do you eat out?

It is possible to try to control your fat consumption when you eat out (see Chapter 11, "Dining Out"), but unless you follow the chef around the kitchen, you can never be really sure how much fat he is using. For the sobering truth about eating out, see pages

76–82, "Fat City," and RESTAURANT FOODS and FAST FOODS in the Food Tables.

Write down the number of meals you eat out (or carry in). Be sure to include the muffin you ate at the coffee bar and the pizza delivered to you at work. If you are eating out twice a week or more, you may find your weight loss has hit a wall. You can tear down the wall. Prepare food at home as much as you can. Take the advice offered in Chapter 9, "Eating In," and Chapter 10, "Cooking Up a Low-Fat Storm." You'll be eating more food, tastier food, and healthier food.

Some of you have no choice about eating out. You are on the road almost every day. Read and memorize the tips in Chapter 12, "Man About Town," as well as in Chapter 11, "Dining Out." For the rest of you, for the sake of your health and weight-loss goals, try to limit your dining out to a rare event.

2. Do you really know what you are eating?

It is very easy to think you have cut way down on your fat, but if you don't write down everything you eat honestly and accurately, you may be consuming more fat than you realize. Perhaps you go to a fast-food restaurant and order a grilled chicken sandwich. You assume it has only 33 fat calories because that is the cost of a chicken breast (13 fat calories) plus a bun (20 fat calories). However, a quick glance at the Food Tables shows you that a grilled chicken fillet sandwich actually contains 153 fat calories. What you considered a good choice suddenly becomes a poor choice. You really need to keep track because fat accumulates as fast as your Visa bill. (To order a handy Passbook for recording your food intake and exercise, see the order form at the back of the book.)

3. Are you eating enough nutritious food?

One of the reasons men are so successful at losing weight is that they are not afraid to eat. But you need to eat a lot of the right foods — low-fat, nutritious food, not high-fat or empty calories. If you fulfill the minimum nutritional requirements as suggested by the base of the Food Guide Pyramid, and make sure most of the food you eat is fiber-rich, you will be a success at losing fat. Besides being chock-full of vitamins and minerals, these foods have a lot of bulk and will keep you full.

4. Are you exercising aerobically for at least 30 minutes every day?

Exercise is an essential part of fat loss. The more you exercise, the greater your energy needs. To supply the fuel to satisfy these additional needs, your body will burn fat from the fat stores (if you are eating a low-fat, nutrient-dense, fiber-rich diet) and you will lose weight. In addition, the more muscle you build by exercising aerobically, the more fat you will burn. You can lose without exercising, but it is much slower and much less permanent.

5. Are you eating portions of processed foods that are too big?

Foods such as pasta, low-fiber cereal, bagels, etc., may be included in a healthy diet, but because they are so processed and fiber-free you can easily overeat them. Their calories add up quickly to very large amounts that will be burned in preference to fat. *You* have to control the amount you eat because these foods are not filling and thus self-limiting, as fiber-rich carbohydrates are. Two cups of pasta are okay, but 4 are too much. You need not go without, but don't go overboard.

6. Are you eating too many "low-fat" foods.

Foods labeled "low-fat" or "nonfat" are sometimes neither. The two "low-fat" muffins you pick up each morning for breakfast may contain as many as 150 fat calories. Unless you know the ingredients and amounts, be suspicious of so-called low-fat food with no nutrition labeling.

Losing Too Much?

Q. If I keep following *Choose to Lose Weight-Loss Plan for Men*, will I eventually become emaciated and waste away to nothing?

A. You only wish! The Fat Budget you determined is the maximum amount of fat you should consume to reach your goal weight and to stay there.

Q. I have reached my goal weight, and my family tells me I am too thin.

A. It is often difficult for overweight people to see their loved ones or friends succeed at losing weight when they haven't had the discipline to make any changes themselves. When they insist that you have become too thin or too fanatical about fat, ignore them. You are *not* too thin. You need to eat a healthy diet for your health. It is all too easy to be convinced that you need to relax and return to your old high-fat, unhealthy eating habits. Stick to your guns. You'll feel great and be much healthier if you continue to keep eating the *Choose to Lose Weight-Loss Plan for Men* way for the rest of your life.

Too Little Fat?

Q. I have cut down my fat intake to almost nothing. Is it dangerous to eat too little fat?

A. First of all, it is hard to believe you are eating no fat. Have you been keeping track? Honestly? You are probably eating a lot more fat than you think.

Second, a low-low-low-low-fat diet is not dangerous. In fact, it can be very healthy if it is filled with nutrient-dense, fiber-rich calories and not empty calories. Mainland Chinese eat a 10% fat diet, and they are much healthier than we are. If you are eating according to the recommendations of the Food Guide Pyramid, you are probably getting adequate fat.

The only problem with eating almost no fat is that it usually accompanies a starvation approach and becomes a short-term solution. Soon you're off *Choose to Lose Weight-Loss Plan for Men* and back to old high-fat habits.

Eating Enough Healthy Food?

Q. I seem to be doing a lousy job of eating according to the Food Guide Pyramid and eating enough calories.

A. Nancy Ochsner of Woodland Park, Colorado, thought of this clever way to make sure you are meeting the recommendations of the Food Guide Pyramid: Each morning place your fruit, vegetable, grain, and dairy requirements for the day on a plastic tray in the refrigerator and make sure you have emptied it by the end of the day.

If you can't accumulate enough total calories, ask yourself: Am I eating real, full meals at breakfast, lunch, and dinner, or am I skipping breakfast, eating a bagel for lunch, and grabbing a bowl of lettuce from a salad bar for dinner? Follow our example: Every night for dinner we have soup, a chicken, turkey, or fish entrée on rice, and two or more vegetables — sometimes one is sweet potato or white potato. Do you see why we have no trouble accumulating enough calories? Are you including healthy snacks? We enjoy 8 cups of air-popped popcorn every evening. Try harder and you will reach and surpass your minimum daily total caloric intake in no time.

The Scale: Throw It Out

Q. You suggest throwing away your scale, but how do you measure your progress if you don't weigh yourself?

A. A scale is a poor judge of your progress. If you are exercising, you will be building muscle. Muscle has weight. In fact, the muscle you are building may be heavier than the fat you are losing, so your weight on the scale may not change and could even increase. But in the long run the muscle you are building will help you burn fat and you will lose weight. Moreover, short-term fluctuations in weight are often due to water retention or loss. Your fat loss will be evident by the way your clothes fit.

When people weigh themselves, they lose sight of why they are trying to lose weight. They fixate on the goal and forget the reason they are making changes. Weighing 160 pounds is not what is important. What is important is eating lots of low-fat, nutrient-dense, fiber-rich foods and exercising aerobically every day.

Cholesterol

Q. I have high blood cholesterol. Will it hurt me to follow *Choose to Lose Weight-Loss Plan for Men?*

A. Lowering your blood cholesterol is actually a side effect of following the *Choose to Lose Weight-Loss Plan for Men.* This is because by reducing total fat you will automatically reduce saturated fat, which is the main culprit in raising blood cholesterol. To learn everything you need to know about heart disease, diet, and cholesterol, read our book *Eater's Choice: A Food Lover's Guide to Lower Cholesterol.* We also recommend cooking the delicious, nutritious recipes from *Eater's Choice Low-Fat Cookbook* to keep your cholesterol low, your body lean, and your taste buds in ecstasy.

Diet Drugs

Q. What's so wrong with having a crutch like a diet drug to lose weight?

A. Everything. Most diet pills act on the brain to curb your hunger so you eat less food. First, we know that eating does not make you fat if you are making low-fat, nutrient-dense, fiber-rich choices. So why curb your appetite?

Second, eating is essential for life. Fruits, vegetables, whole grains, nonfat dairy, and low-fat meats contain vitamins, minerals, and fiber that you need for good health. You need food to fuel your body. You need to eat to keep up your metabolism. Eating is not to be avoided; it is to be enjoyed. It is healthy (and natural) to be hungry and eat.

Third, diet drugs have been shown to be extremely dangerous. In general, the real guinea pigs for the drugs are the people taking them. The new FDA fast-track approach to drug approval means diet pills are put on the market without being tested long enough or carefully enough to see if they are truly safe or effective. When enough people die or get sick, the drugs are taken off the market. Fenfluramine and dexfenfluramine were pulled off the market because people who were taking them began to experience heart problems. Even before the pills were put on the American market it was known that they cause a fatal disease called primary pulmonary hypertension. They probably cause some Alzheimer's-like neurological damage in everyone who takes them. Ignoring the recommendation of a panel of experts, the FDA recently approved the diet drug Meridia, which causes high blood pressure in some people and may increase the risk of stroke and heart disease.

Orlistat (Xenical) is a new kind of diet pill. It acts in the intestine by preventing absorption of about one-third of the fat you eat. But it causes loss of vitamins and in the presence of a high-fat diet causes abdominal pain, gas, urgency, and diarrhea. These side effects can be minimized by eating a low-fat diet. But as you know, eating a low-fat diet by itself results in weight loss. Orlistat is unnecessary as well as dangerous and expensive.

Fourth, diet drugs are expensive.

Fifth, if you stop taking diet drugs, you will gain back all the weight you lost (if you lost any weight).

Most Important: Even if the pills were safe, which is probably not possible, a drug would never give you the benefits of eating nutritious, low-fat foods and exercising — the pleasure of eating delicious food, the contentment of feeling full and satisfied, a reduction of risks for chronic diseases, more energy, better balance, and a sense of well-being, strength, and independence.

Olestra: Fat Substitute

Q. What is olestra, and are olestra-filled foods the answer to a high-fat snack addict's prayer?

A. Olestra (Olean®) is a man-made fat molecule composed of sugar and vegetable oil that is too large to be absorbed by the intestine. So instead of being absorbed and then distributed to the fat stores, it just passes through.

Even though it sounds like the perfect solution for those who want to get the fat taste without fat consequences, eating olestra-filled foods has many drawbacks.

- Olestra may cause gastrointestinal problems such as diarrhea, abdominal cramping, and nausea. These side effects have been so severe as to cause hospitalization.
- Olestra may cause hives.
- When olestra passes through the body, it takes with it the fat-soluble vitamins A, E, D, and K and carotenoids. This loss may have long-term health consequences. Carotenoids are substances found in fruits and vegetables that appear to reduce the risk of cancer, heart disease, and macular degeneration (a common cause of blindness in the elderly).
- For those people who take a blood-thinning medication such as coumadin, olestra may be dangerous.
- Equally as important, the long-term effects of eating olestra have not been measured. According to Dr. Henry Blackburn, a professor of public health at the University of Minnesota and one of the 5 advisers on the FDA Advisory Committee of 20 who voted against recommending olestra's approval, the lack of long-term clinical trials with adequate numbers of humans and the insufficient follow-up on cancer findings in one mouse study made him "unable to arrive at a reasonable certainty of no harm."
- Even if olestra did not have potential health problems, you would need to carefully monitor your intake of olestra-filled, fat-free snack foods. Just like overdosing on high-sugar, fat-free foods, eating too many olestra-filled foods will push out more nutritious foods, and the hundreds of empty calories consumed will be burned in preference to stored fat.
- In addition, these fat-free, fatty-tasting foods will keep up your high-fat taste so you will never lose your taste for high-fat foods.

Choose to Lose for Women

Q. Can my wife follow *Choose to Lose Weight-Loss Plan for Men?*

A. Certainly. However, she might want to purchase our other weight-loss book, *Choose to Lose: A Food Lover's Guide to Permanent Weight Loss,* instead. The basic strategies are the same in both books, but *Choose to Lose Weight-Loss Plan for Men* is written specifically for men. *Choose to*

Lose may speak to her more directly. If she decides to follow *Choose to Lose Weight-Loss Plan for Men*, she will find tables to determine her Fat Budget in Appendix B.

Diet Drinks

Q. I've always chosen diet Coke to avoid the calories. I know that total calories don't make you fat, but can I really drink regular Cola without gaining weight?

A. Neither diet drinks nor regular sodas are fattening. However, if you drink 6-pack (780 calories) after 6-pack (780 + 780 = 1560 total calories) of regular soft drinks, you accumulate so many total calories that your body will burn them instead of fat in your fat stores. This will stall your weight loss.

   Both drinks are poor choices. They contribute nothing to your health and can harm your teeth. Diet drinks have the added disadvantage of containing unhealthy additives. When thirsty, try the best drink choices instead — skim milk, water, and real fruit juices.

Jello and Lettuce Leaves

Q. I love to eat. How can I stay on this plan if I have to eat jello and lettuce leaves?

A. We hate to be rude, BUT DIDN'T YOU READ THIS BOOK?!!! We never eat lettuce leaves and jello. We eat *Grainy Mustard Chicken* and *Turkey Bayou* and *Chili Non Carne. Choose to Lose Weight-Loss Plan for Men* is all about eating lots of delicious food. Low-fat cooking need never be dull. Low-fat cooking can be sublime.

Vegetables

Q. I hate vegetables. Can I follow *Choose to Lose Weight-Loss Plan for Men* without eating them?

A. No! Vegetables are loaded with vitamins, minerals, and fiber as well as all sorts of anti-cancer fighters we don't even have names for. Vegetables fill you up. They add variety to your life. You *must* eat vegetables. You may *think* you don't like vegetables because you remember your mom's mushy overcooked broccoli. Or perhaps eating vegetables was part of a youthful power struggle that you never resolved. Now that you are *open to new things*, give vegetables a chance. You may and probably will find that you love them. Try steaming fresh vegetables until they are crisp but tender. Try vegetables you haven't eaten before. Bake butternut squash or whip sweet potatoes with orange juice. Be open. If you want to live a long, healthy life, you need to eat vegetables.

High-Fat Taste

Q. Will I ever get over my craving for high-fat foods?

A. It is hard to believe, but you can lose your high-fat taste. Consider the lineman who gave up fast-food restaurants but decided to treat himself to a quarter-pounder for his birthday. He unwrapped the sandwich but found it so greasy he couldn't bring himself to eat it. It takes about 12 weeks to change your tastes. If, however, you are constantly subjecting yourself to high-fat foods or high-fat-tasting nonfat foods, you may never give up the taste for fat.

Portion Control

Q. Your underlying message is to "Eat! Eat! Eat!" Do you really mean it?

A. We want you to "Eat! Eat! Eat!" nutrient-dense, fiber-rich foods so you keep up your metabolism, consume enough vitamins, minerals, and fiber for good health, and are satisfied and not hungry. But we want you to use sense. First, we don't want you to eat empty calories like nonfat cakes, crackers, and cookies. Save these for a splurge, just like a high-fat treat. Second, when a food has some redeeming value but is highly processed, like bagels or pretzels or spaghetti, you need to put on the brakes yourself because these foods don't have enough bulk to be self-limiting. One or two bagels is an okay amount, but more is too much. Two cups of spaghetti, maybe 3, is okay. More is too much. Two large pretzels are enough. More is too much. When you eat a fiber-rich food like potatoes, you don't have to be careful because your body says, "ENOUGH!"

Behavior Modification: Chewing Each Biteful 100 Times

Q. What about all these behavioral modification techniques you hear about to help you eat more slowly? Why doesn't *Choose to Lose Weight-Loss Plan for Men* use them?

A. These slowdown techniques were devised to limit the amount of high-fat food people crammed into their mouths. If you are eating nutrient-dense, fiber-rich, low-fat food, it doesn't matter how fast you eat. Ron and Nancy Goor are speed-eaters, and they are both lean. There is, however, a downside to eating so fast. When your host or hostess has spent an hour preparing a dish and you vacuum it down in 30 seconds, she has a right to feel annoyed.

Young Children

Q. If I feed my young children a low-fat diet, will it stunt their growth?

A. Obesity in children is a growing problem (no pun intended). Children are getting fatter and fatter because of our ultra-high-fat food system and lack of exercise. You will be giving your children a precious gift when you follow *Choose to Lose Weight-Loss Plan for Men* and make significant lifestyle changes that include them.

You can't start early enough. The American Heart Association recommends that all children above the age of 2 years eat a low-fat diet because heart disease begins in childhood. The plaque that clogs your arteries and gives you a heart attack at age 55 started accumulating when you were very young.

Food tastes and habits are developed at a young age. Teach your children to eat healthfully, and you will help ensure that they will have a healthy adulthood.

If you worry that following *Choose to Lose Weight-Loss Plan for Men* will stunt your children's growth — don't. If your children eat a low-fat diet with lots of nutrient-dense, fiber-rich food, they will achieve their growth potential. Our two sons, Alex and Dan, were raised on a low-fat diet and are 6 feet 3 inches and 6 feet 4 inches, respectively. Only Michael Jordan would consider their growth stunted.

Water Quota

Q. You always see people on diets walking around with "big sippers." Why isn't water part of *Choose to Lose Weight-Loss Plan for Men?*

A. Drinking 8 glasses of water is de rigueur for many diets for two reasons. The first is that when you eat a low-calorie, high-protein diet, you need to flush out the excess nitrogen waste from your kidneys to prevent kidney disease and kidney failure.

The second reason is to fill you up because on low-calorie diets you are always starving. We recommend instead that when you are hungry, you eat real food, which provides you with vitamins, minerals, and fiber, rather than take a few unsatisfying sips from your water jug.

In addition, when you eat loads of fruits and vegetables, you are getting lots of water because these foods are mostly water.

Starvation Diets

Q. What's wrong with starvation diets?

A. Most guys think starving is a bad idea because it makes them weak, irritable, and HUNGRY. Would it surprise you to know that eating too few calories also makes you lose muscle and slows down your BMR?

Many diets for men allot a total of about 1500 calories. Let's say your body needs 2500 total calories to provide the energy for your basal metabolism plus your physical activity, but you are eating only 1500 total calories. Unlike the federal government, your body cannot operate on a deficit. To function, your body needs 1000 more calories than the 1500 you are consuming. Where does it find them? The carbohydrate stores are too paltry to consider. The only large stores of energy are fat and protein in the muscle. Which of the two will your body raid?

Wouldn't it be great if those 1000 calories were pulled from your fat stores? No such luck. Your body holds on to fat like a drowning man clings to a life raft. Fat is the stored energy of last resort, saved for times of famine. The energy the body prefers to burn is protein released from the breakdown of your muscle. If you're not exercising (and who would have the energy to exercise on a 1500-calorie diet?), you do not replace the muscle; you just lose it.

So now, on your 1500-calorie diet, not only are you too weak to stand without help, have lost all your friends because you're cranky and mean, and are chewing on chair legs for sustenance, you find that your muscles are withering away too. What's more, those muscles would have helped you burn fat.

Let's say you stick to this low-cal diet for a few weeks. You might even lose weight, but you lose weight because you are losing muscle and muscle has weight. So even though you weigh less, you are actually fatter (i.e., a higher percentage of your weight is fat). And since you are starving, you quickly give up this nonsense and eat. You don't eat a bushel of carrots either. You eat all those high-fat foods you craved while you were dieting. With less muscle to burn fat and a slower BMR, you gain weight and end up heavier and fatter. With most men, this is their first and last attempt to lose weight.

The only permanent and healthy way to lose weight is to lose fat. The only permanent and healthy way to lose fat is to eat low-fat, nutrient-dense, fiber-rich food and exercise.

The Yo-yo Syndrome

Q. How do you get off the yo-yo roller coaster?

A. Yo-yoing refers to the practice of following starvation diets again . . .
and again . . . and again, with the result that each time more muscle
is lost, weight is gained back faster, and the dieter ends up heavier
and fatter, with a slower metabolism and less muscle to protect him
against future weight gain.

For those of you who have been caught up in the Yo-yo Syndrome, don't despair. By following *Choose to Lose Weight-Loss Plan for
Men*, you can reverse the damage inflicted by starvation diets and
lack of exercise. You can rev up your metabolism and lose fat and
weight.

17. *Choose to Lose Weight-Loss Plan* for Life

NOW THE BALL is in your court. You have all the information and the skills needed to make significant lifestyle changes. It's your choice and you can do it. Just remember the three important strategies.

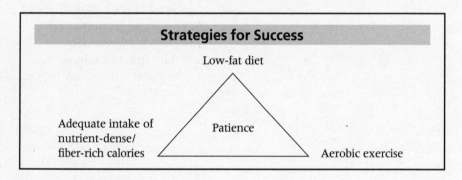

Strategies for Success

Low-fat diet

Adequate intake of nutrient-dense/ fiber-rich calories

Patience

Aerobic exercise

STRATEGIES FOR SUCCESS

1. Eat a Low-Fat Diet

Use your Fat Budget to put all foods in perspective and make wise food choices. Eat under your Fat Budget — it's a ceiling, not a goal — but be sure to include an occasional high-fat favorite so you don't feel deprived. Use the Food Tables and nutrition labels to determine the fat calories in foods so you know exactly what you are eating.

2. Eat Lots of Nutrient-Dense, Fiber-Rich Foods

To be successful for a lifetime, it is of utmost importance that you are not hungry. You must eat lots of food. Of course this recommendation does not include lots of high-fat food or empty calories. Only if you eat enough calories of fruits, vegetables, whole grains, low- or nonfat dairy, and low-fat meats will you consume enough vitamins, minerals, and fiber for long-term health. Eat real, full, delicious meals so you are content and satisfied. *Choose to Lose Weight-Loss Plan for Men* is for the long term.

3. Exercise Aerobically Every Day (Walking Is Fine)

Aerobic exercise builds and preserves muscle and muscle burns fat. Exercise expands your energy needs, so if you are eating a low-fat, nutrient-dense, fiber-rich diet, your body supplies the energy by burning fat from your fat stores, and you lose weight. Aerobic exercise is essential for long-term health. Add strength training and stretching, and you'll be in great condition to live a long and full life.

Keep Track

To help you fulfill these strategies, keep a food record. It is the only way you will truly know if you are eating within your Fat Budget, if you are eating enough calories to maximize your BMR, consume adequate amounts of vitamins, minerals, and fiber, and be full and happy, and if you are meeting the recommendations of the Food Guide Pyramid so you know you are eating a balanced diet.

Forever

Remember: *Choose to Lose Weight-Loss Plan for Men* is not a sometime thing; it is forever. Make your goal to incorporate the three *Choose to Lose Weight-Loss Plan for Men* strategies into your life . . . forever, and you will be a huge success.

PREDICTORS OF SUCCESS

Here is a list of Predictors of Success. Follow them, and you will be a success.

✓ Focus on health, not weight loss.
✓ Focus on body size changes, not scale changes.
✓ Replace high-fat foods with low-fat foods.
✓ Eat enough total calories by eating more fruits, vegetables, whole grains, and low- or nonfat dairy.
✓ Exercise aerobically at least 30 minutes every day.
✓ Eat real, full meals.

✓ Eat within your Fat Budget.
✓ Budget in an occasional high-fat splurge.
✓ Eat out rarely.
✓ Cook or have someone cook for you. Prepare recipes from *Eater's Choice Low-Fat Cookbook* or other low-fat cookbooks.
✓ Have patience!

MEASURING SUCCESS

Fat Loss

How do you measure your success? You probably think that weighing yourself on a scale every day is the best way to see your progress. We recommend that you THROW AWAY YOUR SCALE. Give it to someone you want to drive crazy. *Choose to Lose Weight-Loss Plan for Men* is not about weight loss. It is about fat loss. (Rest assured, if you lose fat, you will lose weight.)

The only weight loss that is meaningful and permanent and has long-term health benefits is fat loss. If you reduce your intake of fat, eat lots of nutritious total calories, and exercise aerobically every day to build and preserve your muscle, you will lose fat. But the scale does not distinguish among water loss,* muscle loss, and fat loss.

In the first few weeks of following *Choose to Lose Weight-Loss Plan for Men*, you will be losing fat and building muscle. This muscle has weight. Actually, muscle is heavier than fat. In the long run added muscle will help you burn fat. In the short run, because the muscle you are building may weigh as much as the fat you are losing, the scale may not show a loss.

A more accurate and positive way to measure your fat-loss progress is to see how you fit into your clothes. Fitting into a smaller pair of pants indicates that you are losing fat and building lean muscle mass, which is just as important as losing pounds. In fact, it is more important, because the greater your muscle mass, the greater your metabolic capacity to burn fat and the more weight you will lose in the future.

Health, Stamina, Energy, Joie de Vivre, Etc.

Choose to Lose Weight-Loss Plan for Men is about fat-loss success, but it is about much more. When you can jump out of bed each morning burst-

---

* It takes 4 grams of water to store 1 gram of carbohydrate. When you follow a low-carbohydrate diet, you reduce your carbohydrate stores, and thus the weight you lose is mostly water. Drink two large glasses of water, and you've gained the weight back.

ing with energy, that's *Choose to Lose Weight-Loss Plan for Men* success. When you walk 3 miles and don't feel tired, that's *Choose to Lose Weight-Loss Plan for Men* success. When you eat a meal and don't suffer heartburn, that's *Choose to Lose Weight-Loss Plan for Men* success. When you see that your cholesterol level and blood pressure levels have plummeted, that's *Choose to Lose Weight-Loss Plan for Men* success. When you are proud to be seen in a bathing suit or shorts, that's *Choose to Lose Weight-Loss Plan for Men* success. When you look forward to seeing your great-grandchildren graduate from college, that's *Choose to Lose Weight-Loss Plan for Men* success.

Choose to Lose Weight-Loss Plan for Men success can be measured in increased stamina, endurance, energy, self-esteem, love of life, and long-term good health. *Choose to Lose Weight-Loss Plan for Men* will make and keep you thin, *and* it will make a tremendous impact on the quality of your life. You just have to do it.

We wish you the best. Good luck!

E-mail (goor@choicediets.com), write (PO Box 2053, Rockville MD 20847–2053), or call (1-888-897-9360) us and tell us how you are doing!

FOOD TABLES

CONTENTS

Can't find a food?
Use the Food Tables Index, pages 391–401.

28 grams = 1 ounce

INTRODUCTION TO THE FOOD TABLES

The Food Tables in *Choose to Lose Weight-Loss Plan for Men* list total calories, fat calories, and saturated-fat calories for thousands of foods. You will find both generic foods, such as vegetables, meat, and fruit, and commercial foods, such as frozen dinners and potato chips.

Although *Choose to Lose Weight-Loss Plan for Men* is all about reducing total fat, we have also listed saturated-fat calories in case you are interested in lowering your blood cholesterol. Saturated fat is the culprit that raises blood cholesterol levels and your risk for heart disease. Although in most cases reducing total fat will automatically reduce saturated fat, there are certain instances where also knowing saturated fat will help you make healthier choices. For example, both olive oil, the most heart-healthy of all the fats, and butter, a highly heart-risky food, are 100 percent fat and fattening. A tablespoon of olive oil, which has 119 total fat calories, has only 16 sat-fat calories. A tablespoon of butter has 100 fat calories but has 65 sat-fat calories. By using the Food Tables, you can quickly see that butter is a poorer choice because it is very saturated.

Because products are constantly changing, always look at nutrition labels for the most up-to-date nutrition information.

For more information on using the Food Tables, read pages 39–44, Chapter 5, "Keeping Track."

BEVERAGES

| | | CALORIES | | |
FOOD	AMOUNT	TOTAL	FAT	SAT-FAT
ALCOHOLIC				
Amaretto di Saronno	1 fl oz	82	0	0
Anisette	1 fl oz	92	0	0
Beer & Ale	12 fl oz	145–165	0	0
Lite	12 fl oz	70–110	0	0
Bourbon	1 fl oz	70	0	0
Brandy	1 fl oz	65	0	0
Bloody Mary	5 fl oz	120	0	0
Brandy Alexander	3 fl oz	254	52	32
Brandy, liqueur, all				
fruit flavors	1 fl oz	88–100	0	0
Champagne	5 fl oz	125	0	0
Cherry Heering	1 fl oz	80	0	0
Crème de banane	1 fl oz	95	0	0
Crème de cacao	1 fl oz	100	0	0
Crème de cassis	1 fl oz	90	0	0
Crème de menthe	1 fl oz	95	0	0
Daiquiri	2 fl oz	120	0	0
banana	3 fl oz	155	2	0
Drambuie	1 fl oz	110	0	0
Eggnog	8 fl oz	340	170	100
Gimlet	2 fl oz	110	0	0
Gin	1 fl oz	75	0	0
Gin and tonic	8 fl oz	195	0	0
Grasshopper	3 fl oz	295	52	32
Irish coffee	8 fl oz	210	99	60
Kahlúa	1 fl oz	105	0	0
Manhattan	4 fl oz	290	0	0
Martini	3 fl oz	225	0	0
Piña colada	6 fl oz	392	105	85
Port	4 fl oz	185	0	0
Rob Roy	3 fl oz	195	0	0

BEVERAGES

FOOD	AMOUNT	CALORIES TOTAL	FAT	SAT-FAT
Rum	1 fl oz	65	0	0
Rye	1 fl oz	70	0	0
Scotch	1 fl oz	70	0	0
Screwdriver	6 fl oz	160	0	0
Sherry				
cream	4 fl oz	185	0	0
dry	4 fl oz	140	0	0
Sloe gin	1 fl oz	180	0	0
Sloe gin fizz	4 fl oz	70	0	0
Stinger	2 fl oz	145	0	0
Tequila	1 fl oz	80	0	0
Tequila sunrise	7 fl oz	220	0	0
Vermouth				
dry	1 fl oz	65	0	0
sweet	1 fl oz	75	0	0
Vodka	1 fl oz	65	0	0
Whiskey	1 fl oz	65–80	0	0
Whiskey sour	1 fl oz	130	0	0
White Russian	3.5 oz	290	26	16
Wine				
red	4 fl oz	85–100	0	0
rosé	4 fl oz	90–130	0	0
white	4 fl oz	85–100	0	0
Mixers				
grenadine	1 fl oz	65	0	0
Snap-E-Tom	6 fl oz	38	0	0
CARBONATED DRINKS				
Club soda	12 fl oz	0	0	0
Cola type	12 fl oz	160	0	0
Ginger ale	12 fl oz	125	0	0
Lemon-lime	12 fl oz	150	0	0
Orange, grape	12 fl oz	180	0	0
COCOA				
Hershey's cocoa	1 tbsp	45	5	0
Hershey's chocolate				
milk mix	3 tbsp	90	0	0
made with whole				
milk	6 fl oz	135	58	34
made with 2% milk	6 fl oz	113	35	20
made with skim milk	6 fl oz	87	5	0
Hershey Hot Cocoa				
Collection				
Chocolate Raspberry	1 env. (35 g)	150	25	5

BEVERAGES

| FOOD | AMOUNT | CALORIES | | |
		TOTAL	FAT	SAT-FAT
Hershey Hot Cocoa Collection (cont.)				
Dutch Chocolate	1 env. (35 g)	150	25	0
Fat-Free	1 env. (25 g)	90	0	0
Good Night Kisses	1 env. (35 g)	150	30	9
Nestlé Carnation				
Double Chocolate				
Meltdown	1 env. (35 g)	150	30	23
Fat-Free	1 env. (8 g)	25	0	0
Rich Chocolate	1 env. (28 g)	120	30	18
Nestlé Quick				
Chocolate	2 tbsp (22 g)	90	5	5
Strawberry	2 tbsp (22 g)	90	0	0
Safeway Hot Cocoa Mix	1 packet (28 g)	110	15	0
Swiss Miss				
Chocolate Sensations	1 env. (34 g)	150	35	14
Cocoa & Cream	1 env. (34 g)	150	45	27
Marshmallow Lovers	1 env. cocoa + 1 env.			
	marshmallow (34 g)	140	25	9
COFFEE (for coffee bar coffees, *see* **RESTAURANT FOODS**)				
Nescafé Cappuccino	1 env. (27 g)	110	20	5
International Coffees (General Foods)				
Cafe Français	8 fl oz prep.	60	30	9
Cafe Vienna	8 fl oz prep.	70	20	5
French Vanilla Cafe	8 fl oz prep.	60	25	5
Italian Cappuccino	8 fl oz prep.	60	15	5
Swiss Mocha	8 fl oz prep.	60	20	5
FRUIT DRINKS				
Noncarbonated				
canned	6 fl oz	85–100	0	0
frozen	6 fl oz	80	0	0
HOT CHOCOLATE				
Without whipped				
cream	8 fl oz	232	122	72
With whipped cream	¼ cup	334	221	133
INSTANT BREAKFAST SHAKES				
Carnation				
Creamy Milk Chocolate	1 env. (37 g)	130	10	5
Creamy Milk Chocolate				
(sugar-free)	1 env. (21 g)	70	10	5
Ovaltine (all types)	4 tbsp (21 g)	80	0	0
Postum	1 tsp (3 g)	10	0	0

BEVERAGES

FOOD	AMOUNT	CALORIES		
		TOTAL	FAT	SAT-FAT
SOYBEAN DRINKS				
Soy Protein Drink	8 fl oz	90	**50**	9
Soy Drink Light	8 fl oz	90	**20**	5
TEA				
Tea	8 fl oz	0	**0**	0

Dairy drinks (milk): *see* **DAIRY AND EGGS;** (milk shakes, etc.), **FAST FOODS.**
Fruit juices: *see* **FRUITS AND FRUIT JUICES.**

DAIRY AND EGGS

FOOD	AMOUNT	CALORIES		
		TOTAL	FAT	SAT-FAT
BUTTER				
Regular	1 pat	36	**36**	23
	1 tbsp	100	**100**	65
	1 stick (½ cup)	813	**813**	515
Whipped	1 tbsp	67	**67**	38
	1 stick (½ cup)	542	**542**	344
light	1 tbsp	35	**30**	25

Margarine and other butter substitutes: *see* **FATS AND OILS.**

FOOD	AMOUNT	CALORIES		
CHEESE				
American	1 oz	106	**80**	50
Blue	1 oz	100	**73**	48
Bonbel (Laughing Cow)	1 oz	70	**50**	36
Brie	1 oz	100	**70**	54
Camembert	1 oz	90	**70**	27
Cheddar	1 oz	114	**85**	54
shredded	¼ cup	110	**80**	54
Colby	1 oz	112	**82**	54
Cottage cheese				
4% fat	½ cup	110	**45**	23
2% fat	½ cup	102	**20**	14
1% fat	½ cup	90	**10**	7
dry curd	½ cup	80	**9**	4
Cream cheese				
regular	1 tbsp	52	**48**	26
with salmon or strawberries	2 tbsp	100	**80**	54
soft	2 tbsp	100	**90**	63
whipped	1 tbsp	37	**34**	19
Edam	1 oz	101	**71**	45

DAIRY AND EGGS

FOOD	AMOUNT	TOTAL	FAT	SAT-FAT
		CALORIES		
Feta	1 oz	75	**54**	38
with basil & tomato	1 oz	80	**60**	36
Farmer				
Friendship	1 oz	40	**27**	18
May-Bud	1 oz	90	**63**	41
Goat cheese (chèvre)	1 oz (1" cube)	80	**50**	41
Gouda	1 oz	101	**70**	45
Gruyère	1 oz	117	**83**	48
Limburger	1 oz	93	**69**	43
Mascarpone	2 tbsp	120	**120**	90
Monterey	1 oz	106	**77**	45
Mozzarella				
whole milk	1 oz	80	**50**	36
fresh, handmade	1 oz	90	**60**	41
shredded	1 oz	90	**65**	42
part skim	1 oz	72	**45**	27
Muenster	1 oz	104	**77**	49
Neufchâtel	1 oz	74	**60**	38
Parmesan	1 tbsp	23	**14**	9
	1 oz	129	**77**	49
Port du Salut	1 oz	100	**72**	43
Provolone	1 oz	100	**68**	44
Ricotta				
whole milk	½ cup	216	**145**	93
part skim	½ cup	171	**88**	55
Romano	1 oz	110	**70**	49
Roquefort	1 oz	105	**78**	49
String	1 oz	80	**50**	36
handmade	1 oz	90	**60**	54
Swiss	1 oz	107	**70**	45
Tilsit	1 oz	96	**66**	43

CHEESE, FAT-FREE

FOOD	AMOUNT	TOTAL	FAT	SAT-FAT
All brands	1 slice (21 g)	25–30	**0**	0
Cream cheese	2 tbsp	30	**0**	0
Mozzarella-type, shredded	¼ cup (28 g)	45	**0**	0

CHEESE, REDUCED-CALORIE OR LITE

FOOD	AMOUNT	TOTAL	FAT	SAT-FAT
Alouette Lite Herbs & Garlic	2 tbsp	60	**35**	27
Bonbel Light Wedge (Laughing Cow)	1 piece (28 g)	50	**30**	18
Cheddar, shredded				
Kraft ⅓ Less Fat	¼ cup (31 g)	90	**50**	36
Sargento	¼ cup (28 g)	70	**40**	18
Cream cheese				
Philadelphia ⅓ Less Fat	2 tbsp (30 g)	70	**60**	36

DAIRY AND EGGS

FOOD	AMOUNT	CALORIES		
		TOTAL	FAT	SAT-FAT
Monterey jack				
Kraft	28 g	80	**45**	27
Dorman's	1 slice (43 g)	120	**60**	41
Mozzarella	¼ cup (28 g)	60	**30**	18
Ricotta	¼ cup (62 g)	75	**35**	18
Rondelé Soft Spreadable Lite	2 tbsp	60	**35**	23
String cheese (Poly-O)	1 piece (28 g)	80	**50**	36
Weight Watchers, all	1 slice (21 g)	50	**20**	0
CHEESE SPREADS				
Alouette				
Garlic & Spices	2 tbsp	70	**60**	41
Spinach	2 tbsp	60	**50**	32
Boursin	2 tbsp	120	**110**	45
Cheez Whiz (Kraft)	2 tbsp (33 g)	100	**70**	45
Rondelé Soft Spreadable				
Black pepper & garden				
vegetable	2 tbsp	90	**80**	54
Garlic & herbs	2 tbsp	100	**80**	54
CREAM				
Half-and-half	1 tbsp	20	**15**	10
Light, coffee or table	1 tbsp	29	**26**	16
	1 cup	469	**417**	260
Nondairy				
frozen				
Rich's Coffee Rich	1 tbsp	25	**15**	0
powdered				
Coffee-Mate	1 tsp	10	**5**	5
	1 env. (3 g)	15	**10**	10
flavored	1⅓ tbsp	60	**25**	23
refrigerated				
Coffee-Mate				
fat-free	1 tbsp	10	**0**	0
Lite	1 tbsp	20	**10**	0
flavored	1 tbsp	40	**20**	0
fat-free	1 tbsp	25	**0**	0
Farm Rich				
fat-free	1 tbsp	10	**0**	0
light	1 tbsp	10	**5**	0
original	1 tbsp	20	**15**	0
International Delight				
all flavors	1 tbsp	35	**10**	0
fat-free	1 tbsp	30	**0**	0
Sour cream	2 tbsp	60	**50**	36
	1 cup	480	**400**	288

DAIRY AND EGGS

| FOOD | AMOUNT | CALORIES | | |
		TOTAL	FAT	SAT-FAT
Sour cream (cont.)				
light	2 tbsp (30 g)	35	**25**	14
no fat	2 tbsp (30 g)	20	**0**	0
Whipping cream				
heavy, fluid	1 cup	821	**792**	493
whipped	½ cup	205	**198**	123
light, fluid	1 cup	699	**665**	416
nondairy (Cool Whip)	2 tbsp (8 g)	25	**15**	14
	½ cup	200	**120**	108
Pressurized topping				
Whipped Light	2 tbsp (10 g)	30	**20**	14
Reddi Whip	2 tbsp (8 g)	20	**15**	9
MILK				
1% fat	1 cup	100	**20**	14
2% fat	1 cup	120	**45**	27
Buttermilk, nonfat	1 cup	80	**0**	0
Chocolate				
2% milk	1 cup	190	**45**	27
whole milk (Nestlé Quick)	1 cup	230	**70**	45
Condensed, sweetened	1 tbsp	62	**15**	9
Evaporated				
skim	1 cup	200	**0**	0
	2 tbsp	25	**0**	0
whole	1 cup	300	**160**	100
	2 tbsp	40	**20**	14
Nonfat				
dry	¼ cup	109	**2**	1
instant	to make 1 qt	326	**6**	4
Skim	1 cup	80	**0**	0
Whole	1 cup	150	**75**	45
dry	¼ cup	159	**77**	48
YOGURT				
Custard-style				
Yoplait custard style				
all flavors	6 oz	190	**30**	18
Yoplait Adventure Pack				
all flavors	4 oz	120	**20**	14
Low-fat yogurt				
Breyers 99% Fat Free				
Black Cherry	8 oz	230	**15**	9
Blueberry	8 oz	220	**15**	9
Peach	8 oz	230	**15**	9
Peaches 'n' Cream	8 oz	240	**15**	9
Raspberry à la Mode	8 oz	220	**15**	9
Strawberry	8 oz	220	**15**	9

DAIRY AND EGGS

| FOOD | AMOUNT | CALORIES | | |
		TOTAL	FAT	SAT-FAT
Low-fat yogurt (cont.)				
Strawberry à la Mode	8 oz	280	25	14
Strawberry Cheese Cake	8 oz	230	20	9
Breyers 99% fat-free Smooth & Creamy				
Black Cherry Parfait	8 oz	230	20	9
Classic Strawberry	8 oz	230	15	9
Raspberries 'n' Cream	8 oz	230	15	9
Strawberry Cheesecake	8 oz	240	15	9
Colombo Low Fat				
all flavors	8 oz	120	40	23
Dannon Low Fat				
Danimals (all flavors)	4.4 oz	140	10	0
Double Delights				
Chocolate Cheesecake	6 oz	220	10	5
all other flavors	6 oz	170	10	5
French Vanilla with fruit	8 oz	270	30	14
Fruit on the bottom,				
all flavors	8 oz	240	25	14
Premium Low-Fat	8 oz	150	35	23
Dannon Sprinkl'ins				
Magic Crystals (vanilla)	4.1 oz	110	10	5
Rainbow Sprinkles	4.1 oz	130	10	5
La Yogurt 99% Fat Free				
all flavors except White				
Chocolate Almond	6 oz	170	15	9
White Chocolate Almond	6 oz	170	25	18
La Yogurt Sabor Latino				
all flavors	6 oz	180	15	9
Safeway Lucerne	8 oz	250	25	14
plain	8 oz	160	35	23
all other flavors	8 oz	250	25	14
Yoplait	6 oz	190	30	18
Trix	4 oz	120	20	14
Yoplait Original 99% Fat-Free	6 oz	180	15	9
Nonfat yogurt				
Breyers Light	8 oz	130	0	0
fruit flavors	8 oz	220	0	0
other flavors	8 oz	170	0	0
Colombo Classic				
vanilla	8 oz	170	0	0
All other flavors	8 oz	200	0	0
Colombo Light				
Key Lime Pie	8 oz	100	0	0
Dannon Light	8 oz	100	0	0
with toppings	8 oz	140	0	0

DAIRY AND EGGS

FOOD	AMOUNT	CALORIES TOTAL	FAT	SAT-FAT
Nonfat yogurt (cont.)				
chunky fruit	6 oz	160	**0**	0
blended (all flavors)	4.4 oz	110	**0**	0
Horizon Organic	6 oz	110	**0**	0
Lucerne Light				
all flavors	6 oz	90	**0**	0
Lucerne Nonfat Pre-Stirred				
all flavors	8 oz	180	**0**	0
SnackWell's				
Double Chocolate	6 oz	190	**0**	0
Milk Chocolate Almond	6 oz	160	**0**	0
Milk Chocolate Cheesecake	6 oz	160	**0**	0
Milk Chocolate				
Peanut Butter	6 oz	180	**0**	0
Stonyfield Farm				
all flavors	8 oz	160	**0**	0
Weight Watchers				
Ultimate 90, all				
flavors	8 oz	90	**0**	0
Yoplait Light, all flavors	6 oz	90	**0**	0
EGG, CHICKEN (*see also* **FROZEN FOODS**)				
Whole, large	1 egg	79	**50**	15
white	1 white	16	**0**	0
yolk	1 yolk	63	**50**	15
EGG, DUCK				
Preserved	1 egg (55 g)	100	**60**	23
EGG SUBSTITUTE				
Egg Beaters (Fleischmann's)	¼ cup (60 g)	30	**0**	0
Healthy Choice Egg Product	¼ cup (56 g)	25	**5**	0
Scramblers (Morningstar Farms)	¼ cup (57 g)	35	**0**	0
Simply Eggs	½ cup (117 g)	80	**20**	9
	3 tbsp (50 g)	35	**10**	0

FAST FOODS

FOOD	AMOUNT	CALORIES TOTAL	FAT	SAT-FAT
ARBY'S				
Bacon platter	1	593	**297**	83
Baked potato, plain	1	355	**0**	0

FAST FOODS

FOOD	AMOUNT	CALORIES		
		TOTAL	FAT	SAT-FAT
Baked potato (cont.)				
Broccoli & Cheddar	1	571	**180**	45
Deluxe	1	736	**324**	144
Margarine & Sour Cream	1	578	**216**	81
Biscuit				
Bacon	1	318	**162**	39
Ham	1	323	**150**	36
Plain	1	280	**135**	30
Sausage	1	460	**288**	85
Blueberry muffin	1	230	**81**	18
Cheesecake	1 serving (87 g)	320	**207**	126
Chicken sandwiches				
Breaded Chicken Fillet	1 (205 g)	536	**252**	45
Chicken Breast	1	445	**207**	27
Chicken Cordon Bleu	1 (240 g)	623	**297**	72
Chicken Fingers	2 pieces (102 g)	290	**144**	18
Grilled Chicken Barbecue	1	388	**117**	27
Grilled Chicken Deluxe	1	430	**180**	36
Roast Chicken Club	1 (241 g)	546	**279**	81
Roast Chicken Deluxe	1	433	**198**	45
Roast Chicken Santa Fe	1 (182 g)	436	**198**	54
Chocolate Chip Cookie	1 (27 g)	125	**54**	18
Cinnamon Nut Danish	1	360	**99**	9
Croissant				
Bacon & egg	1	430	**270**	139
Butter	1	260	**140**	94
Ham & cheese	1	345	**186**	109
Mushroom & cheese	1	495	**340**	137
Plain	1	220	**108**	63
Sausage & egg	1	520	**353**	167
Egg platter	1	460	**216**	65
Fish Fillet Sandwich	1 (220 g)	529	**243**	63
French Toastix	1 serving	430	**189**	45
Fries				
Cheddar Cheddar Curly fries	1 order	333	**162**	36
Curly fries	1 order (100 g)	300	**135**	27
Home-style French fries	1 order (71 g)	246	**119**	27
Ham 'n Cheese Sandwich	1 (169 g)	359	**126**	45
Ham platter	1	518	**234**	72
Light sandwiches				
Roast Beef Deluxe	1 (182 g)	296	**90**	27
Roast Chicken Deluxe	1 (195 g)	276	**54**	18
Roast Turkey Deluxe	1 (195 g)	260	**63**	18
Panini sandwiches				
Roast Beef & Havarti	1 (423 g)	847	**306**	180

FAST FOODS

FOOD	AMOUNT	CALORIES		
		TOTAL	**FAT**	**SAT-FAT**
Panini sandwiches (cont.)				
Roast Chicken & Pesto	1 (388 g)	855	**342**	108
Sicilian Meat & Cheese	1 (361 g)	825	**324**	126
Polar Swirl				
Butterfinger	1 (11.6 oz)	457	**162**	72
Heath	1 (11.6 oz)	543	**198**	45
Oreo	1 (11.6 oz)	482	**198**	90
Peanut Butter Cup	1 (11.6 oz)	517	**216**	72
Snickers	1 (11.6 oz)	511	**170**	63
Potato cakes	2 cakes (85 g)	204	**108**	20
Roast beef sandwiches				
Arby's Melt with Cheddar	1	368	**162**	36
Arby Q	1 (182 g)	431	**162**	54
Bac'n Cheddar Deluxe	1	539	**306**	90
Beef 'n Cheddar	1 (189 g)	487	**252**	81
Giant	1 (228 g)	555	**252**	99
Junior	1	324	**126**	45
Regular	1 (154 g)	388	**171**	63
Special	1 (126 g)	324	**126**	45
Super	1 (247 g)	523	**243**	81
Salads				
Chef salad (no dressing)	1	205	**86**	35
Roast chicken salad (no dressing)	1 (408 g)	149	**18**	5
Garden salad (no dressing)	1	61	**5**	0
Side salad (no dressing)	1 (142 g)	25	**3**	0
Sauces & Dressings				
Arby's Sauce	1 packet (14 g)	15	**2**	0
Bleu Cheese Dressing	1 packet (56 g)	290	**281**	54
Buttermilk Ranch	1 packet	349	**347**	50
Cheddar Cheese Sauce	1 packet (21 g)	35	**27**	9
Honey French Dressing	1 packet (56 g)	280	**207**	27
Horsey Sauce	1 packet (14 g)	60	**45**	9
Italian, light	1 packet	23	**10**	1
Mayonnaise	1 packet (14 g)	110	**108**	63
Red Ranch Dressing	1 packet (14 g)	75	**54**	9
Tartar Sauce	1 tbsp	70	**70**	9
Thousand Island Dressing	1 packet (56 g)	260	**234**	36
Sausage platter	1	640	**370**	120
Shakes				
Chocolate	12 oz	451	**108**	27
Jamocha	12 oz	384	**90**	27
Vanilla	12 oz	360	**108**	36
Vanilla nonfat	455 g	470	**18**	14

FAST FOODS

FOOD	AMOUNT	CALORIES		
		TOTAL	FAT	SAT-FAT
Soups				
Boston Clam Chowder	1 cup	190	81	27
Cream of Broccoli	1 cup	160	72	36
Lumberjack Mixed Vegetable	1 cup	90	36	18
Old-Fashioned Chicken Noodle	1 cup	80	18	0
Potato with Bacon	1 cup	170	63	27
Wisconsin Cheese	1 cup	281	162	63
Sub Roll Sandwiches				
French Dip	1	475	198	72
Hot Ham 'n Swiss	1	500	207	63
Italian	1	675	324	117
Philly Beef 'n Swiss	1	755	423	135
Roast Beef	1	700	378	126
Triple Cheese Melt	1	720	405	144
Turkey	1	550	243	63
Turnover				
Apple	1	330	126	63
Blueberry	1	320	180	57
Cherry	1	320	117	45
ARTHUR TREACHER'S				
Chicken, fried	1 serving	369	198	36
Chicken patties	2 patties (136 g)	369	194	32
Chicken sandwich	1 (156 g)	413	173	27
Chips (French fries)	1 serving	276	117	18
Cod fillet, "Bake 'n Broil"	1 serving (142 g)	245	128	NA
Chowder	1 serving	112	45	18
Cole slaw	1 serving (85 g)	123	74	10
Fish, broiled	5 oz	245	126	NA
Fish, fried	2 pieces (148 g)	355	180	27
Fish sandwich	1 (156 g)	440	216	38
French fries "Chips"	1 serving (114 g)	276	119	21
Hushpuppy "Krunch Pup"	1 piece (57 g)	203	133	33
Krunch Pup (batter-fried hot dog)	1	203	135	36
Lemon Luv (fried pie)	1 serving (85 g)	276	126	20
Shrimp, fried	1 serving (116 g)	381	220	30
BURGER KING				
Big King Sandwich	1 (226 g)	660	390	162
Biscuit				
with Bacon, Egg, & Cheese	1 (171 g)	510	280	90
with Sausage	1 (151 g)	590	360	117
BK Big Fish Sandwich	1 (252 g)	720	387	81
BK Broiler Chicken Sandwich	1 (247 g)	530	230	45
Blueberry mini muffins	1 serving	292	126	27
Breakfast Buddy with sausage, egg, & cheese	1	255	144	54

FAST FOODS

FOOD	AMOUNT	CALORIES		
		TOTAL	FAT	SAT-FAT
Broiled Chicken Salad, no dressing	1 (302 g)	190	**90**	45
Cheeseburger	1 (138 g)	380	**170**	81
Deluxe	1	390	**207**	72
Double	1 (210 g)	600	**320**	153
Bacon	1 (218 g)	640	**350**	162
Bacon deluxe	1	584	**342**	144
Chicken Sandwich	1 (229 g)	710	**390**	81
Chicken Tenders	8 pieces (123 g)	350	**200**	63
Croissan'wich				
Bacon, Egg, & Cheese	1	350	**216**	72
Ham, Egg, & Cheese	1	350	**198**	63
Sausage, Egg, & Cheese	1 (176 g)	600	**410**	144
Danish				
Apple cinnamon	1	390	**117**	27
Cheese	1	406	**144**	45
Dipping Sauces				
Barbecue, honey	1 serving (28 g)	35–90	**0**	0
Ranch	1 serving (28 g)	171	**162**	27
French Fries, Medium	1 serving (116 g)	400	**190**	72
French Toast Sticks	1 serving (141 g)	500	**240**	63
Garden Salad	1 (215 g)	100	**45**	27
Hamburger, regular	1 (126 g)	330	**140**	54
Burger Buddies	1 serving	349	**153**	63
Deluxe	1	344	**171**	54
Double Whopper	1 (351 g)	870	**500**	171
with Cheese	1 (375 g)	960	**570**	216
Whopper	1 (270 g)	640	**350**	99
with Cheese	1 (294 g)	730	**410**	144
Whopper Jr.	1 (164 g)	420	**220**	72
with Cheese	1 (177 g)	460	**250**	90
Hash Browns, small	1 serving (75 g)	240	**140**	54
Ocean Catch fish fillet sandwich	1	479	**297**	72
Onion Rings	1 serving (124 g)	310	**130**	18
Pies				
Dutch Apple	1 serving (113 g)	300	**140**	27
Cherry	1	360	**117**	36
Lemon	1	290	**72**	27
Salads				
Chef	1	178	**81**	36
Chunky chicken	1	142	**36**	9
Side	1 (133 g)	60	**25**	18
Scrambled Egg Platter				
croissant, hash browns	1 serving	549	**306**	81
with bacon	1 serving	610	**351**	99
with sausage	1 serving	768	**477**	135

FAST FOODS

FOOD	AMOUNT	CALORIES		
		TOTAL	FAT	SAT-FAT
Shakes				
Chocolate, medium	284 g	320	**60**	36
with Syrup	341 g	440	**60**	36
Strawberry, medium, with syrup	341 g	420	**50**	36
Vanilla, medium	284 g	300	**50**	36
Speciality Sandwiches				
Chicken	1	688	**360**	72
Ham & Cheese	1	471	**216**	81
Whaler Sandwich	1	488	**243**	54
with cheese	1	530	**270**	72
CARL'S JR.				
Barbecue Chicken Sandwich	1	310	**54**	14
Breakfast Burrito	1	430	**234**	108
Breakfast Quesadilla	1	300	**126**	54
Carl's Catch Fish Sandwich	1	560	**270**	63
Chicken Club Sandwich	1	550	**261**	72
Cheese Danish	1	400	**198**	45
Cheeseburger				
Western Bacon Cheeseburger	1	870	**315**	144
Double	1	970	**513**	243
Cheesecake, Strawberry Swirl	1 piece (3.5 oz)	300	**153**	81
Chicken Stars	6 pieces	230	**126**	27
Chocolate Cake	1 piece (3 oz)	300	**90**	24
Chocolate Chip Cookie	1	370	**171**	72
Cinnamon Rolls	1 order	420	**117**	36
CrissCut Fries, large	1 serving	550	**306**	81
English Muffin with Margarine	1	230	**90**	14
French Fries, regular	1 serving	370	**180**	63
French Toast Dips	1 order	410	**225**	54
Fudge Moussecake	1 piece	400	**207**	99
"Great Stuff" potato				
Bacon & Cheese	1	630	**261**	63
Broccoli & Cheese	1	530	**198**	45
Plain	1	290	**0**	0
Sour Cream & Chive	1	430	**126**	27
Hamburger	1	200	**72**	36
Big Burger	1	470	**180**	72
Famous Big Star	1	610	**342**	99
Super Star	1	820	**477**	180
Hash Brown Nuggets	1 order	270	**153**	36
Hot & Crispy Sandwich	1	400	**198**	45
Hotcakes with margarine	1 serving	510	**216**	45
Muffin				
Blueberry	1	340	**126**	18
Bran	1	370	**117**	18

FAST FOODS

FOOD	AMOUNT	CALORIES		
		TOTAL	FAT	SAT-FAT
Onion Rings	1 order	520	**234**	54
Roast Beef Club Sandwich	1	620	**306**	99
Roast Beef Deluxe Sandwich	1	540	**234**	90
Salad-to-Go				
Charbroiled Chicken	1	260	**81**	45
Garden	1	50	**27**	14
Santa Fe Chicken Sandwich	1	530	**270**	63
Scrambled Eggs	1 order (3.6 oz)	160	**99**	36
Shakes, regular	1	350	**63**	36
Shakes				
Chocolate, small	1 (13.5 oz)	390	**63**	45
Strawberry, small	1 (13.5 oz)	400	**63**	45
Vanilla, small	1 (13.5 oz)	330	**72**	45
Sunrise Sandwich	1	370	**189**	54
Teriyaki Chicken Sandwich	1	330	**54**	18
Turkey Club Sandwich	1	530	**207**	54
Zucchini	1 order	380	**207**	54
CHICK-FIL-A				
Chargrilled Chicken Sandwich	1 (150 g)	280	**30**	9
Chargrilled Chicken Club				
Sandwich	1 (232 g)	390	**110**	45
Cheesecake, plain	1 slice (88 g)	270	**190**	81
with blueberry topping	1 slice (122 g)	350	**173**	NA
with strawberry topping	1 slice (122 g)	343	**173**	NA
Chick-Fil-A-Nuggets				
8-pack	1 serving (110 g)	290	**130**	27
12-pack	1 serving (170 g)	430	**200**	40
Chicken Salad Sandwich	1 (167 g)	320	**40**	18
Chicken Sandwich	1 (167 g)	290	**80**	18
Chick-n-Strips	1 serving (119 g)	230	**70**	18
Cole Slaw	1 serving (79 g)	130	**50**	9
Fudge Nut Brownie	1 (74 g)	350	**140**	27
Grilled 'n Lites	2 skewers	97	**18**	NA
Hearty Breast of Chicken Soup	1 serving (215 g)	110	**10**	0
Icedream	1 (127 g)	140	**35**	9
Lemon Pie	1 slice (99 g)	280	**200**	54
Salads				
Carrot & Raisin	1 (76 g)	150	**20**	0
Chargrilled Chicken Garden	1 (397 g)	170	**30**	9
Chicken Salad Plate	1 (468 g)	290	**40**	0
Chick-n-Strips	1 (451 g)	290	**80**	18
Tossed	1 (130 g)	70	**0**	0
Waffle Potato Fries	1 serving (85 g)	290	**90**	36
CHURCH'S FRIED CHICKEN				
Apple pie	1 (3 oz)	300	**171**	NA

FAST FOODS

FOOD	AMOUNT	CALORIES		
		TOTAL	FAT	SAT-FAT
Biscuits	1	250	**148**	NA
Cajun Rice	1 order (88 g)	130	**63**	NA
Catfish, fried	3 pieces	201	**108**	NA
Chicken breast fillet sandwich	1	608	**306**	NA
Chicken nuggets				
regular	6 pieces	330	**171**	NA
spicy	6 pieces	312	**153**	NA
Cole slaw	1 serving	83	**63**	NA
Corn on the cob	1 ear	190	**49**	NA
with butter oil	1 ear	237	**81**	NA
Dinner roll	1	83	**18**	NA
Fish fillet sandwich	1	430	**162**	NA
French fries, regular	3 oz	256	**117**	NA
Fried chicken				
Breast	1 serving	278	**153**	NA
Leg	1 serving	147	**81**	NA
Thigh	1 serving	305	**198**	NA
Wing	1 serving	303	**180**	NA
Hush puppies	2 pieces	156	**54**	NA
Mashed potatoes & gravy	1 order	90	**30**	NA
Pecan pie	1 serving	367	**180**	NA
DAIRY QUEEN				
Banana Split	1	510	**99**	72
BBQ beef sandwich	1	225	**36**	9
Breaded chicken fillet sandwich	1	430	**180**	36
with Cheese	1	480	**225**	63
Buster Bar	1	460	**261**	81
Butterfinger Blizzard				
regular	1	750	**234**	NA
small	1	520	**162**	NA
Cheese Dog	1	290	**162**	72
Chicken Breast Fillet Sandwich	1	430	**180**	36
with Cheese	1	480	**225**	63
Chicken Strip Basket				
with BBQ Sauce	1 order	810	**333**	81
with Gravy	1 order	860	**378**	99
Chili Dog	1	280	**144**	54
Chili 'n Cheese Dog	1	330	**189**	81
Chocolate Chip Cookie Dough Blizzard				
regular	1	950	**324**	NA
small	1	660	**216**	NA
Chocolate cone				
regular	1	350	**99**	72
small	1	230	**63**	45

FAST FOODS

| FOOD | AMOUNT | CALORIES | | |
		TOTAL	FAT	SAT-FAT
Chocolate cone, Dipped				
regular	1	510	225	140
small	1	340	144	90
Chocolate Dilly Bar	1	210	117	54
Chocolate Mint Dilly Bar	1	190	108	NA
Chocolate Sandwich Cookie Blizzard				
regular	1	640	207	NA
small	1	520	162	NA
Double Delight	1 serving	490	180	NA
DQ Caramel & Nut Bar	1	260	117	NA
DQ Frozen Cake Slice	1	380	162	72
DQ Frozen Heart Cake	1/10 cake	270	81	NA
DQ Frozen Log Cake	1/8 cake	280	81	NA
DQ Frozen 8" Round Cake	1/8 cake	340	108	NA
DQ Frozen 10" Round Cake	1/12 cake	360	108	NA
DQ Frozen Sheet Cake	1/20 cake	350	108	NA
DQ Fudge Bar	1	50	0	0
DQ Homestyle Burgers				
Bacon Double Cheeseburger	1	610	324	162
Cheeseburger	1	340	153	72
Deluxe Double Cheeseburger	1	540	279	144
Deluxe Double Hamburger	1	440	198	90
Double Cheeseburger	1	540	279	144
Hamburger	1	290	108	45
Ultimate Burger	1	670	387	171
DQ Lemon Freez'r	1/2 cup	80	0	0
DQ Nonfat Yogurt	1/2 cup	100	0	0
DQ Sandwich	1	140	36	18
DQ Soft Serve				
Chocolate	1/2 cup	150	45	NA
Vanilla	1/2 cup	140	41	NA
DQ Treatzza Pizza				
Heath	1/8 pizza	180	63	NA
M&M's	1/8 pizza	190	63	NA
Peanut Butter Fudge	1/8 pizza	220	90	NA
Strawberry-Banana	1/8 pizza	180	54	NA
DQ Vanilla Orange Bar	1	60	0	0
Fish Fillet Sandwich	1	370	144	32
with Cheese	1	420	189	54
Float	1	410	63	41
Freeze	1	500	108	72
French fries				
large	1 order	390	162	36
regular	1 order	300	126	27
small	1 order	210	90	18
Garden salad, no dressing	1	200	117	63

FAST FOODS

FOOD	AMOUNT	CALORIES		
		TOTAL	FAT	SAT-FAT
Grilled Chicken Fillet Sandwich	1	310	**90**	23
Heath Blizzard				
regular	1	820	**324**	153
small	1	560	**207**	99
Heath Breeze				
regular	1	680	**189**	54
small	1	450	**108**	27
Hot Fudge Brownie Delight	1	710	**261**	126
Malt				
Chocolate				
regular	1	1060	**225**	NA
small	1	880	**198**	NA
Vanilla				
small	1	610	**126**	72
Mr. Misty Float	1	390	**63**	41
Mr. Misty Freeze	1	500	**108**	70
Mr. Misty Kiss	1	70	**0**	0
Mr. Misty				
regular	1	290	**0**	0
small	1	250	**0**	0
Nutty Double Fudge	1	580	**198**	90
Onion Rings, regular	1 order	240	**108**	23
Parfait	1 serving	430	**72**	47
Peanut Buster	1 serving	730	**288**	90
QC Chocolate Big Scoop	1	250	**126**	90
QC Vanilla Big Scoop	1	250	**126**	90
Reese's Peanut Butter Cup Blizzard				
regular	1	790	**297**	NA
small	1	590	**216**	NA
Shakes				
Chocolate				
regular	1	770	**180**	111
small	1	540	**126**	72
Vanilla				
regular	1	600	**144**	90
small	1	520	**126**	72
Starkiss	1	80	**0**	0
Strawberry Blizzard				
regular	1	570	**144**	99
small	1	400	**100**	72
Strawberry Breeze				
regular	1	460	**9**	5
small	1	320	**5**	0
Strawberry Shortcake	1 order	430	**126**	NA
Strawberry Waffle Cone Sundae	1	350	**108**	45

FAST FOODS

		CALORIES		
FOOD	AMOUNT	TOTAL	FAT	SAT-FAT
Sundae				
Chocolate				
regular	1	410	**90**	58
small	1	300	**63**	45
Toffee Dilly Bar with Heath Pieces	1	210	**108**	NA
Vanilla cone				
child's	1	140	**36**	27
large	1	410	**108**	72
regular	1	350	**90**	63
small	1	230	**60**	45
Yogurt Cup, regular	1	230	**5**	0
Yogurt Strawberry Sundae, regular	1	300	**5**	0
DOMINO'S PIZZA				
Breadsticks	1	78	**30**	6
Buffalo Wings				
Barbeque	1 order (10 pcs)	501	**219**	59
	1 wing	50	**22**	6
Hot	1 order (10 pcs)	449	**215**	59
	1 wing	45	**22**	6
Cheesy Bread	1 piece	103	**49**	17
Deep Dish Pizza				
6" small pizza				
Cheese only	1 serving (215 g)	595	**247**	95
with Anchovies	1 serving	640	**265**	99
with Bacon	1 serving	677	**310**	117
with Beef	1 serving	639	**283**	110
with Cheddar	1 serving	681	**310**	135
with Extra Cheese	1 serving	654	**287**	118
with Ham	1 serving	612	**253**	97
with Italian Sausage	1 serving	639	**309**	108
with Olives	1 serving	605	**256**	96
with Pepperoni	1 serving	645	**288**	111
all other toppings	1 serving	597	**247**	95
12" medium pizza (8 slices)				
Cheese only	2 slices (180 g)	477	**194**	76
with Anchovies	2 slices	500	**203**	78
with Bacon	2 slices	559	**257**	98
with Beef	2 slices	533	**238**	94
with Cheddar	2 slices	534	**236**	103
with Extra Cheese	2 slices	525	**228**	97
with Ham	2 slices	495	**201**	78
with Italian Sausage	2 slices	532	**233**	92
with Olives	2 slices	490	**204**	77
with Pepperoni	2 slices	552	**255**	100
all other toppings	2 slices	479	**194**	76

FAST FOODS

| FOOD | AMOUNT | CALORIES | | |
		TOTAL	FAT	SAT-FAT
Deep Dish Pizza (cont.)				
14" large pizza (12 slices)				
Cheese only	2 slices (173 g)	455	178	70
with Anchovies	2 slices	478	187	72
with Bacon	2 slices	530	219	90
with Beef	2 slices	499	214	85
with Cheddar	2 slices	503	213	92
with Extra Cheese	2 slices	500	210	90
with Ham	2 slices	472	184	72
with Italian Sausage	2 slices	499	209	83
with Olives	2 slices	466	187	71
with Pepperoni	2 slices	521	232	91
all other toppings	2 slices	457	178	70
Hand-Tossed Pizza				
12" medium pizza (8 slices)				
Cheese only	2 slices (149 g)	347	96	47
with Anchovies	2 slices	370	105	49
with Bacon	2 slices	429	159	69
with Beef	2 slices	403	140	65
with Cheddar	2 slices	404	138	74
with Extra Cheese	2 slices	395	130	68
with Ham	2 slices	365	103	49
with Italian Sausage	2 slices	402	135	63
with Olives	2 slices	359	106	49
with Pepperoni	2 slices	422	157	71
all other toppings	2 slices	349	96	47
14" large pizza (12 slices)				
Cheese only	2 slices (137 g)	317	98	43
with Anchovies	2 slices	340	107	45
with Bacon	2 slices	392	139	63
with Beef	2 slices	361	134	58
with Cheddar	2 slices	365	133	65
with Extra Cheese	2 slices	362	130	63
with Ham	2 slices	334	104	45
with Italian Sausage	2 slices	361	129	56
with Olives	2 slices	329	108	44
with Pepperoni	2 slices	383	152	64
all other toppings	2 slices	320	98	43
Thin Crust Pizza				
12" medium pizza (4 slices)				
Cheese only	1 slice (106 g)	271	106	47
with Anchovies	1 slice	294	115	49
with Bacon	1 slice	353	169	69
with Beef	1 slice	327	150	65
with Cheddar	1 slice	328	148	74
with Extra Cheese	1 slice	319	140	68

FAST FOODS

| FOOD | AMOUNT | CALORIES | | |
		TOTAL	FAT	SAT-FAT
Thin Crust Pizza (cont.)				
with Ham	1 slice	289	113	49
with Italian Sausage	1 slice	326	145	63
with Olives	1 slice	283	116	48
with Pepperoni	1 slice	346	167	71
all other toppings	1 slice	273	106	47
14" large pizza (6 slices)				
Cheese only	1 slice (99 g)	253	99	44
with Anchovies	1 slice	276	108	46
with Bacon	1 slice	328	140	64
with Beef	1 slice	297	135	59
with Cheddar	1 slice	301	134	66
with Extra Cheese	1 slice	298	131	64
with Ham	1 slice	270	105	46
with Italian Sausage	1 slice	297	130	57
with Olives	1 slice	264	109	45
with Pepperoni	1 slice	319	153	65
all other toppings	1 slice	255	99	44
DUNKIN' DONUTS				
Cookies				
Chocolate chunk	1	200	90	47
with nuts	1	210	99	45
Oatmeal pecan raisin	1	200	81	38
Croissant	1	310	171	37
Almond	1	420	234	46
Chocolate	1	440	261	94
Donuts				
Apple Crumb	1 (85 g)	250	90	25
Apple filled with cinnamon				
sugar	1 (79 g)	250	99	20
Bavarian filled with chocolate	1	240	99	NA
Blueberry filled	1 (68 g)	210	72	15
Boston Kreme	1 (79 g)	240	99	22
Chocolate Kreme	1 (68 g)	250	126	26
Dunkin'	1 (60 g)	240	126	26
Jelly filled	1 (68 g)	220	81	15
Lemon filled	1 (79 g)	260	108	22
Peanut	1 (105 g)	480	261	49
Sugared Jelly Stick	1 (85 g)	310	108	23
Vanilla Kreme	1 (68 g)	250	108	23
Glazed coffee roll	1 (79 g)	280	108	21
Glazed cruller	1 (68 g)	260	99	20
Glazed French cruller	1 (40 g)	140	72	16
Rings				
Buttermilk cake	1 (99 g)	410	180	55

FAST FOODS

FOOD	AMOUNT	CALORIES		
		TOTAL	FAT	SAT-FAT
Rings (cont.)				
Cake, plain	1 (57 g)	262	162	33
Chocolate coconut	1 (96 g)	420	216	72
Chocolate-frosted cake	1 (65 g)	280	144	31
Chocolate-frosted yeast	1 (54 g)	200	90	17
Cinnamon cake	1 (62 g)	260	135	29
Coconut-coated cake	1 (88 g)	360	189	68
Glazed buttermilk	1 (74 g)	290	126	29
Glazed chocolate	1 (77 g)	320	162	21
Glazed whole-wheat ring	1 (71 g)	280	135	28
Glazed yeast ring	1 (54 g)	200	81	18
Powdered cake	1 (62 g)	270	144	30
Sugared cake	1 (60 g)	270	162	34
Vanilla-frosted yeast	1 (57 g)	200	81	16
Mini Doughnuts				
Cake	1 (31 g)	100	54	11
Chocolate glazed	1 (31 g)	122	63	12
Cinnamon cake	1 (26 g)	116	63	14
Coconut	1 (34 g)	140	72	27
Coffee roll	1 (23 g)	78	27	6
Eclair	1 (37 g)	114	45	10
Muffins				
Apple 'n spice	1 (96 g)	300	72	15
Banana nut	1 (94 g)	310	90	18
Blueberry	1 (102 g)	280	72	14
Bran with raisins	1 (105 g)	310	81	11
Corn	1 (96 g)	340	108	15
Cranberry nut	1 (96 g)	290	81	16
Oat bran	1 (96 g)	330	99	14
Muffins, lowfat				
Apple 'n spice	1 (99 g)	220	14	0
Banana	1 (99 g)	240	14	0
Blueberry	1 (99 g)	220	14	0
Cherry	1 (99 g)	230	14	0
Cranberry-orange	1 (99 g)	230	14	0
Munchkins				
Butternut cake	1 (17 g)	70	27	9
Coconut cake	1 (17 g)	70	36	14
Glazed cake	1 (17 g)	60	27	5
Glazed chocolate	1 (20 g)	70	27	6
Glazed yeast	1 (14 g)	50	18	4
Jelly-filled yeast	1 (14 g)	50	18	4
Plain cake	1 (14 g)	50	27	5
Powdered cake	1 (14 g)	50	27	5

HARDEE'S

FOOD	AMOUNT	CALORIES		
Apple turnover	1	270	108	36

FAST FOODS

		CALORIES		
FOOD	AMOUNT	TOTAL	FAT	SAT-FAT
Bagel				
Bacon	1	280	81	34
Bacon & egg	1	330	108	41
Bacon, egg, & cheese	1	375	144	68
Egg	1	250	54	24
Egg & cheese	1	295	90	NA
Plain	1	200	27	5
Sausage	1	350	144	59
Sausage & egg	1	400	171	68
Sausage, egg, & cheese	1	445	207	86
Big Cookie	1	280	108	36
Big Country Breakfast				
Bacon	1	820	441	117
Country ham	1	670	342	81
Ham	1	620	297	63
Sausage	1	1000	594	180
Big Twin	1	450	225	99
Biscuit	1	257	112	29
Bacon	1	360	189	36
Bacon & egg	1	570	297	81
Bacon, egg, & cheese	1	610	333	99
Canadian Rise 'n Shine	1	570	288	99
Cheese	1	304	142	NA
Chicken	1	510	225	63
Cinnamon 'n Raisin	1	370	162	45
Country ham	1	430	198	54
Country ham & egg	1	400	198	36
Ham	1	400	180	54
Ham & egg	1	370	171	36
Ham, egg & cheese	1	540	270	90
Jelly	1	440	189	NA
'n Gravy	1	510	252	81
Rise 'n Shine	1	390	189	54
Sausage	1	510	279	90
Sausage & egg	1	630	360	99
Steak	1	580	288	90
Steak & egg	1	550	288	72
Ultimate omelet	1	570	297	99
Breadstick	1	150	36	0
Cheeseburger	1	310	126	63
Cravin' Bacon	1	690	414	144
Quarter-pound Double	1	470	243	126
Mesquite Bacon	1	370	162	NA
Mushroom 'n Swiss	1	520	243	117
The Boss	1	570	297	NA
Chicken Fillet Sandwich	1	480	162	36

FAST FOODS

FOOD	AMOUNT	CALORIES		
		TOTAL	FAT	SAT-FAT
Coleslaw	114 g (4 oz)	240	180	27
Combo sub	1	380	54	27
Cool Twist cone	1	180	18	9
Cool Twist sundae				
hot fudge	1	290	54	27
strawberry	1	210	18	9
Fisherman's Fillet Sandwich	1	560	243	63
French fries				
Crispy Curls	1 order	300	144	27
large	1 order	430	162	45
medium	1 order	350	135	36
small	1 order	240	90	27
Fried chicken				
Breast	1	370	135	36
Chicken Stix	6 pieces	210	81	18
Leg	1	170	63	18
Thigh	1	330	135	36
Wing	1	200	72	18
Frisco Breakfast Ham Sandwich	1	500	225	72
Frisco Chicken Sandwich	1	680	369	90
Frisco Club Sandwich	1	670	378	108
Grilled Chicken Breast Sandwich	1	350	99	18
Hamburger	1	270	99	45
Big Deluxe	1	530	270	117
Frisco Burger	1	760	450	162
The Works Burger	1	530	270	NA
Ham Sub	1	370	63	36
Hash Rounds, regular	1 order	230	126	27
Hot dog	1	290	144	36
Hot Ham 'n Cheese Sandwich	1	350	117	54
Marinated Chicken Grill	1	340	90	18
Mashed potatoes	114 g (4 oz)	70	9	5
Muffin				
Blueberry	1	400	153	36
Oatbran raisin	1	410	144	27
Pancakes, 3, plain	1 order	280	18	9
with 2 strips of bacon	1 order	350	81	27
with 1 sausage patty	1 order	430	144	54
Roast Beef Sandwich				
big	1	460	216	81
regular	1	320	144	54
Roast Beef Sub	1	370	45	27
Salads				
Chef salad	1	200	117	72
Garden, no dressing	1	220	117	63
Grilled chicken, no dressing	1	150	27	9

FAST FOODS

FOOD	AMOUNT	CALORIES		
		TOTAL	FAT	SAT-FAT
Salads (cont.)				
Potato salad	1 small	260	**171**	27
Side, no dressing	1	25	**9**	5
Shrimp 'n Pasta Salad	1 serving	362	**261**	NA
Shakes				
Chocolate	1	370	**45**	27
Peach	1	390	**36**	27
Strawberry	1	420	**36**	27
Vanilla	1	350	**45**	27
Turkey Club Sandwich	1	390	**144**	36
Turkey sub	1	390	**63**	36
JACK IN THE BOX				
Apple turnover	1	350	**171**	36
Bacon & Cheddar Potato Wedges	1 order	800	**522**	144
Breakfast Jack	1	280	**108**	45
Cheeseburger	1	320	**135**	54
Bacon bacon	1	710	**405**	135
Double	1	450	**216**	108
Ultimate	1	1030	**711**	234
Cheesecake	1 piece	310	**162**	81
Chocolate Chip Cookie Dough	1 piece	360	**162**	72
Chicken and mushroom sandwich	1	438	**162**	45
Chicken Caesar Sandwich	1	490	**234**	54
Chicken Fajita Pita	1	280	**81**	27
Chicken Sandwich	1	400	**162**	36
Chicken strips	4 pieces	290	**117**	27
Chicken Supreme Sandwich	1	620	**324**	99
Chicken Teriyaki Bowl	1	670	**36**	9
Chicken wings	6 pieces	846	**396**	96
Country Fried Steak Sandwich	1	450	**225**	63
Crescent				
Sausage	1	670	**432**	171
Supreme	1	570	**324**	135
Curly fries	1 order	360	**180**	45
Dipping sauces				
Buttermilk House	1 oz	130	**117**	45
Tartar	1 oz	150	**135**	9
all others	1 oz	40	**0**	0
Double fudge cake	1 piece	288	**81**	20
Egg rolls	3 pieces	440	**216**	63
Fish Supreme Sandwich	1	590	**306**	54
French fries				
jumbo	1 order	400	**171**	45
regular	1 order	350	**153**	36
small	1 order	220	**99**	23
super scoop	1 order	590	**261**	63

FAST FOODS

| FOOD | AMOUNT | CALORIES | | |
		TOTAL	FAT	SAT-FAT
Grilled Chicken Fillet Sandwich	1	430	171	45
Guacamole	28 g (1 oz)	50	36	5
Hamburger	1	276	108	37
Colossus	1	1100	756	252
Grilled Sourdough burger	1	670	387	144
Ham & Swiss burger	1	638	351	NA
Jumbo Jack	1	590	324	99
with Cheese	1	680	396	144
Mushroom burger	1	477	243	NA
Outlaw burger	1	720	360	153
Quarter-pound burger	1	510	243	90
Sourdough Jack	1	690	414	144
Swiss & bacon burger	1	643	387	NA
Hash browns	1 order	170	108	27
Jumbo Jack	1	584	306	99
with Cheese	1	677	360	126
Milk shakes				
Chocolate, regular	1	390	54	32
Strawberry, regular	1	330	63	36
Vanilla, regular	1	350	63	36
Mini chimichangas	4 pieces	571	252	77
Moby Jack	1	444	225	NA
Old-fashioned Patty Melt	1	713	414	133
Monterey Roast Beef Sandwich	1	540	270	81
Onion rings	1 order	380	207	54
Pancake platter	1	400	108	27
Really Big Chicken Sandwich	1	900	504	126
Salad				
Chef salad	1	325	162	76
Garden chicken	1	200	81	36
Pasta seafood salad	1 serving	394	198	NA
Side	1	70	36	23
Taco salad	1	503	279	121
Scrambled egg				
platter	1	560	288	78
pocket	1	430	189	72
Shakes				
Chocolate	1	330	63	39
Oreo Cookie Ice Cream	1	740	324	NA
Strawberry	1	320	63	39
Vanilla	1	320	54	32
Sirloin Steak Sandwich	1	517	207	45
Sourdough Breakfast Sandwich	1	380	180	63
Spicy Crispy Chicken Sandwich	1	560	243	45
Stuffed Jalapeños				
7 pieces	1 order	530	279	117
10 pieces	1 order	750	396	162

FAST FOODS

| FOOD | AMOUNT | CALORIES | | |
		TOTAL	FAT	SAT-FAT
Supreme nachos	1 serving	718	360	NA
Taco				
regular	1	190	99	36
super	1	280	153	54
Toasted raviolis	7 pieces	537	252	72
Tortilla chips	1 serving	139	54	NA
Ultimate Breakfast Sandwich	1	620	315	99
KFC (KENTUCKY FRIED CHICKEN)				
BBQ baked beans	1 serving (156 g)	190	25	9
Biscuit	1 (56 g)	180	80	23
Chicken Little Sandwich	1	169	90	18
Chunky Chicken Pot Pie	1 (368 g)	770	378	117
Coleslaw	1 serving (142 g)	142	80	14
Corn on the cob	1 serving (162 g)	150	15	0
Cornbread	1 (56 g)	228	117	18
Green beans	1 serving (132 g)	45	15	5
Hot Wings	6 pcs (135 g)	471	297	72
Kentucky Fried Chicken				
Colonel's Rotisserie Gold Chicken				
Quarter-breast & wing	1 serving (176 g)	335	168	49
without skin & wing	1 serving (116 g)	199	53	15
Quarter-thigh & leg	1 serving (145 g)	333	213	59
without skin	1 serving (116 g)	217	110	32
Crispy Strips				
Colonel's	3 (92 g)	261	142	33
Spicy Buffalo	3 (120 g)	350	170	36
Extra Tasty Crispy Chicken				
Breast	1 (168 g)	470	250	63
Drumstick	1 (67 g)	190	100	27
Thigh	1 (118 g)	370	220	54
Whole Wing	1 (55 g)	200	120	36
Hot & Spicy Chicken				
Breast	1 (180 g)	530	310	72
Drumstick	1 (64 g)	190	100	27
Thigh	1 (107 g)	370	240	63
Whole Wing	1 (55 g)	210	130	36
Original Recipe Chicken				
Breast	1 (153 g)	400	220	54
Drumstick	1 (61 g)	140	80	18
Thigh	1 (91 g)	250	160	41
Whole Wing	1 (47 g)	140	90	23
Tender Roast Chicken				
Breast with skin	1 (139 g)	251	97	27
without skin	1 (118 g)	169	39	11
Drumstick with skin	1 (55 g)	97	39	11
without skin	1 (38 g)	67	22	6

FAST FOODS

FOOD	AMOUNT	CALORIES		
		TOTAL	FAT	SAT-FAT
Kentucky Fried Chicken (cont.)				
Thigh with skin	1 (90 g)	207	126	34
without skin	1 (59 g)	106	50	15
Whole Wing with skin	1 (50 g)	121	69	19
Kentucky Nuggets	6 pieces	284	162	54
Macaroni & cheese	1 serving (153 g)	180	70	27
Mashed potatoes with gravy	1 serving (136 g)	120	50	9
Mean Greens	1 serving (152 g)	70	30	9
Original Recipe Chicken Sandwich	1 (206 g)	497	201	43
Potato Salad	1 serving (160 g)	230	130	18
Potato Wedges	1 serving (135 g)	180	70	36
Value BBQ Flavored Chicken Sandwich	1 (149 g)	256	74	9
LONG JOHN SILVER'S				
Baked Chicken with light herb	1 order	120	36	11
dinner	1 order	550	135	29
Baked Fish with lemon crumb	1 order (3 pcs)	150	9	5
dinner	1 order	570	108	19
Baked shrimp	1 order	120	45	NA
Batter-dipped chicken	1 piece (57 g)	120	50	14
Batter-dipped chicken sandwich, no sauce	1 piece	280	72	19
Batter-dipped clams	85 g	300	150	36
Batter-dipped fish sandwich, no sauce	1 piece (153 g)	320	120	32
Batter-dipped fish	1 piece (84 g)	170	100	24
Batter-dipped shrimp	1 piece (11 g)	35	20	5
Battered-fried shrimp	1 piece	47	27	6
dinner	1 serving	711	405	NA
Breaded clams	1 order	526	279	46
Breaded oyster	1 piece	60	27	NA
Breaded shrimp	1 order	388	207	21
platter	1 order	962	513	NA
Cheese sticks	45 g	160	80	36
Chicken nuggets dinner	6 pieces	699	405	NA
Chicken Planks	2 pieces	240	108	29
with fries	2 pieces	490	234	51
with fries, coleslaw, 2 hush puppies	3 pieces	890	396	86
for kids, incl. fries and hush puppy	2 pieces	560	261	57
Chocolate chip cookie	1	230	81	51
Chowders				
Clam	1 serving (6.6 oz)	128	45	16
Seafood chowder	1 cup	140	54	18
Seafood gumbo	1 cup	120	72	19

FAST FOODS

		CALORIES		
FOOD	**AMOUNT**	**TOTAL**	**FAT**	**SAT-FAT**
Clams with fries, coleslaw, 2 hush				
puppies	1 dinner	980	**468**	99
Coleslaw	1 order (96 g)	140	**60**	9
Combination entrees, with fries, slaw, 2 hush puppies				
1 fish + 2 chicken	1 order	950	**441**	99
2 fish + 8 shrimp	1 order	1140	**585**	127
2 fish + 5 shrimp + 1 chicken	1 order	1160	**585**	128
2 fish + 4 shrimp + clams (3 oz)	1 order	1240	**630**	137
Corn cobbette	1 piece (111 g)	140	**70**	14
Crispy fish	1 piece	150	**72**	20
with fries, coleslaw, and 2 hush				
puppies	3 pieces	980	**450**	102
Fish				
for kids, incl. fries and hush				
puppy	1 piece	500	**252**	52
Fish and chicken				
for kids, incl. fries and hush				
puppy	1 piece each	620	**306**	67
with fries	1 piece each	550	**288**	61
Fish & Fryes				
2 pieces fish	1 order	651	**324**	72
3 pieces fish	1 order	853	**432**	91
Fish & More, with fries, coleslaw,				
& 2 hush puppies	2 pieces	890	**432**	91
Fish dinner, fried, 3-piece	1 order	1180	**630**	NA
Fish sandwich, homestyle	1 order	510	**198**	44
Flavorbaked chicken	74 g	110	**30**	9
with rice, green beans, and				
baked potato	1 piece	448	**68**	NA
with rice and side salad	1 piece	275	**63**	NA
Flavorbaked chicken sandwich	1 (165 g)	290	**90**	18
Flavorbaked fish	1 piece (65 g)	90	**25**	9
with rice, green beans, and				
baked potato	2 pieces	518	**86**	NA
with rice and side salad	2 pieces	345	**81**	NA
Flavorbaked fish and chicken combo				
with rice, baked potato, and				
green beans	1 piece each	538	**90**	NA
Flavorbaked fish sandwich	1 (170 g)	320	**120**	63
Fries	1 order (85 g)	250	**130**	23
Green beans	1 order (99 g)	30	**5**	0
Hush puppy	1 piece (23 g)	60	**20**	0
Oatmeal raisin cookie	1	160	**90**	18
Ocean Chef Salad	1	110	**9**	4
Oyster dinner	1 order	789	**405**	NA

FAST FOODS

FOOD	AMOUNT	CALORIES		
		TOTAL	FAT	SAT-FAT
Pies				
Apple	1 piece	320	117	41
Cherry	1 piece	360	117	40
Lemon	1 piece	340	81	27
Pineapple cream cheese cake	1 piece (991 g)	310	162	81
Popcorn				
chicken	94 g	250	120	32
fish	102 g	290	130	36
shrimp	94 g	280	130	36
Regular chicken classic wrap	1 (312 g)	730	320	63
Rice pilaf	1 order (85 g)	140	25	9
Salads, no dressing				
Garden	1	45	0	0
Grilled chicken	1	140	20	5
Ocean chef	1	130	20	0
Side	1	25	0	0
Scallop dinner	1 order	747	405	NA
Saltines crackers	2	25	9	NA
Seafood platter	1 order	976	522	NA
Seafood salad	1	380	279	46
Shrimp with fries, coleslaw, & 2				
hush puppies	10 pieces	840	423	87
Tartar sauce	1	50	45	9
Ultimate fish sandwich	1 (182 g)	430	190	63
Walnut brownie	1	440	198	49
MCDONALD'S				
Apple Bran Muffin, lowfat	1	300	30	5
Arch Deluxe	1	550	280	99
with bacon	1	590	310	108
Bacon, Egg, & Cheese Biscuit	1	470	250	72
Baked apple pie	1	260	120	32
Big Mac	1	560	280	90
Biscuit	1	290	130	27
Breakfast Burrito	1 order	320	180	63
Cheeseburger	1	320	120	54
Chicken McNuggets				
4 pieces	1 order	190	100	23
6 pieces	1 order	290	150	32
9 pieces	1 order	430	230	45
Cinnamon roll	1	400	180	45
Cookies				
Chocolate chip	1	170	90	54
McDonaldland	1 pkg	180	45	9
Crispy Chicken Deluxe	1	500	220	36

FAST FOODS

FOOD	AMOUNT	CALORIES		
		TOTAL	FAT	SAT-FAT
Danish				
Apple	1	360	140	45
Cheese	1	410	200	72
Cinnamon raisin	1	430	198	63
Iced cheese	1	390	198	54
Raspberry	1	400	144	45
Egg McMuffin	1 order	290	110	41
English muffin	1 order	140	20	0
Fish Fillet Deluxe	1	560	250	54
Fries				
small	1 order	210	90	14
large	1 order	450	200	36
super size	1 order	540	230	41
Grilled Chicken Deluxe	1	440	180	27
Hamburger	1	130	70	14
Hash browns	1 order	144	81	26
Hotcakes	1 order	310	60	14
with syrup and 2 pats of				
margarine	1 order	510	140	27
McChicken	1	490	261	45
McD.L.T.	1 order	680	396	133
McLean Deluxe	1	340	108	41
with cheese	1	400	144	63
Quarter Pounder	1	420	190	72
with cheese	1	530	270	117
Salads & dressings				
Caesar dressing	1 pkg	160	130	27
Croutons	1 pkg	50	10	0
Fat-free herb vinaigrette	1 pkg	50	0	0
Garden salad	1	35	0	0
Grilled Chicken Salad Deluxe	1	120	10	0
Ranch dressing	1 pkg	230	180	27
Red French Reduced Calorie	1 pkg	160	70	9
Sauces				
Barbeque, Sweet 'n Sour, Honey	1 pkg	45–50	0	0
Honey mustard	1 pkg	50	40	5
Hot mustard	1 pkg	60	30	0
Light mayonnaise	1 pkg	40	35	5
Sausage	1	170	150	45
Sausage Biscuit	1	470	280	81
with egg	1	550	330	90
Sausage McMuffin	1	360	210	72
with egg	1	440	260	90
Scrambled eggs	2	160	110	32
Shakes				
Chocolate	1 small	360	80	54

FAST FOODS

FOOD	AMOUNT	CALORIES		
		TOTAL	**FAT**	**SAT-FAT**
Shakes (cont.)				
Strawberry	1 small	360	**80**	54
Vanilla	1 small	360	**80**	54
Soft serve and cone	1 serving	189	**45**	20
Sundae & toppings				
Hot caramel	1	360	**90**	54
Hot fudge	1	340	**90**	54
Strawberry	1	290	**70**	45
nuts	1 serving	40	**30**	0
Vanilla reduced-fat ice cream cone	1	150	**40**	27
PIZZA HUT				
Bigfoot pizza				
Cheese	2 slices	372	**108**	54
Pepperoni	2 slices	410	**126**	54
Pepperoni, mushroom, & Italian sausage	2 slices	428	**144**	72
Hand-tossed pizza, medium				
Beef	2 slices	520	**162**	72
Cheese	2 slices	470	**126**	72
Ham	2 slices	426	**90**	54
Italian sausage	2 slices	534	**198**	90
Meat Lovers	2 slices	628	**198**	108
Pepperoni	2 slices	476	**144**	72
Pepperoni Lovers	2 slices	612	**252**	108
Pork topping	2 slices	536	**180**	90
Super Supreme	2 slices	592	**234**	90
Supreme	2 slices	568	**216**	90
Veggie Lovers	2 slices	432	**108**	54
Pan pizza, medium				
Beef	2 slices	572	**234**	90
Cheese	2 slices	522	**198**	90
Ham	2 slices	478	**162**	54
Italian sausage	2 slices	586	**270**	90
Meat Lovers	2 slices	680	**324**	126
Pepperoni	2 slices	530	**216**	72
Pepperoni Lovers	2 slices	664	**306**	126
Pork topping	2 slices	588	**252**	90
Super Supreme	2 slices	646	**306**	108
Supreme	2 slices	622	**270**	108
Veggie Lovers	2 slices	486	**180**	54
Personal pan pizza				
Pepperoni	1 pizza	637	**252**	90
Supreme	1 pizza	722	**306**	108
Thin 'n Crispy pizza, medium				
Beef	2 slices	458	**198**	90
Cheese	2 slices	410	**144**	72

FAST FOODS

FOOD	AMOUNT	CALORIES TOTAL	FAT	SAT-FAT
Thin 'n Crispy pizza, medium (cont.)				
Ham	2 slices	368	126	54
Italian sausage	2 slices	472	216	90
Meat Lovers	2 slices	576	234	108
Pepperoni	2 slices	430	180	72
Pepperoni Lovers	2 slices	578	288	126
Pork topping	2 slices	474	216	90
Super Supreme	2 slices	540	252	108
Supreme	2 slices	514	234	90
Veggie Lovers	2 slices	372	126	54
POPEYE'S CHICKEN				
Apple pie	1 slice	290	144	NA
Biscuit	1	250	135	NA
Cajun rice	111 g	150	50	NA
Cole slaw	114 g	149	100	NA
Corn on the cob	1	127	27	NA
French fries	1 order	240	108	NA
Fried chicken				
Breast, mild or spicy	1 (105 g)	270	144	NA
Leg, mild or spicy	1 (48 g)	120	66	NA
Tender, mild or spicy	1 (34 g)	110	63	NA
Thigh, mild or spicy	1 (88 g)	300	204	NA
Wing, mild or spicy	1 (45 g)	160	96	NA
Fried shrimp	1 order (79 g)	250	148	NA
Nuggets	1 order	410	288	NA
Onion rings	1 order	310	174	NA
Potatoes & gravy	108 g	100	54	NA
Red beans & rice	167 g	270	153	NA
ROY ROGERS				
Baked beans	1 order (142 g)	160	18	9
Baked potato	1 (110 g)	130	9	0
with margarine	1 (124 g)	240	117	18
Big Breakfast Platter with ham	1 (267 g)	710	351	99
Big Country Breakfast Platter				
with bacon	1 (217 g)	740	387	117
with sausage	1 (274 g)	920	540	171
Biscuit	1 (83 g)	390	189	54
Bacon & egg	1 (121 g)	470	234	72
Bacon	1 (89 g)	420	207	63
Cinnamon 'n raisin	1 (80 g)	370	162	45
Ham & cheese	1 (127 g)	450	216	72
Ham, egg, & cheese	1 (159 g)	500	243	90
Sausage & egg	1 (149 g)	560	315	99
Sausage	1 (118 g)	510	279	90
Biscuits 'n Gravy	1 order (221 g)	510	252	81

FAST FOODS

FOOD	AMOUNT	CALORIES		
		TOTAL	FAT	SAT-FAT
Cheeseburger	1 (140 g)	393	**198**	108
¼ lb cheeseburger	1 (149 g)	480	**261**	153
Bacon	1 (156 g)	520	**297**	162
Cheesesteak Sandwich	1 (216 g)	580	**324**	126
Chicken soup	1 order (302 g)	225	**63**	18
Chili	1 order (288 g)	295	**135**	63
Coleslaw	1 order (142 g)	295	**225**	36
Fish Sandwich	1 (186 g)	490	**189**	45
French fries				
large	1 order (173 g)	430	**162**	45
regular	1 order (142 g)	350	**135**	36
Fried chicken				
Breast	1 piece (148 g)	370	**135**	36
Leg	1 piece (69 g)	170	**63**	18
Thigh	1 piece (121 g)	330	**135**	36
Wing	1 piece (66 g)	200	**72**	18
Gold Rush Chicken Sandwich	1 (190 g)	558	**270**	81
Grilled Chicken Sandwich	1 (213 g)	294	**72**	27
Gravy	43 g	20	**5**	5
Hamburger	1 (126 g)	343	**162**	81
¼ lb burger	1 (135 g)	412	**225**	126
Mashed potatoes	1 order (142 g)	92	**5**	5
Nuggets	6 pieces (113 g)	290	**162**	36
Roast beef sandwich	1 (192 g)	329	**90**	27
¼ Roy Roaster				
Dark meat, with skin	1 piece (144 g)	490	**306**	90
without skin	1 piece (111 g)	190	**90**	27
White meat, with skin	1 piece (175 g)	500	**261**	81
without skin	1 piece (134 g)	190	**54**	18
Salads				
Garden	1 (278 g)	110	**45**	27
Grilled Chicken	1 (378 g)	221	**81**	36
Side	1 (140 g)	20	**5**	5
Sourdough ham, egg, & cheese	1 (193 g)	480	**216**	81
Strawberry shortcake	1 order (171 g)	440	**171**	45
Sundaes				
Hot fudge	1 (168 g)	320	**90**	45
Strawberry	1 (158 g)	260	**54**	27
3 pancakes	1 order (137 g)	280	**18**	9
with 1 sausage	1 order (176 g)	430	**144**	54
with 2 bacon	1 order (151 g)	350	**81**	27
Vanilla frozen yogurt cone	1 (118 g)	180	**36**	27

SUBWAY
Cookies

Brazil nut & chocolate chips	1	230	**108**	NA
Chocolate chip	1	210	**90**	NA

FAST FOODS

		CALORIES		
FOOD	AMOUNT	TOTAL	FAT	SAT-FAT
Cookies (cont.)				
Chocolate chip/M&M	1	210	**90**	NA
Chocolate chunk	1	210	**90**	NA
Oatmeal raisin	1	200	**72**	NA
Peanut butter	1	220	**108**	NA
Sugar	1	230	**108**	NA
White chip macadamia nut	1	230	**108**	NA
6-inch cold sandwiches (include meat/poultry/seafood, onions, lettuce, tomatoes, pickles, green peppers, olives)				
BLT				
wheat bread	198 g	327	**95**	27
white bread	191 g	311	**93**	27
Classic Italian BMT				
wheat bread	253 g	460	**194**	63
white bread	246 g	445	**193**	72
Cold-Cut Trio				
wheat bread	253 g	378	**118**	36
white bread	246 g	362	**116**	36
Ham				
wheat bread	239 g	302	**48**	9
white bread	232 g	287	**47**	9
Roast beef				
wheat bread	239 g	303	**42**	9
white bread	232 g	288	**41**	9
Spicy Italian				
wheat bread	239 g	482	**222**	81
white bread	232 g	467	**220**	81
Subway Club				
wheat bread	253 g	312	**45**	9
white bread	246 g	297	**43**	9
Subway Seafood & Crab				
wheat bread	253 g	430	**174**	27
made with light mayo	253 g	347	**89**	18
white bread	246 g	415	**172**	27
made with light mayo	246 g	332	**88**	18
Tuna				
wheat bread	253 g	542	**291**	45
made with light mayo	253 g	391	**135**	18
white bread	246 g	527	**289**	45
made with light mayo	246 g	376	**134**	18
Turkey breast				
wheat bread	239 g	289	**36**	9
white bread	232 g	273	**34**	9
Turkey breast & ham				
wheat bread	239 g	295	**42**	9
white bread	232 g	280	**41**	9

FAST FOODS

FOOD	AMOUNT	CALORIES		
		TOTAL	FAT	SAT-FAT
6-inch cold sandwiches (cont.)				
Veggie Delite				
wheat bread	182 g	237	**25**	0
white bread	175 g	222	**24**	0
6-inch hot sandwiches (include meat/poultry/seafood, onions, lettuce, tomatoes, pickles, green peppers, olives)				
Chicken taco sub (values include cheese)				
wheat bread	293 g	436	**144**	45
white bread	286 g	421	**143**	45
Meatball				
wheat bread	267 g	419	**145**	54
white bread	260 g	404	**144**	54
Pizza sub (values incl. cheese)				
wheat bread	257 g	383	**196**	81
white bread	250 g	448	**194**	81
Roasted chicken breast				
wheat bread	253 g	348	**54**	9
white bread	246 g	332	**52**	9
Steak & cheese (values incl. cheese)				
wheat bread	264 g	398	**88**	54
white bread	257 g	383	**86**	54
Subway Melt (values incl. cheese)				
wheat bread	258 g	382	**107**	45
white bread	251 g	366	**106**	45
Deli Style Sandwiches (include deli roll, meat/poultry/seafood, onions, lettuce, tomatoes, pickles, green peppers, olives)				
Bologna	171 g	292	**104**	36
Ham	171 g	234	**40**	9
Roast beef	180 g	245	**40**	9
Tuna	178 g	354	**161**	27
made with light mayo	178 g	279	**84**	18
Turkey breast	180 g	235	**35**	9
Optional fixin's for sandwiches				
bacon	2 slices (8 g)	45	**36**	9
cheese	2 triangles (11 g)	41	**27**	18
light mayo	1 tsp (5 g)	18	**18**	0
mayo	1 tsp (5 g)	37	**36**	9
oil	1 tsp (5 g)	45	**45**	9
Breads				
Deli style roll	62 g	185	**26**	9
6" wheat bread	77 g	215	**22**	0
12" wheat bread	154 g	430	**45**	9
6" white bread	70 g	200	**21**	0
12" white bread	140 g	400	**42**	9
Salads (values do not include salad dressing)				
BLT	276 g	140	**76**	27

FAST FOODS

		CALORIES		
FOOD	AMOUNT	TOTAL	FAT	SAT-FAT
Salads without salad dressing (cont.)				
Chicken taco (includes cheese)	370 g	250	**126**	45
Classic Italian BLT	331 g	274	**176**	63
Cold-Cut Trio	330 g	191	**100**	27
Ham	316 g	116	**30**	9
Meatball	345 g	233	**127**	45
Pizza (includes cheese)	335 g	277	**177**	72
Roast beef	316 g	117	**24**	9
Roasted chicken breast	331 g	162	**35**	9
Steak & cheese (includes cheese)	342 g	212	**69**	45
Subway Club	331 g	126	**26**	9
Subway Melt	336 g	195	**89**	36
Subway Seafood & Crab	331 g	244	**155**	27
made with light mayo	331 g	161	**71**	9
Tuna	331 g	356	**272**	45
made with light mayo	331 g	205	**117**	18
Turkey breast	316 g	102	**17**	9
Turkey breast & ham	316 g	109	**24**	9
Veggie Delite	260 g	51	**7**	0
TACO BELL				
Border Wraps				
Chicken Fajita Wrap	1 order (227 g)	470	**200**	54
Chicken Fajita Wrap Supreme	1 order (255 g)	520	**230**	72
Steak Fajita Wrap	1 order (227 g)	470	**190**	54
Steak Fajita Wrap Supreme	1 order (255 g)	510	**220**	72
Veggie Fajita Wrap	1 order (227 g)	420	**170**	45
Veggie Fajita Wrap Supreme	1 order (255 g)	470	**200**	63
Breakfast				
Breakfast Cheese Quesadilla	1 order (156 g)	380	**190**	81
Breakfast Quesadilla with Bacon	1 order (170 g)	450	**240**	99
Breakfast Quesadilla with				
Sausage	1 order (170 g)	430	**230**	90
Country Breakfast Burrito	1 order (114 g)	270	**130**	45
Double Bacon & Egg Burrito	1 order (177 g)	480	**250**	81
Fiesta Breakfast Burrito	1 order (99 g)	280	**140**	54
Grande Breakfast Burrito	1 order (177 g)	420	**200**	63
Hash Brown Nuggets	1 order (99 g)	280	**160**	45
Burrito				
7-Layer Burrito	1 order (284 g)	530	**200**	63
Bacon Cheeseburger Burrito	1 order (241 g)	570	**280**	108
Bean Burrito	1 order (199 g)	380	**110**	36
Big Beef Burrito Supreme	1 order (298 g)	520	**210**	90
Big Chicken Burrito Supreme	1 order (255 g)	510	**210**	63
Burrito Supreme	1 order (255 g)	440	**170**	72
Chicken Club Burrito	1 order (227 g)	540	**290**	90

FAST FOODS

| FOOD | AMOUNT | CALORIES | | |
		TOTAL	FAT	SAT-FAT
Burrito (cont.)				
Chili Cheese Burrito	1 order (142 g)	330	120	54
Grilled Chicken Burrito	1 order (199 g)	410	140	41
Nachos and Sides				
Big Beef Nachos Supreme	1 order (199 g)	450	220	72
Choco Taco Ice Cream Dessert	1 order (114 g)	310	150	90
Cinnamon Twists	1 order (28 g)	140	50	0
Mexican rice	1 order (135 g)	190	80	32
Nachos	1 order (99 g)	320	170	36
Nachos BellGrande	1 order (312 g)	770	360	99
Pintos 'n Cheese	1 order (128 g)	190	80	36
Sauces and Condiments				
Burger Sauce	14 g	60	45	9
Cheddar cheese	7 g	30	20	14
Club Sauce	14 g	80	70	9
Fajita Sauce	14 g	70	60	9
Guacamole	21 g	35	30	0
Nacho Cheese Sauce	57 g	120	90	23
Sour cream	21 g	40	35	23
Three-Cheese Blend	7 g	25	15	9
all other sauces are fat-free				
Specialties				
Big Beef MexiMelt	1 order (135 g)	290	140	63
Cheese Quesadilla	1 order (121 g)	350	160	81
Chicken Quesadilla	1 order (170 g)	410	190	90
Mexican Pizza	1 order (220 g)	570	320	90
Taco Salad with Salsa	1 order (539 g)	850	470	135
without shell	1 order (468 g)	420	200	99
Tostada	1 order (177 g)	300	130	45
Taco	1 order (78 g)	180	90	36
BLT Soft Taco	1 order (128 g)	340	210	72
Double Decker Taco	1 order (163 g)	340	130	45
Double Decker Taco Supreme	1 order (199 g)	390	170	72
Grilled Chicken Soft Taco	1 order (128 g)	240	110	32
Grilled Steak Soft Taco	1 order (128 g)	230	90	23
Grilled Steak Soft Taco Supreme	1 order (163 g)	290	130	45
Soft Taco	1 order (99 g)	220	90	41
Soft Taco Supreme	1 order (142 g)	260	120	63
Taco Supreme	1 order (114 g)	220	120	63
WENDY'S				
Baked potato, plain	1 (284 g)	284	0	0
Bacon & cheese	1 (380 g)	530	160	36
Broccoli & cheese	1 (411 g)	470	130	23
Cheese	1 (383 g)	570	210	72
Chili & cheese	1 (439 g)	630	220	81

FAST FOODS

| FOOD | AMOUNT | CALORIES | | |
		TOTAL	FAT	SAT-FAT
Baked potato (cont.)				
Sour cream & chives	1 (314 g)	380	60	36
Sour cream	1 pkt (28 g)	60	50	32
Whipped margarine	1 pkt (14 g)	60	60	14
Big Bacon Classic sandwich	1 (282 g)	580	270	108
Breaded chicken	1 fillet (99 g)	230	100	23
Sandwich	1 (208 g)	440	160	32
Chicken club sandwich	1 (216 g)	470	180	36
Cheeseburger				
Double	1	590	297	128
Jr. cheeseburger	1 (130 g)	320	120	54
Bacon	1 (166 g)	380	170	63
Deluxe	1 (180 g)	360	150	54
Kid's meal	1 (123 g)	320	120	54
Chicken nuggets				
5 piece	75 g	210	130	27
4 piece, kid's	60 g	170	100	23
Barbeque sauce	1 pkt (28 g)	45	0	0
Honey mustard	1 pkt (28 g)	130	100	18
Spicy Buffalo Wing sauce	1 pkt (28 g)	25	10	0
Sweet & sour sauce	1 pkt (28 g)	50	0	0
Chili				
large	1 (340 g)	310	60	23
small	1 (227 g)	210	54	18
cheddar cheese, shredded	2 tbsp (17 g)	70	50	32
Saltine crackers	2 (6 g)	25	5	0
Chocolate chip cookie	1 (57 g)	270	110	54
Chow mein noodles	¼ cup	74	36	5
Cole slaw	½ cup	90	72	18
Country fried steak sandwich	1	460	234	63
Fish sandwich	1	460	225	42
French fries				
biggie	1 order (159 g)	470	200	32
medium	1 order (130 g)	390	170	27
small	1 order (91 g)	270	120	18
Frosty dairy dessert				
large	1 (369 g)	540	120	81
medium	1 (298 g)	440	100	63
small	1 (227 g)	330	80	45
Fruit-flavored drink	12 fl oz	110	0	0
Grilled chicken	1 fillet (82 g)	110	25	9
sandwich	1 (189 g)	310	70	14
Hamburger	1 (133 g)	360	150	54
with everything	1 (219 g)	420	180	63
Double	1	520	243	96

FAST FOODS

FOOD	AMOUNT	CALORIES		
		TOTAL	FAT	SAT-FAT
Hamburger (cont.)				
Jr. hamburger	1 (118 g)	270	90	32
Kid's meal	1 (111 g)	270	90	32
Hot chocolate	6 fl oz (170 g)	80	25	0
Pitas				
Chicken Caesar	1 (237 g)	490	160	45
Classic Greek	1 (234 g)	440	180	72
Garden ranch chicken	1 (283 g)	480	160	36
Garden veggie	1 (257 g)	400	150	32
Pita dressings				
Caesar vinaigrette	1 tbsp (17 g)	70	60	9
Garden ranch	1 tbsp (16 g)	50	40	9
Salads, without dressing				
Caesar side salad	1 (89 g)	100	35	14
Deluxe garden	1 (270 g)	110	50	9
Grilled chicken Caesar	1 (262 g)	260	80	27
Grilled chicken salad	1 (338 g)	200	70	14
Side salad	1 (262 g)	60	25	0
Taco salad	1 (468 g)	468	380	90
Salad dressings (2 tbsp = 1 ladle)				
Blue cheese	2 tbsp (28 g)	180	170	32
French	2 tbsp (28 g)	120	90	14
fat-free	2 tbsp (28 g)	35	0	0
Italian Caesar	2 tbsp (28 g)	150	140	23
reduced fat, reduced calorie	2 tbsp (28 g)	40	30	0
Hidden Valley ranch	2 tbsp (28 g)	100	90	14
reduced fat	2 tbsp (28 g)	60	50	9
Salad oil	1 tbsp (14 g)	120	120	18
Thousand Island	2 tbsp (28 g)	90	80	14
Wine vinegar	1 tbsp (14 g)	0	0	0
Soft breadstick	1 (44 g)	130	30	5
Spicy chicken	1 fillet (104 g)	210	80	14
sandwich	1 (213 g)	410	130	23
Sunflower seeds and raisins	2 tbsp	140	90	67
Taco chips	15 (42 g)	210	100	14
Turkey ham	¼ cup	35	18	4
WHITE CASTLE				
Breakfast sandwich	1	340	220	NA
Cheese sticks	1 order	290	150	NA
Cheeseburger	1	160	85	NA
bacon	1	200	115	NA
double	1	285	165	NA
Chicken rings	1 order	310	190	NA
Chicken sandwich	1	190	70	NA
Chocolate shake	1	220	60	NA

FAST FOODS

| FOOD | AMOUNT | CALORIES | | |
		TOTAL	FAT	SAT-FAT
Fish sandwich	1	160	60	NA
French fries	1 order	115	50	NA
Hamburger	1	135	65	NA
double	1	235	125	NA
Onion chips	1 order	180	80	NA

FATS AND OILS

| FOOD | AMOUNT | CALORIES | | |
		TOTAL	FAT	SAT-FAT
ANIMAL FATS				
Beef tallow	1 tbsp	116	116	58
Butter				
regular	1 pat	36	36	23
	1 tbsp	100	100	65
	1 stick	813	813	515
whipped	1 tsp	23	23	12
	1 tbsp	67	67	38
Chicken fat	1 tbsp	115	115	34
Duck fat	1 tbsp	115	115	39
Goose fat	1 tbsp	115	115	32
Lard (pork)	1 tbsp	116	116	45
Mutton tallow	1 tbsp	116	116	55
Turkey fat	1 tbsp	115	115	34
BUTTER SUBSTITUTES				
Butter Buds Sprinkles	1 tsp (2 g)	8	0	0
Molly McButter	1 tsp (2 g)	5	0	0
MARGARINES				
Stick				
Brummel & Brown	1 tbsp (14 g)	90	90	18
Fleischmann's	1 tbsp (14 g)	90	90	14
Lower Fat	1 tbsp (14 g)	50	50	9
I Can't Believe It's Not Butter	1 tbsp (14 g)	90	90	18
Imperial	1 tbsp (14 g)	90	90	18
Land O Lakes	1 tbsp (14 g)	100	100	18
Country Morning Blend	1 tbsp (14 g)	100	100	23
Light	1 tbsp (14 g)	50	50	27
Blue Bonnet	1 tbsp (14 g)	70	70	14
Parkay	1 tbsp (14 g)	90	90	14
Promise	1 tbsp (14 g)	90	90	23
Shedd's Spread Country Crock				
Churn Style	1 tbsp (14 g)	80	80	18
Spreadable Stick	1 tbsp (14 g)	80	80	14

FATS AND OILS

| FOOD | AMOUNT | CALORIES | | |
		TOTAL	FAT	SAT-FAT
Squeeze				
I Can't Believe It's Not Butter	1 tbsp (14 g)	80	**80**	14
Parkay	1 tbsp (14 g)	70	**70**	14
Tub				
Brummel & Brown	1 tbsp (14g)	50	**50**	9
Fleischmann's				
Soft spread	1 tbsp (14 g)	80	**80**	14
Lower Fat	1 tbsp (14 g)	40	**40**	0
I Can't Believe It's Not Butter	1 tbsp (14 g)	90	**90**	18
Light	1 tbsp (14 g)	50	**45**	9
Land O Lakes	1 tbsp (14 g)	100	**100**	18
Spread with sweet cream	1 tbsp (10 g)	80	**80**	18
Parkay				
Soft	1 tbsp (14 g)	90	**90**	18
Spread	1 tbsp (14 g)	60	**60**	14
Promise	1 tbsp (14 g)	80	**80**	18
Buttery Light	1 tbsp (14 g)	50	**50**	9
Ultra 70% less fat	1 tbsp (14 g)	30	**30**	0
Ultra Fat-Free	1 tbsp (14 g)	5	**0**	0
Shedd's Spread Country Crock	1 tbsp (14 g)	60	**60**	14
Light	1 tbsp (14 g)	50	**50**	9
Churn Style	1 tbsp (14 g)	60	**60**	14
Smart Beat, Super Light	1 tbsp (14 g)	20	**20**	0
OILS				
Canola	1 tbsp	120	**120**	9
Cocoa butter	1 tbsp	120	**120**	73
Coconut	1 tbsp	120	**120**	106
Corn	1 tbsp	120	**120**	15
Cottonseed	1 tbsp	120	**120**	32
Olive	1 tbsp	119	**119**	16
Palm	1 tbsp	120	**120**	60
Palm kernel	1 tbsp	120	**120**	100
Peanut	1 tbsp	119	**119**	21
Safflower	1 tbsp	120	**120**	11
Sesame	1 tbsp	120	**120**	17
Soybean	1 tbsp	120	**120**	18
Sunflower	1 tbsp	120	**120**	13
Walnut	1 tbsp	120	**120**	11
SALAD DRESSINGS & SPREADS				
Balsamic & Basil Vinaigrette				
Ken's	2 tbsp	110	**110**	14
Balsamic Vinaigrette				
Newman's Own	2 tbsp	90	**80**	9
Blue cheese				
Chunky (Hellmann's)	2 tbsp	140	**130**	27
Chunky (Ken's)	2 tbsp	140	**140**	27

FATS AND OILS

| FOOD | AMOUNT | CALORIES | | |
		TOTAL	FAT	SAT-FAT
Blue cheese (cont.)				
Chunky (Wish-Bone)	2 tbsp	170	150	23
Chunky, Fat-Free (Wish-Bone)	2 tbsp	35	0	0
Free (Kraft)	2 tbsp	45	0	0
Regular (Kraft)	2 tbsp	130	120	23
Safeway Select	2 tbsp	150	140	18
Burgundy Basil Vinaigrette				
(Ken's)	2 tbsp	70	45	0
Caesar				
Classic (Kraft)	2 tbsp	110	90	18
Classic (Wish-Bone)	2 tbsp	110	90	18
Creamy (Hellmann's)	2 tbsp	170	160	27
Fat-Free (Hidden Valley)	2 tbsp	30	0	0
Free Classic (Kraft)	2 tbsp	45	0	0
Gourmet Caesar (Good Seasons)	2 tbsp prepared	150	140	0
Italian Free (Kraft)	2 tbsp	25	0	0
Lite (Ken's)	2 tbsp	70	60	5
Regular (Hellmann's)	2 tbsp	100	80	9
Regular (Ken's)	2 tbsp	170	160	23
Roasted Garlic (Safeway Select)	2 tbsp	150	130	14
California				
Safeway	2 tbsp	110	80	9
Catalina				
⅓ less fat (Kraft)	2 tbsp	80	40	5
Free (Kraft)	2 tbsp	35	0	0
Regular (Kraft)	2 tbsp	130	100	14
Coleslaw Dressing				
Hidden Valley	2 tbsp	150	140	14
Kraft	2 tbsp	150	110	14
Creamy Roasted Garlic				
Fat-Free (Wish-Bone)	2 tbsp	40	0	0
French				
Country, Lite (Ken's)	2 tbsp	90	50	0
Creamy (Kraft)	2 tbsp	160	140	23
Deluxe (Wish-Bone)	2 tbsp	120	100	14
Fat-Free	2 tbsp	30	0	0
Fat-Free (Hellmann's)	2 tbsp	45	0	0
Free (Kraft)	2 tbsp	45	0	0
Honey & Bacon (Hidden Valley)	2 tbsp	150	110	5
Garlic & Herb (Good Seasons)	2 tbsp prepared	140	140	0
Honey Dijon				
Fat-Free (Ken's)	2 tbsp	40	0	0
Free (Kraft)	2 tbsp	45	0	0
Light (Hidden Valley)	2 tbsp	35	0	0
Regular (Kraft)	2 tbsp	140	120	23

FATS AND OILS

FOOD	AMOUNT	CALORIES		
		TOTAL	**FAT**	**SAT-FAT**
Honey Mustard				
Lite (Ken's)	2 tbsp	70	**40**	0
Italian				
Creamy (Ken's)	2 tbsp	80	**60**	5
Creamy (Wish-Bone)	2 tbsp	110	**90**	14
Fat-Free (Ken's)	2 tbsp	10	**0**	0
Fat-Free (Wish-Bone)	2 tbsp	10	**0**	0
Free (Kraft)	2 tbsp	20	**0**	0
Herb & Cheese, Fat-Free				
(Hidden Valley)	2 tbsp	30	**0**	0
Light (Newman's Own)	2 tbsp	45	**35**	0
Lite (Wish-Bone)	2 tbsp	15	**5**	0
Parmesan & Herb (Safeway				
Select)	2 tbsp	140	**130**	14
Regular (Good Seasons)	2 tbsp prepared	140	**140**	0
Regular (Kraft)	2 tbsp	120	**110**	14
Regular (Safeway)	2 tbsp	90	**70**	9
Regular (Wish-Bone)	2 tbsp	80	**70**	9
Zesty Italian (Good Seasons)	2 tbsp prepared	140	**140**	0
Zesty Italian (Kraft)	2 tbsp	110	**100**	9
Mayonnaise				
Hellman's				
Regular	1 tbsp (15 g)	100	**100**	14
Low-Fat	1 tbsp (15 g)	25	**10**	0
Kraft				
Regular	1 tbsp	100	**100**	18
Free	1 tbsp (15 g)	10	**0**	0
Light	1 tbsp (15 g)	50	**45**	9
Mayonnaise substitute				
Miracle Whip (Kraft)				
Regular	1 tbsp	70	**60**	9
Light	1 tbsp	35	**25**	0
Free	1 tbsp	15	**0**	0
Nacho Cheese Ranch (Hidden				
Valley)	2 tbsp	130	**120**	NA
Olive Oil & Vinegar				
Newman's Own	2 tbsp	150	**150**	23
Olive Oil Vinaigrette				
Ken's	2 tbsp	60	**50**	5
Oriental				
Wish-Bone	2 tbsp	70	**45**	5
Oriental Sesame (Good Seasons)	2 tbsp prepared	150	**140**	NA
Parmesan, Creamy				
Low-Fat (Hidden Valley)	2 tbsp	30	**0**	0
Romano (Kraft)	2 tbsp	170	**160**	14
Peppercorn Free (Kraft)	2 tbsp	50	**0**	0

FATS AND OILS

| FOOD | AMOUNT | CALORIES | | |
		TOTAL	FAT	SAT-FAT
Pizza Ranch (Hidden Valley)	2 tbsp	140	130	NA
Potato Salad Dressing (Marzetti)	2 tbsp	150	130	23
Ranch				
⅓ less fat (Kraft)	2 tbsp	110	100	14
Caesar (Kraft)	2 tbsp	110	90	18
Cucumber (Kraft)	2 tbsp	140	130	18
Cucumber Ranch (Kraft)	2 tbsp	60	45	9
Fat-Free (Wish-Bone)	2 tbsp	40	0	0
Garlic! (Hidden Valley)	2 tbsp	130	120	14
Light (Hidden Valley)	2 tbsp	80	60	5
Light (Ken's)	2 tbsp	100	90	5
Original (Hidden Valley)	2 tbsp	140	130	23
Original with Bacon, fat-free (Hidden Valley)	2 tbsp	50	0	0
Original, fat-free (Hidden Valley)	2 tbsp	30	0	0
Peppercorn Free (Kraft)	2 tbsp	45	0	0
Regular (Kraft)	2 tbsp	170	170	27
Regular (Wish-Bone)	2 tbsp	160	150	23
Safeway	2 tbsp	140	140	9
Super Creamy (Hidden Valley)	2 tbsp	140	130	23
Raspberry				
Safeway Select	2 tbsp	130	100	9
Raspberry Walnut Vinaigrette, Lite (Ken's)	2 tbsp	80	50	0
Red Wine Vinaigrette				
Regular (Wish-Bone)	2 tbsp	90	45	5
Fat-Free (Wish-Bone)	2 tbsp	35	0	0
Red Wine & Herb				
Fat-Free (Hidden Valley)	2 tbsp	45	0	0
Russian				
Wish-Bone	2 tbsp	110	50	9
Salsa Zesty Garden (Kraft)	2 tbsp	70	60	NA
Sandwich Spread (Kraft)	1 tbsp	50	35	5
Reduced fat	1 tbsp	35	25	0
Slaw Dressing (Marzetti)	2 tbsp	170	140	23
Fat-Free	2 tbsp	45	0	0
Sun-Dried Tomato & Spices (Safeway Select)	2 tbsp	130	90	9
Sun-Dried Tomato Vinaigrette, Fat-Free (Ken's)	2 tbsp	60	0	0
Tangy Tomato Bacon (Kraft)	2 tbsp	130	100	9
Taco Ranch (Hidden Valley)	2 tbsp	130	120	NA
Thousand Island				
Fat-Free (Wish-Bone)	2 tbsp	35	0	0
Free (Kraft)	2 tbsp	40	0	0

FATS AND OILS

FOOD	AMOUNT	CALORIES		
		TOTAL	FAT	SAT-FAT
Thousand Island (cont.)				
Regular (Kraft)	2 tbsp	110	**90**	14
Safeway	2 tbsp	120	**100**	14
SHORTENINGS				
Crisco	1 tbsp	110	**110**	27
Flair	1 tbsp	100	**100**	45

FISH AND SHELLFISH

Unless otherwise noted, fish is baked, steamed, or broiled with *no added fat.* If fish is baked in butter or margarine and you are keeping track of total fat, for each teaspoon of butter or margarine you use, add 33 total calories to the total calories listed for each fish and 33 fat calories to the fat calories listed for each fish. If you are keeping track of saturated fat, for each teaspoon of butter you use, add 33 total calories to the total calories listed for each fish and 22 sat-fat calories to the sat-fat calories listed for each fish. For margarine, add 33 total calories to the total calories listed for each fish and 18 sat-fat calories to the sat-fat calories listed for each fish. *See also* **FROZEN, MICROWAVE AND REFRIGERATED FOODS, FAST FOODS,** and **RESTAURANT FOODS.**

*Remember that most of the following calorie figures are for **only 1 ounce** of seafood!*

FOOD	AMOUNT	CALORIES		
		TOTAL	FAT	SAT-FAT
Abalone				
raw	1 oz	30	**2**	0
cooked, fried	1 oz	54	**17**	4
Anchovy				
raw	1 oz	37	**12**	3
canned in oil, drained	5 anchovies (20 g)	42	**17**	4
	1 oz	60	**25**	6
Bass				
Freshwater, raw	1 oz	32	**9**	2
	1 fillet (79 g)	90	**26**	6
Striped, raw	1 oz	27	**6**	1
	1 fillet (159 g)	154	**33**	7
Bluefish				
raw	1 oz	35	**11**	2
	1 fillet (150 g)	186	**57**	12
Burbot, raw	1 oz	25	**2**	0
	1 fillet (116 g)	104	**8**	2
Butterfish, raw	1 oz	41	**20**	9
	1 fillet (32 g)	47	**23**	10

FISH AND SHELLFISH

		CALORIES		
FOOD	AMOUNT	TOTAL	FAT	SAT-FAT
Carp				
raw	1 oz	36	14	3
	1 fillet (218 g)	276	110	21
cooked, dry heat	1 oz	46	18	4
Catfish, channel				
breaded and fried	1 oz	65	34	8
	1 fillet (87 g)	199	104	26
raw	1 oz	33	11	3
	1 fillet (79 g)	92	30	7
Caviar, black and red	1 tbsp	40	26	15
	1 oz	71	45	27
Cisco (lake herring)				
raw	1 oz	28	5	1
	1 fillet (79 g)	78	14	3
smoked	1 oz	50	30	4
Clams				
raw, cherrystones or littlenecks	9 large or 20 small (180 g)	133	16	1
	1 oz	22	3	0
breaded and fried	1 oz	57	28	7
	20 small clams (188 g)	379	189	45
canned, drained solids	1 oz	42	5	0
	½ cup	118	14	1
cooked, moist heat	1 oz	42	5	0
	20 small clams (90 g)	133	16	2
fritters	1 fritter	124	54	NA
Cod, Atlantic				
raw	1 oz	23	2	0
	1 fillet (231 g)	190	14	3
baked	1 oz	30	2	0
	1 fillet (180 g)	189	14	3
canned	1 oz	30	2	1
dried and salted	1 oz	81	6	0
Cod, Pacific, raw	1 oz	23	2	0
	1 fillet (116 g)	95	7	1
Crab				
Alaska King, steamed	1 oz	27	4	0
	1 leg (172 g)	129	18	2
Alaska King, imitation, made from surimi	1 oz	29	3	1
Blue				
raw	1 oz	25	3	0
	1 crab (21 g)	18	2	0
cooked, moist heat	1 oz	27	4	1

FISH AND SHELLFISH

		CALORIES		
FOOD	AMOUNT	TOTAL	FAT	SAT-FAT
Crab (cont.)				
canned	1 oz	28	3	0
	½ cup	67	7	2
Crab cakes	1 cake	93	41	8
	1 oz	44	19	4
Chesapeake Bay Deluxe Crab				
Cakes, frozen	1 oz	65	41	NA
Dungeness, raw	1 oz	24	2	0
Nutri Sea Crab Sticks	1 oz	29	3	NA
Nutri Sea King Crab	1 oz	31	3	NA
Sea Legs Crabmeat Salad Style	1 oz	27	3	NA
Crayfish				
raw	1 oz	25	3	0
	8 crayfish (27 g)	24	2	0
steamed	1 oz	32	3	0
Croaker, Atlantic				
raw	1 oz	30	8	3
	1 fillet (79 g)	83	22	8
breaded and fried	1 oz	63	32	9
	1 fillet (87 g)	192	99	27
Cusk, raw	1 oz	25	2	0
Cuttlefish, raw	1 oz	22	2	0
Dolphinfish, raw	1 oz	24	2	0
	1 fillet (204 g)	174	13	3
Drum, freshwater, raw	1 oz	34	13	3
	1 fillet (198 g)	236	88	20
Eel				
raw	1 oz	52	30	6
baked	1 oz	67	38	8
	1 fillet (159 g)	375	214	43
Flatfish (flounder or sole)				
raw	1 oz	26	3	1
	1 fillet (163 g)	149	17	4
baked or steamed	1 oz	33	4	1
	1 fillet (127 g)	148	17	4
Gefilte fish	1 piece	35	7	2
	1 oz	24	4	1
Grouper				
raw	1 oz	26	3	1
	1 fillet (259 g)	238	24	5
baked or steamed	1 oz	33	3	1
	1 fillet (202 g)	238	24	5
Haddock				
raw	1 oz	25	2	0
	1 fillet (193 g)	168	12	2

FISH AND SHELLFISH

		CALORIES		
FOOD	**AMOUNT**	**TOTAL**	**FAT**	**SAT-FAT**
Haddock (cont.)				
baked or steamed	1 oz	32	2	0
	1 fillet (150 g)	168	12	2
smoked	1 oz	33	2	0
Halibut, Atlantic and Pacific				
baked or steamed	1 oz	40	7	1
	½ fillet (159 g)	223	42	6
Herring, Atlantic				
raw	1 oz	45	23	5
	1 fillet (184 g)	291	150	34
baked or steamed	1 oz	57	30	7
canned	1 oz	59	35	7
in tomato sauce	1 herring (37 g)	97	52	10
pickled	1 oz	65	39	6
	1 herring	112	68	9
	1 piece (15 g)	33	21	3
smoked, kippered	1 oz	60	33	7
	1 fillet (40 g)	87	45	10
Herring, Pacific, raw	1 oz	55	35	8
Lobster, Northern				
raw	1 oz	26	2	0
	1 lobster (150 g)	136	12	1
cooked, moist heat	1 oz	28	2	0
	1 cup	142	8	1
Newburg (with butter, eggs, sherry, cream)	1 cup	485	239	160
Salad (with mayonnaise)	½ cup or 4 oz	286	149	NA
Lox (smoked salmon)	1 oz	33	11	2
Mackerel, Atlantic				
raw	1 oz	58	35	8
	1 fillet (112 g)	229	140	33
baked or steamed	1 oz	74	45	11
	1 fillet (88 g)	231	141	33
Mackerel, Jack, canned	1 cup	296	108	30
Mackerel, King, raw	1 oz	30	9	1
	½ fillet (198 g)	207	36	6
Mackerel, Pacific and Jack, raw	1 oz	44	20	6
	1 fillet (225 g)	353	160	46
Mackerel, Spanish				
raw	1 oz	39	16	5
	1 fillet (187 g)	260	106	31
baked or steamed	1 oz	45	16	5
	1 fillet (146 g)	230	83	24
Milkfish, raw	1 oz	42	17	4
Monkfish, raw	1 oz	21	4	1

FISH AND SHELLFISH

FOOD	AMOUNT	CALORIES		
		TOTAL	FAT	SAT-FAT
Mullet, striped				
raw	1 oz	33	10	3
	1 fillet (119 g)	139	41	12
baked	1 oz	42	12	4
	1 fillet (93 g)	139	41	12
Mussels, Blue				
raw	1 oz	24	6	1
	1 cup	129	30	6
Ocean perch, Atlantic				
raw	1 oz	27	4	1
	1 fillet (64 g)	60	9	1
baked	1 oz	34	5	1
	1 fillet (50 g)	60	9	1
breaded and fried	1 fillet	185	99	NA
Octopus, raw	1 oz	23	3	1
Oysters, Eastern				
raw	6 medium (84 g)	58	19	5
	1 cup	170	55	14
breaded and fried	1 oz	56	32	8
	6 medium (88 g)	173	100	25
canned	1 oz	19	6	2
	½ cup	85	28	7
steamed	1 oz	39	13	3
	6 medium (42 g)	58	19	5
stew (2 parts milk, 1 part oyster)	1 cup	233	139	80
Oyster, Pacific, raw	1 oz	23	6	1
	1 medium (50 g)	41	10	2
Pike, Northern				
raw	1 oz	25	2	0
	½ fillet (198 g)	175	12	2
baked	1 oz	32	2	0
	½ fillet (155 g)	176	12	2
Pike, Walleye, raw	1 oz	26	3	1
	1 fillet (159 g)	147	17	4
Pollock, Atlantic, raw	1 oz	26	2	0
	½ fillet (193 g)	177	17	2
Pollock, Walleye				
raw	1 oz	23	2	0
	1 fillet (77 g)	62	6	1
baked	1 oz	32	3	1
	1 fillet (60 g)	68	6	1

FISH AND SHELLFISH

FOOD	AMOUNT	CALORIES TOTAL	FAT	SAT-FAT
Pompano, Florida				
raw	1 oz	47	24	9
	1 fillet (112 g)	184	95	35
baked	1 oz	60	31	11
	1 fillet (88 g)	185	96	36
Pout, ocean, raw	1 oz	22	2	1
	½ fillet (176 g)	140	14	5
Rockfish, Pacific				
raw	1 oz	27	4	1
	1 fillet (191 g)	180	27	6
baked	1 oz	34	5	1
	1 fillet (149 g)	180	27	6
Roughy, Orange, raw	1 oz	36	18	0
Sablefish				
raw	1 oz	55	39	8
	½ fillet (193 g)	377	266	56
smoked	1 oz	72	51	10
Salmon, Atlantic, raw	1 oz	40	16	3
Salmon, Chinook				
raw	1 oz	51	27	6
smoked	1 oz	33	11	2
Salmon, Chum				
raw	1 oz	34	10	2
canned	1 oz	40	14	4
Salmon, Coho				
raw	1 oz	41	15	3
Salmon, Pink				
raw	1 oz	33	9	1
canned	1 oz	39	15	4
Salmon, Sockeye				
raw	1 oz	48	22	4
canned, drained	1 oz	40	14	4
Salmon, smoked (lox)	1 oz	33	11	2
Sardines, Atlantic, canned in oil,				
drained	1 oz	59	29	3
	2 sardines (24 g)	50	25	3
	1 can (3¼ oz)	192	95	13
Sardines, Pacific, canned in				
tomato sauce, drained	1 oz	51	31	8
	1 sardine (38 g)	68	41	11
Scallops				
raw	1 oz	25	2	0
	2 large or 5 small (30 g)	26	2	0
breaded, fried	1 oz	61	28	6
	2 large (31 g)	67	31	7

FISH AND SHELLFISH

		CALORIES		
FOOD	AMOUNT	TOTAL	FAT	SAT-FAT
Scallops (cont.)				
steamed	1 oz	32	4	1
Scup, raw	1 oz	30	7	2
	1 fillet (64 g)	67	16	4
Sea bass				
raw	1 oz	27	5	1
	1 fillet (129 g)	125	23	6
baked	1 oz	35	7	2
	1 fillet (101 g)	125	23	6
Sea trout, raw	1 oz	29	9	3
	1 fillet (238 g)	248	77	22
Shad				
raw	1 oz	56	35	8
	1 fillet (184 g)	362	228	52
baked	1 oz	57	29	NA
Shark				
raw	1 oz	37	11	2
batter-dipped and fried	1 oz	65	35	8
Sheepshead				
raw	1 oz	31	6	2
	1 fillet (238 g)	257	52	13
baked	1 oz	36	4	1
	1 fillet (186 g)	234	27	6
Shrimp				
raw	1 oz	30	4	1
	4 large (28 g)	30	4	1
breaded, fried	1 oz	69	31	5
	4 large (30 g)	73	33	6
canned	1 oz	34	5	1
	½ cup	77	11	2
Cocktail (Sau-Sea)	½ cup	90	0	0
steamed	1 oz	28	3	1
	4 large (22 g)	22	2	1
Smelt, Rainbow				
raw	1 oz	28	6	1
baked	1 oz	35	8	2
Snapper				
raw	1 oz	28	3	1
	1 fillet (218 g)	217	26	6
baked	1 oz	36	4	1
	1 fillet (170 g)	217	26	6
Sole (see Flatfish)				
Spiny Lobster, raw	1 oz	32	4	1
	1 lobster (209 g)	233	28	4
Spot, raw	1 oz	35	12	4
	1 fillet (64 g)	79	28	8

FISH AND SHELLFISH

		CALORIES		
FOOD	AMOUNT	TOTAL	FAT	SAT-FAT
Squid (calamari)				
raw	1 oz	26	4	1
fried	1 oz	50	19	5
Sturgeon				
raw	1 oz	30	10	2
baked	1 oz	38	13	3
smoked	1 oz	48	11	3
Sucker, White, raw	1 oz	26	6	1
	1 fillet (159 g)	147	33	6
Sunfish, Pumpkinseed, raw	1 oz	25	2	0
	1 fillet (48 g)	43	3	0
Surimi	1 oz	28	2	0
Swordfish				
raw	1 oz	34	10	3
baked	1 oz	44	13	4
Tilefish				
raw	1 oz	27	6	1
	½ fillet (193 g)	184	40	8
baked	1 oz	42	12	2
	½ fillet (150 g)	220	63	12
Trout, Rainbow				
raw	1 oz	33	9	2
	1 fillet (79 g)	93	24	5
baked	1 oz	43	11	2
	1 fillet (62 g)	94	24	5
Tuna				
raw	1 oz	41	12	3
baked	1 oz	52	16	4
canned, drained				
solid white in water	1 oz	35	5	2
chunk light in oil	1 oz	55	25	4
canned, undrained				
solid white in oil	1 can (6 oz)	450	300	55
Tuna salad	½ cup	190	85	14
Turbot, European, raw	1 oz	27	8	2
	½ fillet (204 g)	194	54	14
Whelk				
raw	1 oz	39	1	0
steamed	1 oz	78	2	0
Whitefish				
raw	1 oz	38	15	2
	1 fillet (198 g)	266	104	16
smoked	1 oz	30	2	1
Whiting				
raw	1 oz	26	3	1
	1 fillet (92 g)	83	11	2

FISH AND SHELLFISH

| FOOD | AMOUNT | CALORIES | | |
		TOTAL	FAT	SAT-FAT
Whiting (cont.)				
baked	1 oz	33	**4**	1
	1 fillet (72 g)	83	**11**	2
Wolffish, Atlantic, raw	1 oz	27	**6**	1
	½ fillet (153 g)	147	**33**	5
Yellowtail, raw	1 oz	41	**13**	3
	½ fillet (187 g)	273	**88**	22

FROZEN, MICROWAVE, AND REFRIGERATED FOODS

| FOOD | AMOUNT | CALORIES | | |
		TOTAL	FAT	SAT-FAT
APPETIZERS				
Cocktail Beef Franks (Cohen's)	7 (89 g)	320	**240**	81
Eggrolls				
Beef Steak Teriyaki (Lo-An)	1 (78 g)	140	**35**	9
Chicken & Shrimp (Lo-An)	1 (78 g)	140	**35**	9
Chicken Munchers Mini				
Eggrolls (La Choy)	6 eggrolls (85 g)	210	**80**	23
Egg Roll Bites (Matlaw's)	2 pieces (28 g)	45	**5**	0
Lobster (Lo-An)	1 (78 g)	150	**35**	9
Pork (Chung's)	2 (168 g)	400	**180**	45
Shrimp Munchers Mini				
Eggrolls (La Choy)	6 eggrolls (85 g)	190	**60**	14
Shrimp (Lo-An)	1 (78 g)	150	**45**	9
Vegetable (Barney's)	3 (81 g)	140	**35**	14
White Meat				
Chicken (Chung's)	2 (168 g)	340	**100**	14
White Meat Chicken (Lo-An)	1 (78 g)	140	**35**	NA
Potato Knishes	1 knish (210 g)	436	**150**	36
Puffs				
Mushroom Puffs (Mother's)	2 pieces (66 g)	190	**100**	18
Potato Puff (Manischewitz)	5 pieces (92 g)	340	**180**	45
Spinach & Potato Puff				
(Manischewitz)	5 pieces (92 g)	320	**180**	45
Spinach Puffs (Mother's)	2 pieces (66 g)	200	**100**	18
Quiche				
Petite Quiche Appetizers	6 (128 g)	370	**200**	90
Turnover				
Beef (Manischewitz)	4 pieces (85 g)	300	**190**	54
BREADS				
New York Brand				
Texas Garlic Toast	1 slice (40 g)	170	**90**	18
with cheese	1 slice (48 g)	190	**100**	36

FROZEN, MICROWAVE, AND REFRIGERATED FOODS

		CALORIES		
FOOD	AMOUNT	TOTAL	FAT	SAT-FAT
BREADS (cont.)				
Pepperidge Farm				
Five Cheese & Garlic				
Cheese Bread	2 ¼" slices (56 g)	200	**90**	41
Garlic Toast	1 slice (40 g)	160	**90**	14
Mozzarella Garlic Cheese				
Bread	2 ¼" slices (56 g)	200	**90**	45
Sourdough Garlic Bread	2 ½" slices (50 g)	170	**60**	9
BREAKFAST FOODS				
Blintzes				
Empire Kosher				
Apple	2 (124 g)	220	**50**	14
Cherry	2 (124 g)	200	**35**	9
Golden				
Blueberry	1 (62 g)	90	**9**	0
Cherry	1 (62 g)	95	**9**	0
Potato	1 (62 g)	90	**36**	9
Ratner's				
Blueberry Cheese	1 (61 g)	100	**5**	0
Cheese	1 (61 g)	90	**5**	0
jumbo	1 (94.5 g)	133	**6**	5
Cherry	1 (61 g)	100	**5**	0
Potato	1 (61 g)	110	**30**	18
Breakfast Burritos				
Bacon (Great Starts,				
Swanson)	1 pkg (99 g)	250	**100**	36
Breakfast Sandwich				
Great Starts (Swanson)				
Egg, Canadian Bacon &				
Cheese on a Muffin	1 pkg (116 g)	290	**140**	54
French Toast Sticks with				
Syrup	1 pkg (120 g)	320	**90**	45
Pancakes with Bacon	1 pkg (128 g)	400	**180**	63
Pancakes with Sausage	1 pkg (170 g)	490	**230**	99
Sausage, Egg & Cheese on a				
Biscuit	1 pkg (156 g)	460	**250**	99
Scrambled Eggs & Bacon				
with Home-Fried Potatoes	1 pkg (149 g)	290	**170**	81
Scrambled Eggs & Sausage				
with Hashed Brown				
Potatoes	1 pkg (177 g)	360	**230**	90
Morningstar Farms				
Breakfast Links	2 links (45 g)	60	**20**	5
Breakfast Patties	1 patty (38 g)	70	**25**	5
Breakfast Strips	2 strips (16 g)	60	**40**	5
Grillers	1 patty (64 g)	140	**60**	5

FROZEN, MICROWAVE, AND REFRIGERATED FOODS

		CALORIES		
FOOD	**AMOUNT**	**TOTAL**	**FAT**	**SAT-FAT**
Breakfast Sandwich (cont.)				
Weight Watchers Smart Ones				
English Muffin Sandwich	1 (113 g)	210	50	18
Handy Ham & Cheese				
Omelet	1 (113 g)	220	45	23
Croissants				
Original (Sara Lee)	1 (43 g)	170	70	NA
French Toast, Frozen				
Aunt Jemima, all types	2 (118 g)	240	60	18
Breakfast Blast Mini Sticks				
(Swanson)	1 pkg (120 g)	310	130	NA
Downyflake				
Cinnamon Swirl	2 (113 g)	270	50	NA
Plain	2 (113 g)	260	60	NA
Great Starts (Swanson)				
Cinnamon Swirl French				
Toast with Sausage	1 pkg (156 g)	440	250	108
French Toast Sticks	1 pkg (120 g)	320	90	NA
French Toast with Sausage	1 pkg (156 g)	410	230	81
Muffins				
Blueberry (Sara Lee)	1 muffin (64 g)	220	100	NA
Pancakes, Frozen				
Aunt Jemima				
Buttermilk Pancake Batter	½ cup batter			
	(4 4" pancakes)	260	30	9
Low-fat	3 (97 g)	150	15	0
Great Starts (Swanson)				
6 Silver Dollar Pancakes				
with Sausage	1 pkg (106 g)	340	160	81
Hungry Jack (Pillsbury)				
Blueberry	3 (116 g)	270	35	9
Buttermilk	3 (116 g)	270	40	9
Toaster Strudel				
Apple	1 pastry (54 g)	200	80	14
Brown Sugar Cinnamon	1 pastry (54 g)	190	70	14
Cherry	1 pastry (54 g)	190	70	14
Cream Cheese & Blueberry	1 pastry (54 g)	200	90	27
Strawberry	1 pastry (54 g)	200	80	18
Strawberry Kiwi	1 pastry (54 g)	190	70	18
Tropical Wave	1 pastry (54 g)	190	70	14
Wildberry	1 pastry (54 g)	190	70	18
Waffles, Frozen				
Aunt Jemima				
Blueberry	2 waffles (72 g)	190	50	14
Buttermilk	2 waffles (72 g)	200	50	14
Homestyle	2 waffles (72 g)	200	50	14
Low-fat	2 waffles (74 g)	160	15	5

FROZEN, MICROWAVE, AND REFRIGERATED FOODS

		CALORIES		
FOOD	AMOUNT	TOTAL	FAT	SAT-FAT
Waffles, Frozen (cont.)				
Oatmeal	2 waffles (84 g)	200	70	NA
Original	2 waffles (72 g)	200	60	0
Belgian Chef Belgian Waffles	2 waffles (75 g)	170	25	5
Breakfast Blast 5 Waffle Sticks	1 (78 g)	330	150	NA
Downyflake				
Homestyle and Buttermilk	2 waffles (68 g)	170	35	NA
Eggo (Kellogg's)				
Blueberry	2 waffles (78 g)	220	80	14
Buttermilk, Strawberry, or				
Homestyle	2 waffles (78 g)	220	70	14
Common Sense Oat Bran	2 waffles (78 g)	200	60	NA
Fat free	2 waffles (58 g)	120	0	0
Minis (Homestyle)	3 sets of 4 waffles			
	(93 g)	260	80	18
Special K	2 waffles (58 g)	120	0	0
Nutrigrain Eggo				
Apple Cinnamon	2 waffles (78 g)	220	70	14
Banana Bread	2 waffles (78 g)	200	60	9
Cinnamon Twist	3 sets of 4 waffles			
	(92 g)	290	90	18
Multi-bran	2 waffles (78 g)	180	50	9
Nut & Honey	2 waffles (78 g)	240	90	18
Whole Wheat	2 waffles (78 g)	190	60	9
Hungry Jack (Pillsbury)				
Apple Cinnamon	2 waffles (71 g)	200	50	18
Buttermilk	2 waffles (68 g)	190	50	18
Homestyle	2 waffles (68 g)	180	50	18
Mini Funfetti	3 sets of 4 waffles			
	(93 g)	260	70	23
DISHES OR DINNERS				
Amy's				
Burritos				
cheese	1 burrito (170 g)	280	70	23
non-dairy	1 burrito (170 g)	250	95	9
California Veggie Burger	1 burger (72 g)	100	25	0
Enchiladas				
Black Bean, Vegetable	1 enchilada (135 g)	130	40	0
Cheese	1 enchilada (135 g)	210	80	23
Spanish Rice & Beans	1 meal (284 g)	250	70	9
Lasagna				
Tofu Vegetable	1 lasagna (269 g)	300	90	9
Vegetable	1 lasagna (269 g)	300	90	36
Macaroni & Cheese	1 entree (255 g)	390	130	72
Mexican Tamale Pie	1 pie (227 g)	220	30	0

FROZEN, MICROWAVE, AND REFRIGERATED FOODS

		CALORIES		
FOOD	AMOUNT	TOTAL	FAT	SAT-FAT
Amy's (cont.)				
Pot Pies				
Beef	1 pie (198 g)	400	**210**	99
Broccoli	1 pie (213 g)	430	**190**	90
Vegetable	1 pie (213 g)	360	**160**	99
Shepherd's Pie	1 pie (227 g)	160	**35**	0
Veggie Loaf	1 entree (284 g)	260	**50**	5
Authentic Chinese Entrees				
Kung Pao Chicken	1 cup (199 g)	250	**40**	9
Moo Goo Gai Pan	1 cup (199 g)	260	**70**	18
Sweet & Sour Pork	1 cup (199 g)	250	**40**	9
Banquet				
Boneless Pork Riblet Meal	1 meal (283 g)	400	**170**	72
Brown Gravy & Salisbury	1 patty with gravy			
Steaks	(132 g)	230	**150**	72
Chicken Fried Beef Steak				
Meal	1 meal (283 g)	420	**210**	63
Chicken Nugget Meal	1 meal (191 g)	430	**210**	72
Chicken Pot Pie	1 pie (198 g)	380	**200**	81
Country Fried Chicken	3 oz (84 g)	270	**160**	45
Creamy Broccoli, Chicken, &				
Cheese Meal	1 cup (219 g)	280	**130**	63
Fish Stick Meal	1 meal (187 g)	300	**120**	32
Fried Chicken	3 oz (84 g)	280	**160**	45
Fried Chicken Meal	1 meal (255 g)	470	**240**	81
Fried Chicken (The Hearty				
One)	416 g	870	**500**	117
Grilled Chicken Meal	1 meal (280 g)	330	**120**	27
Homestyle Gravy & Sliced	2 slices with gravy			
Turkey	(134 g)	120	**70**	27
Lasagna with Meat Sauce	1 cup (224 g)	350	**100**	45
Potato, Ham, & Broccoli au				
Gratin	⅔ cup (140 g)	220	**120**	45
Salisbury Steak Meal	1 meal (269 g)	380	**220**	81
Salisbury Steak Meal				
(The Hearty One)	1 meal (467 g)	780	**490**	189
Southern Fried Chicken	3 oz (84 g)	280	**160**	45
Turkey (mostly white meat)				
Meal	1 meal (262 g)	280	**90**	23
Turkey (mostly white meat)				
Meal (The Hearty One)	1 meal (481 g)	630	**290**	72
Turkey Pot Pie	1 pie (198 g)	370	**180**	72
Birds Eye Easy Recipe				
Asian Stir Fry	2¼ cups (253 g)			
	as packaged	230	**15**	0
	as prepared	330	**90**	18

FROZEN, MICROWAVE, AND REFRIGERATED FOODS

FOOD	AMOUNT	CALORIES TOTAL	FAT	SAT-FAT
Birds Eye Easy Recipe (cont.)				
Original Stir Fry	2¼ cups (270 g)			
	as packaged	210	**35**	5
	as prepared	300	**100**	25
Primavera	1¾ cups (215 g)			
	as packaged	180	**45**	9
	as prepared	250	**80**	14
Southwestern	1¾ cups (233 g)			
	as packaged	200	**50**	9
	as prepared	270	**70**	14
Teriyaki Stir Fry	2 cups (250 g)			
	as packaged	210	**25**	5
	as prepared	290	**60**	9
Birds Eye Pasta Secrets				
Italian Pesto	2⅓ cups (181 g) frozen or 1 cup cooked	240	**80**	18
Primavera	2⅓ cups (189 g) frozen or 1 cup cooked	230	**90**	27
Three Cheese	2 cups (173 g) froz. or 1 cup cooked	230	**70**	23
White Cheddar	2 cups (180 g) froz. or 1 cup cooked	240	**90**	23
Zesty Garlic	2 cups (167 g) froz. or 1 cup cooked	240	**90**	23
Boca Burger (vegan)	1 burger (71 g)	84	**0**	0
Budget Gourmet				
Beef Pepper Steak with Rice	1 entree (255 g)	270	**70**	23
Cheese Manicotti with Meat Sauce	1 entree (255 g)	350	**170**	81
Escalloped Noodles & Turkey	1 entree (226 g)	320	**150**	63
Fettuccini Alfredo with Four Cheeses	1 entree (226 g)	320	**110**	45
Italian Sausage Lasagna	1 entree (283 g)	410	**190**	81
Macaroni & Cheese (side dish)	1 pkg (163 g)	260	**100**	54
Rice Pilaf with green beans (side dish)	1 pkg (141 g)	220	**90**	27
Rigatoni in Cream Sauce with Broccoli & White Chicken	1 entree (226 g)	250	**60**	32
Roast Beef Supreme	1 entree (255 g)	310	**120**	63
Spinach au Gratin (side dish)	1 pkg (141 g)	160	**110**	63
Stir Fry Rice & Vegetables	1 entree (226 g)	350	**140**	54
Spicy Szechuan Vegetables & Chicken	1 entree (226 g)	290	**80**	27

FROZEN, MICROWAVE, AND REFRIGERATED FOODS

		CALORIES		
FOOD	AMOUNT	TOTAL	FAT	SAT-FAT
Budget Gourmet (cont.)				
Swedish Meatballs	1 entree (283 g)	550	310	162
Three Cheese Lasagna	1 entree (255 g)	330	110	72
Budget Gourmet Low Fat				
Angel Hair Pasta	1 entree (226 g)	230	45	14
Chicken Oriental & Vegetables	1 entree (255 g)	290	70	23
Chinese Style Vegetables & Chicken	1 entree (226 g)	250	60	23
Fettuccini Primavera in Herb Sauce with Chicken	1 entree (255 g)	280	70	32
Glazed Turkey	1 entree (255 g)	250	45	18
Italian Style Vegetables & Chicken	1 entree (226 g)	250	60	23
Linguini with Clams & Shrimp	1 entree (255 g)	280	70	45
Orange Glazed Chicken Breast	1 entree (255 g)	280	30	9
Pasta in Wine & Mushroom Sauce with Chicken	1 entree (255 g)	280	60	18
Penne Pasta with Chunky Tomatoes & Italian Sausage in Sauce	1 entree (226 g)	270	45	14
Rigatoni in Cream Sauce with Broccoli & White Chicken	1 entree (226 g)	250	60	32
Roast Chicken with Herb Gravy	1 meal (283 g)	260	70	32
Spaghetti Marinara	1 entree (226 g)	260	50	9
Ziti Parmesano	1 entree (226 g)	260	60	18
Butterball Chicken Requests				
Italian Style Herb	1 piece (99 g)	190	60	18
Original	1 piece (99 g)	180	60	18
Parmesan	1 piece (99 g)	200	60	27
Celentano				
Broccoli Stuffed Shells	4 shells (280 g)	190	35	9
Cheese Ravioli	6 ravioli (182 g)	360	35	18
Eggplant Parmigiana	½ tray (196 g)	320	190	45
Eggplant Rollettes	1 tray (280 g)	330	130	36
Low Fat Lasagne	1 tray (280 g)	260	25	9
Manicotti	2 pieces (196 g)	310	130	63
Stuffed Shells	3 shells (196 g)	300	130	63
Dinty Moore				
Beef Stew	1 cup (213 g)	190	90	45
Chicken and Dumplings	1 cup (213 g)	200	50	18
Corned Beef Hash	1 cup (213 g)	350	200	81
Don Miguel				
Bean and Cheese Burrito	1 (198 g)	420	120	NA
Bean and Cheese Chimichanga	1 (198 g)	470	160	NA

FROZEN, MICROWAVE, AND REFRIGERATED FOODS

FOOD	AMOUNT	CALORIES		
		TOTAL	FAT	SAT-FAT
Don Miguel (cont.)				
Beef and Cheese Burrito	1 (198 g)	390	100	NA
Chicken and Cheese Burrito	1 (198 g)	410	130	NA
Chicken Burrito	1 (198 g)	360	70	NA
Empire Kosher				
Breaded Mushrooms	7 pieces (81 g)	90	5	0
Breaded Zucchini	7 pieces (83 g)	100	5	0
Chicken Fat	1 tbsp (14 g)	120	120	36
Chicken Pie	1 pie (227 g)	440	190	45
Chicken Nuggets	5 nuggets (85 g)	180	80	14
Chicken Stix	4 stix (88 g)	180	90	18
Ground Turkey	4 oz (112 g)	150	70	18
Potato Pancakes (Latkes)	1 piece (56 g)	100	40	5
Golden				
Potato Pancakes (Latkes)	1 (38 g)	71	27	0
Gorton's				
Butterfly Shrimp	20 (91 g)	240	120	27
Crunchy Golden Breaded Fish Fillets	1 fillet (108 g)	250	130	36
Crunchy Golden Fish Sticks	6 sticks (104 g)	250	120	32
Garlic & Herb Breaded Fish Fillets	1 fillet (104 g)	220	100	27
Lemon Pepper Battered Fish Fillets	1 fillet (104 g)	270	160	45
Parmesan Fish Sticks	2 fillets (104 g)	260	140	36
Southern Fried Fish Fillets	1 fillet (104 g)	230	130	36
Gorton's Grilled Fillets				
Italian Herb	1 fillet (108 g)	130	50	9
all other flavors	1 fillet (108 g)	120	50	9
Gorton's Homestyle Baked Fillets				
Au Gratin	1 fillet (131 g)	130	45	18
Garlic Butter Crumb	1 fillet (131 g)	170	80	14
Primavera	1 fillet (131 g)	120	45	23
Green Giant Create a Meal! Meal Starter				
Beefy Noodle Flavor	1¾ cups (178 g)			
	as packaged	170	15	0
	1¼ cups as prep.	350	130	45
Cheesy Pasta & Vegetable	1¾ cups (176 g)			
	as packaged	230	90	54
	1¼ cups as prep.	440	210	108
Country Chicken Noodle Flavor with Pasta	1¼ cups (176 g)			
	as packaged	130	5	0
	1¼ cups as prep.	280	80	18
Fajita Style	⅓ package (168 g)	140	60	41
	2 fajitas prep.	430	140	54

FROZEN, MICROWAVE, AND REFRIGERATED FOODS

		CALORIES		
FOOD	AMOUNT	TOTAL	FAT	SAT-FAT
Green Giant Create a Meal! Meal Starter (cont.)				
Hearty Vegetable Stew	1¼ cups (186 g)			
	as packaged	130	**5**	0
	1¼ cups as prep.	280	**80**	18
Homestyle Stew	1¼ cups (189 g)			
	as packaged	140	**25**	5
	1 cup as prep.	340	**140**	54
Lo Mein Stir Fry	2⅓ cups (212 g)			
	as packaged	170	**10**	0
	1¼ cups as prep.	320	**60**	14
Oven Roasted Garlic Herb	1¾ cups (184 g)			
	as packaged	160	**0**	0
	1¾ cups as prep.	360	**80**	14
Oven Roasted Homestyle Pot Roast	1¾ cups (191 g)			
	as packaged	150	**5**	0
	2 cups as prep.	370	**120**	27
Oven Roasted Savory Onion	1¾ cups (185 g)			
	as packaged	130	**10**	0
	1¾ cups as prep.	340	**120**	27
Skillet Lasagna	1¾ cups (188 g)			
	as packaged	160	**5**	0
	1¼ cups as prep.	350	**120**	45
Szechuan Stir Fry	1¾ cups (200 g)			
	as packaged	150	**45**	5
	1¼ cups as prep.	310	**130**	27
Teriyaki Stir Fry	1¾ cups (199 g)			
	as packaged	100	**5**	0
	1¼ cups as prep.	230	**50**	9
Green Giant Pasta Secrets				
Alfredo	2 cups (160 g) froz.			
	or 1 cup cooked	260	**90**	27
Garlic Seasoning	2 cups (188 g) froz.			
	or 1 cup cooked	250	**90**	45
Lasagna Style	2 cups (188 g) froz.			
	or 1 cup cooked	260	**90**	27
White Cheddar Sauce	2 cups (181 g) froz.			
	or 1 cup cooked	270	**80**	23
Healthy Choice				
Beef Macaroni	1 meal (240 g)	220	**35**	18
Beef Pepper Steak Oriental	1 meal (269 g)	250	**35**	18
Beef Stroganoff	1 meal (311 g)	310	**60**	27
Beef Tips, Traditional	1 meal (318 g)	260	**50**	27
Breast of Turkey, Traditional	1 meal (298 g)	290	**40**	18
Cacciatore Chicken	1 meal (354 g)	270	**35**	9
Charbroiled Beef Patty	1 meal (311 g)	280	**50**	27
Chicken & Vegetables Marsala	1 meal (326 g)	240	**35**	18

FROZEN, MICROWAVE, AND REFRIGERATED FOODS

		CALORIES		
FOOD	**AMOUNT**	**TOTAL**	**FAT**	**SAT-FAT**
Healthy Choice (cont.)				
Chicken Breast Con Queso				
Burrito	1 meal (299 g)	350	50	23
Chicken Enchilada Suprema	1 meal (320 g)	300	60	27
Chicken Fettuccini Alfredo	1 meal (240 g)	280	60	23
Chicken Parmigiana	1 meal (326 g)	330	70	27
Chicken Teriyaki	1 meal (311 g)	270	50	27
Country Breaded Chicken	1 meal (290 g)	350	80	18
Country Glazed Chicken	1 meal (240 g)	230	35	14
Country Herb Chicken	1 meal (344 g)	320	50	23
Country Inn Roast Turkey	1 meal (283 g)	250	50	18
Country Roast Turkey with				
Mushrooms	1 meal (240 g)	220	35	9
Fiesta Chicken Fajitas	1 meal (198 g)	260	35	9
Ginger Chicken Hunan	1 meal (357 g)	380	45	9
Grilled Chicken Sonoma	1 meal (255 g)	230	35	9
Grilled Chicken with Mashed				
Potatoes	1 meal (226 g)	170	30	14
Grilled Glazed Pork Patty	1 meal (272 g)	300	60	18
Honey Mustard Chicken	1 meal (269 g)	270	35	14
Lemon Pepper Fish	1 meal (303 g)	320	60	18
Macaroni & Cheese	1 meal (255 g)	320	60	23
Meatloaf, Traditional	1 meal (340 g)	320	45	23
Mesquite Chicken BBQ	1 meal (298 g)	310	45	18
Pasta Shells Marinara	1 meal (340 g)	390	70	32
Penne Pasta & Roasted				
Tomato Sauce	1 meal (226 g)	230	45	9
Roasted Chicken	1 meal (311 g)	230	45	23
Salisbury Steak, Traditional	1 meal (326 g)	330	60	27
Sesame Chicken	1 meal (276 g)	240	25	5
Sesame Chicken Shanghai	1 meal (340 g)	300	45	9
Shrimp & Vegetables Maria	1 meal (354 g)	290	45	18
Southwestern Grilled Chicken	1 meal (289 g)	230	60	27
Spaghetti & Sauce with				
Seasoned Beef	1 meal (283 g)	280	50	18
Yankee Pot Roast	1 meal (311 g)	290	60	27
Zucchini Lasagna	1 meal (383 g)	330	15	9
Hormel				
Beef Stew	1 cup (213 g)	190	90	36
Chili, no beans	1 cup (209 g)	220	50	23
Macaroni & Cheese	1 cup (213 g)	270	100	NA
Noodles & Chicken (Hearty				
Helpings)	1 cup (298 g)	250	100	NA
Inland Valley MunchSkin Meals				
Cheese & Potato Potato Skins Kit	2 topped potato skins			
	(113 g)	250	140	63

FROZEN, MICROWAVE, AND REFRIGERATED FOODS

		CALORIES		
FOOD	AMOUNT	TOTAL	FAT	SAT-FAT
Kid Cuisine				
Circus Show Corn Dog	1 meal (249 g)	450	140	45
Cosmic Chicken Nuggets	1 meal (257 g)	500	230	90
Game Time Taco Roll-Ups	1 meal (208 g)	420	160	63
High Flying Fried Chicken	1 meal (286 g)	440	180	81
Magical Macaroni & Cheese	1 meal (300 g)	440	110	45
Pirate Pizza with Cheese	1 meal (226 g)	430	100	45
Wave Rider Waffle Sticks	1 meal (187 g)	380	70	18
Kids Fun Feast (Swanson)				
Chillin' Cheese Pizza	1 pkg (224 g)	350	80	41
Chompin' Chicken Drumlets	1 pkg (255 g)	490	220	81
Frazzlin' Fried Chicken	1 pkg (312 g)	660	320	NA
Frenzied Fish Sticks	1 pkg (198 g)	370	130	45
Munchin' Mini Tacos	1 pkg (204 g)	390	140	54
Razzlin' Rings	1 pkg (340 g)	390	100	45
Roarin' Ravioli	1 pkg (312 g)	440	110	41
Kid's Kitchen (Hormel)				
Beans & Weiners	1 cup (220 g)	310	110	NA
Beefy Mac	1 cup (213 g)	190	50	NA
Kosherific				
Fish Sticks	6 (113 g)	280	130	23
Lean Cuisine				
Baked Chicken	1 pkg (244 g)	230	35	14
Baked Fish	1 pkg (255 g)	270	50	18
Beef Peppercorn	1 pkg (248 g)	220	60	18
Beef Portabello	1 pkg (255 g)	220	60	32
Beef Pot Roast	1 pkg (255 g)	210	60	18
Cheese Cannelloni	1 pkg (258 g)	230	35	18
Cheese Lasagna with Chicken Breast Scaloppini	1 pkg (283 g)	290	70	18
Cheese Ravioli	1 pkg (240 g)	270	60	27
Chicken a l'Orange	1 pkg (255 g)	250	15	5
Chicken & Vegetables	1 pkg (297 g)	250	45	9
Chicken Carbonara	1 pkg (255 g)	280	60	18
Chicken Chow Mein	1 pkg (255 g)	220	35	9
Chicken Enchilada Suiza	1 pkg (255 g)	280	40	14
Chicken Fettuccine	1 pkg (262 g)	280	50	18
Chicken in Wine Sauce	1 pkg (230 g)	210	50	18
Chicken Lasagna	1 pkg (283 g)	270	70	27
Chicken Medallions with Cheese Sauce	1 pkg (265 g)	260	70	27
Chicken Mediterranean	1 pkg (297 g)	270	30	9
Chicken Parmesan	1 pkg (308 g)	220	40	14
Chicken in Peanut Sauce	1 pkg (255 g)	290	50	9
Chicken Piccata	1 pkg (255 g)	270	60	18
Chicken Pie	1 pkg (269 g)	290	80	23

FROZEN, MICROWAVE, AND REFRIGERATED FOODS

		CALORIES		
FOOD	**AMOUNT**	**TOTAL**	**FAT**	**SAT-FAT**
Lean Cuisine (cont.)				
Chicken with Basil Cream Sauce	1 pkg (240 g)	270	60	18
Classic Cheese Lasagna	1 pkg (326 g)	270	35	23
Fettuccini Alfredo	1 pkg (262 g)	300	60	23
Fiesta Chicken	1 pkg (240 g)	250	45	5
Glazed Chicken	1 pkg (240 g)	240	50	9
Glazed Turkey Tenderloins	1 pkg (255 g)	240	40	9
Grilled Chicken & Penne Pasta	1 pkg (265 g)	260	70	27
Grilled Chicken Salsa	1 pkg (251 g)	270	60	23
Herb Roasted Chicken	1 pkg (226 g)	210	40	9
Homestyle Turkey	1 pkg (265 g)	230	40	9
Honey Roasted Chicken	1 pkg (240 g)	290	50	18
Honey Roasted Pork	1 pkg (269 g)	250	50	23
Lasagna with Meat Sauce	1 pkg (297 g)	290	60	32
Macaroni and Cheese	1 pkg (283 g)	290	60	36
Meatloaf	1 pkg (265 g)	250	60	27
Oriental-Style Dumplings	1 pkg (255 g)	300	50	14
Oven Roasted Beef	1 pkg (262 g)	260	70	27
Roasted Turkey Breast	1 pkg (276 g)	270	20	5
Salisbury Steak	1 pkg (269 g)	280	70	36
Southern Beef Tips	1 pkg (248 g)	290	50	18
Spaghetti with Meat Sauce	1 pkg (326 g)	290	45	14
Shrimp & Angel Hair Pasta	1 pkg (283 g)	290	50	9
Swedish Meatballs	1 pkg (258 g)	290	50	23
Three-Bean Chili	1 pkg (283 g)	250	50	18
Vegetable Eggroll	1 pkg (255 g)	340	60	18
Lean Cuisine Great for Lunch				
Alfredo Pasta Primavera	1 pkg (283 g)	290	60	27
Broccoli & Cheddar Cheese				
Sauce over Baked Potato	1 pkg (290 g)	250	80	NA
Cheese Lasagna Casserole	1 pkg (283 g)	270	50	27
Mandarin Chicken	1 pkg (255 g)	250	35	5
Penne Pasta with Tomato				
Basil Sauce	1 pkg (283 g)	270	30	9
Roasted Potatoes with				
Broccoli & Cheddar Cheese				
Sauce	1 pkg (290 g)	260	50	32
Teriyaki Stir-Fry	1 pkg (283 g)	290	30	5
Lean Cuisine Hearty Portions				
Cheese & Spinach Manicotti	1 pkg (439 g)	340	60	23
Chicken & Barbecue Sauce	1 pkg (393 g)	380	50	14
Chicken Florentine	1 pkg (395 g)	420	80	27
Grilled Beef Patty & Gravy				
with Whipped Potatoes	1 pkg (439 g)	370	80	36
Grilled Chicken & Penne Pasta	1 pkg (396 g)	380	60	23
Lasagna	1 pkg (425 g)	440	80	36

FROZEN, MICROWAVE, AND REFRIGERATED FOODS

| FOOD | AMOUNT | CALORIES | | |
		TOTAL	FAT	SAT-FAT
Lean Cuisine Hearty Portions (cont.)				
Roasted Chicken with				
Mushrooms	1 pkg (354 g)	380	**60**	9
Roasted Turkey Breast	1 pkg (396 g)	290	**45**	18
Lo-An Eggrolls (*see* **APPETIZERS: Eggrolls**)				
Mama Lucia				
Italian Style Meatballs	3 (84g)	270	**190**	81
Marie Callender's				
Beef Tips in Mushroom Sauce	1 meal (385 g)	430	**170**	63
Breaded Chicken Parmigiana				
Dinner	1 dinner (454 g)	620	**250**	72
Chicken (White Meat) &				
Broccoli Pot Pie	1 cup (290 g)	710	**440**	117
Chicken Cordon Bleu	1 meal (368 g)	590	**230**	72
Chicken Pot Pie	1 cup (241 g)	520	**290**	72
Chili & Cornbread	1 cup + 1.5 oz			
	cornbread (297 g)	350	**120**	54
Chunky Chicken & Noodles	1 meal (368 g)	520	**270**	99
Country Fried Chicken & Gravy	1 meal (454 g)	620	**270**	81
Fettuccini Primavera with				
Tortellini	1 cup (234 g)	430	**240**	108
Fettuccini with Broccoli &				
Chicken in Alfredo Sauce	1 cup (221 g)	410	**220**	90
Grilled Chicken in Mushroom				
Sauce	1 dinner (397 g)	480	**140**	54
Grilled Turkey Breast Strips &				
Rice Pilaf	1 meal (333 g)	310	**90**	32
Herb Roasted Chicken	1 dinner (397 g)	670	**380**	135
Lasagna with Meat Sauce	1 cup (246 g)	370	**170**	81
Macaroni & Cheese	1 meal (382 g)	510	**160**	81
Meatloaf & Gravy with				
Mashed Potatoes	1 meal (397 g)	540	**270**	108
Sirloin Salisbury Steak &				
Gravy	1 meal (397 g)	550	**220**	99
Spaghetti & Meat Sauce	1 cup + 2 oz garlic			
	bread (290 g)	380	**120**	36
Stuffed Pasta Trio	1 meal (297 g)	380	**160**	81
Swedish Meatballs	1 meal (354 g)	520	**240**	90
Turkey Pot Pie	1 cup (280 g)	600	**320**	81
Turkey with Gravy & Dressing	1 meal (397 g)	500	**170**	81
Matlaw's				
Stuffed Clams	1 clam (71 g)	120	**50**	NA
Michelina's				
Chicken Italiano with				
Parmesan Cheese	1 pkg (213 g)	250	**60**	18
Chili-Mac	1 container (227 g)	270	**80**	27

FROZEN, MICROWAVE, AND REFRIGERATED FOODS

		CALORIES		
FOOD	AMOUNT	TOTAL	FAT	SAT-FAT
Michelina's (cont.)				
Gravy with Egg Noodles and				
Swedish Meatballs	1 pkg (284 g)	360	110	41
Fettuccine Alfredo	1 pkg (269 g)	410	150	72
Four Cheese Lasagna	1 pkg (227 g)	290	70	36
Lasagna with Meat Sauce	1 pkg (255 g)	300	70	32
Linguini with Clams	1 pkg (255 g)	310	30	5
Macaroni & Beef	1 container (227 g)	250	60	23
Macaroni & Cheese	1 container (227 g)	340	120	54
Penne Pollo	1 pkg (255 g)	320	80	36
Pepper Steak & Rice	1 pkg (241 g)	270	40	14
Rigatoni Pomodoro	1 container (227 g)	220	20	0
Salisbury Steak & Gravy	1 pkg (241 g)	300	160	63
Spaghetti Bolognese	1 pkg (255 g)	290	35	9
Wheels & Cheese	1 container (227 g)	300	80	41
Michelina's Lean 'n Tasty				
Black Bean Chili	1 pkg (284 g)	400	45	9
Fettuccine with Creamy Pesto				
Sauce	1 pkg (241 g)	250	60	32
Glazed Chicken	1 pkg (227 g)	280	30	5
Gravy with Egg Noodles &				
Swedish Meat Balls	1 pkg (284 g)	300	60	14
Honey Barbecue Sauce with				
Chicken & Rice	1 pkg (241 g)	300	20	0
Mac & Beef	1 pkg (227 g)	230	50	18
Macaroni & Cheese	1 pkg (227 g)	270	60	32
Penne Arrabiata	1 pkg (255 g)	230	20	0
Penne Pasta with Mushrooms	1 pkg (227 g)	250	50	32
Spaghetti & Meatballs with				
Tomato Sauce	1 pkg (255 g)	290	60	23
Spaghetti with Onions, Green				
Peppers & Mushrooms	1 pkg (255 g)	280	50	9
Teriyaki Chicken with Rice	1 pkg (241 g)	290	25	5
Mrs. Budd's				
Chicken à la King	1 cup (238 g)	420	80	23
Chicken Supreme	1 cup (238 g)	430	100	27
White Meat Chicken Pie				
Fancy Vegetables	1 cup (227 g)	310	140	45
Original Recipe	1 cup (227 g)	330	150	45
Mrs. Paul's				
Deviled Crabs	1 cake (82 g)	170	60	14
Eggplant Parmigiana	½ cup (118 g)	190	100	27
Grilled Salmon				
Creamy Dill	1 fillet (92 g)	90	25	9
Honey Mustard	1 fillet (92 g)	90	15	5

FROZEN, MICROWAVE, AND REFRIGERATED FOODS

		CALORIES		
FOOD	AMOUNT	TOTAL	FAT	SAT-FAT
Mrs. Paul's (cont.)				
Grilled Tuna				
Barbecue	1 fillet (92 g)	100	5	0
Sesame Teriyaki	1 fillet (92 g)	110	15	0
Mrs. Paul's Dream Kitchen				
Crispy Crunchy Fish Fillets	2 fillets (106 g)	240	110	27
Crispy Crunchy Fish Sticks	6 sticks (95 g)	210	90	23
Mrs. Paul's Grilled Fillets				
Garlic Butter	1 fillet (104 g)	130	50	9
Lemon Pepper	1 fillet (104 g)	130	50	9
Mrs. Paul's Premium Fillets				
Flounder	1 fillet (80 g)	170	70	23
Haddock	1 fillet (120 g)	230	100	23
Nancy's Quiche				
Quiche Florentine	1 quiche (170 g)	440	230	108
Quiche Lorraine	1 quiche (170 g)	470	240	108
Petite Quiche Appetizers				
all types	6 (128 g)	370	200	90
Natural Touch				
Garden Veggie Pattie	1 patty (67 g)	100	25	5
Patio Burritos				
Bean & Cheese	1 burrito (142 g)	300	80	41
Beef & Bean	1 burrito (142 g)	320	110	41
Chicken	1 burrito (142 g)	290	70	27
Patio Dinners				
Cheese Enchilada Dinner	1 meal (340 g)	370	110	45
Fiesta Dinner	1 meal (340 g)	350	100	45
Mexican Style Dinner	1 meal (376 g)	470	170	72
Quiche St. Jacques				
Quiche Jardiniere	$\frac{1}{11}$ of 9" diameter quiche (57 g)	160	100	45
Quiche Lorraine	$\frac{1}{11}$ of 9" diameter quiche (57 g)	170	110	54
Quiche Maximilian	$\frac{1}{11}$ of 9" diameter quiche (57 g)	160	110	45
Quiche Provençal	$\frac{1}{11}$ of 9" diameter quiche (57 g)	160	100	45
Ratner's				
Potato Pancakes (Latkes)	1 pancake (43 g)	110	60	27
Rice Gourmet				
Broccoli Chicken Rice Bowl	1 bowl (312 g)	500	220	72
Teriyaki Style Rice Bowl (beef)	1 bowl (312 g)	370	60	14
Teriyaki Style Rice Bowl (chicken)	1 bowl (312 g)	420	45	9
Safeway Select				
Beef Pot Pie	1 cup (213 g)	570	270	63
Chicken & Broccoli Pot Pie	1 cup (241 g)	640	310	90

FROZEN, MICROWAVE, AND REFRIGERATED FOODS

		CALORIES		
FOOD	AMOUNT	TOTAL	FAT	SAT-FAT
Safeway Select (cont.)				
Chicken Pot Pie	1 cup (241 g)	630	350	81
Turkey Pot Pie	1 cup (241 g)	610	310	90
Safeway Select Gourmet Club				
(10 lowfat) Chicken Fillets	2 pieces (142 g)	120	0	0
Boneless Pork Shoulder				
Country Style Ribs	84 g	160	70	23
Cheese & Broccoli Potatoes	1 potato (147 g)	260	90	41
Cheese Cannelloni	1 piece (189 g)	210	60	27
Chicken Breasts	1 fillet (113 g)	225	85	18
Chicken Nuggets	6 nuggets (112 g)	290	180	45
Chicken Strips	4 strips (122 g)	230	120	27
Deluxe Beef Shepherd's Pie	1 cup (227 g)	360	180	81
Deluxe Beef Steak Pot Pie	1 cup (227 g)	400	170	45
Deluxe Chicken Pot Pie	1 cup (227 g)	480	250	63
Extra Lean Roadhouse Beef				
Patties	1 patty (113 g)	130	40	18
Extra Lean Steakhouse Beef				
Patties	1 patty (113 g)	130	45	18
Four Stuffed Baked Potatoes	1 potato (147 g)	280	100	45
Lean Turkey with Beans &				
Salsa	1 cup (235 g)	180	50	9
Lowfat Tuna Noodle Casserole	1 cup (235 g)	320	25	9
Lowfat Turkey Lasagna	1 cup (227 g)	300	30	9
Meat Lasagna	1 cup (227 g)	300	90	45
Six Vegetable Lasagna	1 cup (227 g)	310	150	99
St. Louis Style Pork Spareribs	2 ribs (125 g)	370	210	72
Veal Cannelloni	1 piece (189 g)	250	100	63
Sea Pak				
Clam Strips	1 pkg (141 g)	410	200	36
Jumbo Butterfly Shrimp	4 shrimp (85 g)	200	80	9
Popcorn Shrimp	15 shrimp (85 g)	210	110	18
Spare the Rib				
Pork, no bones	5 oz (140 g)	380	260	72
Stouffer's				
Baked Chicken Breast				
(Homestyle)	1 pkg (251 g)	260	100	54
Breaded Pork Cutlet				
(Homestyle)	1 pkg (283 g)	420	200	90
Cheddar Pasta with Beef &				
Tomatoes	1 pkg (311 g)	500	210	90
Cheese Ravioli	1 pkg (301 g)	380	120	54
Chicken à la King	1 pkg (269 g)	350	110	36
Chicken & Dumplings				
(Homestyle)	1 pkg (283 g)	280	70	32
Chicken Breast in Barbecue				
Sauce (Homestyle)	1 pkg (283 g)	510	210	108

FROZEN, MICROWAVE, AND REFRIGERATED FOODS

FOOD	AMOUNT	CALORIES		
		TOTAL	FAT	SAT-FAT
Stouffer's (cont.)				
Chicken Breast with Mushroom Gravy (Homestyle)	1 pkg (283 g)	360	**130**	63
Chicken Parmigiana (Homestyle)	1 pkg (340 g)	460	**140**	36
Chicken Pie	1 pkg (283 g)	540	**290**	90
	1 cup (250 g)	500	**280**	90
Chili with Beans	1 pkg (248 g)	290	**90**	36
Chunky Beef & Tomatoes (Homestyle)	1 pkg (283 g)	280	**80**	32
Country Style Biscuit	1 pkg (255 g)	510	**260**	72
Creamed Chipped Beef	½ cup (125 g)	160	**100**	27
Escalloped Apples	⅔ cup (158 g)	190	**25**	9
Escalloped Chicken and Noodles	1 pkg (283 g)	430	**240**	45
Fettuccini Alfredo	1 pkg (283 g)	520	**250**	144
Fish Filet (Homestyle)	1 pkg (255 g)	430	**190**	45
Five Cheese Lasagna	1 pkg (304 g)	360	**120**	63
Fried Chicken Breast (Homestyle)	1 pkg (251 g)	400	**150**	54
Green Pepper Steak	1 pkg (297 g)	320	**80**	27
Lasagna Bake with Meat Sauce	1 pkg (290 g)	370	**100**	45
Lasagna with Meat & Sauce	1 cup (215 g)	260	**90**	36
Lasagna with Tomato Sauce & Italian Sausage	1 pkg (308 g)	340	**100**	45
Macaroni and Beef	1 pkg (326 g)	340	**80**	36
Macaroni and Cheese	1 cup (225 g)	320	**140**	63
Macaroni and Cheese with Broccoli	1 pkg (297 g)	360	**150**	72
Meatloaf (Homestyle)	1 pkg (279 g)	390	**180**	99
Roast Turkey Breast (Homestyle)	1 pkg (272 g)	310	**110**	54
Salisbury Steak (Homestyle)	1 pkg (272 g)	380	**160**	72
Sliced Beef Brisket (Homestyle)	1 pkg (283 g)	370	**150**	90
Spaghetti with Meatballs	1 pkg (357 g)	440	**130**	45
Spaghetti with Meat Sauce	1 pkg (272 g)	350	**100**	36
Stuffed Peppers	1 pepper & sauce (220 g)	180	**70**	9
Swedish Meatballs with Pasta	1 pkg (290 g)	480	**210**	81
Tuna Noodle Casserole	1 pkg (283 g)	340	**130**	41
Turkey Tetrazzini	1 pkg (283 g)	360	**150**	63
Veal Parmigiana (Homestyle)	1 pkg (329 g)	430	**150**	45
Vegetable Lasagna	1 pkg (297 g)	440	**180**	54
Welsh Rarebit	¼ cup (62 g)	120	**80**	36

FROZEN, MICROWAVE, AND REFRIGERATED FOODS

		CALORIES		
FOOD	AMOUNT	TOTAL	FAT	SAT-FAT
Stouffer's Family Style Favorites				
Lasagna with Meat Sauce	1 cup (215 g)	270	**80**	41
Macaroni & Cheese	1 cup (255 g)	380	**150**	72
Stouffer's Hearty Portions				
Beef Pot Roast	1 pkg (453 g)	430	**160**	63
Country Fried Beef Steak	1 pkg (453 g)	750	**370**	117
Pork with Roasted Potatoes	1 pkg (453 g)	570	**140**	45
Roast Beef	1 pkg (453 g)	430	**160**	54
Salisbury Steak	1 pkg (453 g)	630	**260**	117
Sliced Turkey Breast	1 pkg (453 g)	570	**240**	63
Swanson Classic Mac & More				
Macaroni & Cheese	1 pkg (170 g)	240	**80**	36
Swanson Dinners				
Beef Pot Pie	1 pkg (198 g)	415	**210**	81
Boneless Pork Rib	1 pkg (298 g)	470	**170**	63
Chicken Nuggets	1 pkg (284 g)	590	**230**	63
Chicken Pot Pie	1 pie (198 g)	410	**200**	81
Country Fried Beef Steak	1 pkg (305 g)	460	**200**	90
Fish 'n Chips	1 pkg (284 g)	490	**180**	36
Fried Chicken				
Dark Portions	1 pkg (312 g)	580	**270**	90
White Portions	1 pkg (312 g)	630	**280**	72
Meatloaf	1 pkg (305 g)	380	**130**	54
Salisbury Steak	1 pkg (312 g)	340	**140**	54
Sirloin Beef Tips	1 pkg (447 g)	450	**140**	NA
Turkey (Mostly White Meat)	1 pkg (333 g)	320	**70**	27
Turkey Pot Pie	1 pie (198 g)	400	**190**	72
Veal Parmigiana	1 pkg (319 g)	390	**160**	72
Yankee Pot Roast	1 pkg (326 g)	250	**40**	14
Swanson Hungry Man				
Beef Pot Pie	1 pkg (397 g)	660	**299**	117
Boneless Chicken	1 pkg (489 g)	630	**200**	54
Boneless Pork Rib	1 pkg (400 g)	770	**340**	117
Chicken Pot Pie	1 pkg (397 g)	650	**320**	126
Country Fried Beef Steak	1 pkg (454 g)	660	**300**	126
Fisherman's Platter	1 pkg (368 g)	650	**230**	54
Fried Chicken (Mostly White Meat)	1 pkg (439 g)	800	**350**	99
Salisbury Steak	1 pkg (461 g)	610	**310**	153
Traditional Pot Roast	1 pkg (454 g)	360	**50**	18
Turkey (Mostly White Meat)	1 pkg (475 g)	510	**130**	36
Turkey Pot Pie	1 pkg (397 g)	650	**310**	117
Taj Gourmet				
Bean Masala	1 pkg (342 g)	330	**50**	5
Chicken Korma	1 pkg (312 g)	330	**80**	18
Chicken Tikka Masala	1 pkg (312 g)	330	**80**	27

FROZEN, MICROWAVE, AND REFRIGERATED FOODS

FOOD	AMOUNT	CALORIES		
		TOTAL	FAT	SAT-FAT
Taj Gourmet (cont.)				
Dal Bahaar	1 pkg (342 g)	330	60	5
Palak Paneer	1 pkg (342 g)	320	60	27
Vegetable Korma	1 pkg (342 g)	300	50	9
Tyson				
Beef Fajitas	3½ fajitas (357 g)	480	120	36
Van De Kamp's				
Baked Breaded Fish Fillets	2 fillets (99 g)	150	25	5
Battered Fish Fillets	1 fillet (75 g)	180	100	14
Breaded Fish Fillets	2 fillets (99 g)	280	170	27
Breaded Fish Sticks	6 sticks (114 g)	290	150	23
Garlic & Herb Baked Breaded Fish Fillets	1 fillet (78 g)	150	45	9
Lemon Pepper Baked Breaded Fish Fillets	1 fillet (78 g)	140	45	9
Weight Watchers Smart Ones				
Angel Hair Pasta	1 entree (255 g)	180	20	0
Bowtie Pasta & Mushrooms Marsala	1 entree (273 g)	270	60	41
Broccoli and Cheese Baked Potato	1 entree (283 g)	250	50	36
Chicken Fettuccini	1 entree (283 g)	300	60	18
Creamy Rigatoni with Broccoli & Chicken	1 entree (255 g)	230	20	5
Fiesta Chicken	1 entree (241 g)	210	20	5
Grilled Salisbury Steak	1 entree (241 g)	250	80	36
Homestyle Macaroni & Cheese	1 entree (255 g)	290	60	27
Hunan Style Rice & Vegetables	1 entree (293 g)	280	70	18
Lasagna Florentine	1 entree (283 g)	200	20	0
Lemon Herb Chicken Piccata	1 entree (241 g)	200	20	5
Macaroni and Cheese	1 entree (255 g)	220	20	5
Pasta & Spinach Romano	1 entree (294 g)	260	70	27
Pasta with Tomato Basil Sauce	1 entree (272 g)	260	60	23
Penne Pasta with Sundried Tomatoes	1 entree (283 g)	280	70	45
Penne Pollo	1 entree (283 g)	290	50	27
Ravioli Florentine	1 entree (241 g)	220	20	5
Roast Turkey Medallions	1 entree (241 g)	180	20	5
Santa Fe Style Rice & Beans	1 entree (283 g)	290	70	36
Shrimp Marinara	1 entree (255 g)	180	20	5
Swedish Meatballs	1 entree (255 g)	300	90	36
Tuna Noodle Casserole	1 entree (269 g)	270	60	23
Yu Sing (Michelina's)				
Chicken Fried Rice	1 pkg (227 g)	360	70	14
Chicken Lo Mein	1 meal (227 g)	230	40	NA
Oriental Beef & Peppers	1 pkg (227 g)	290	60	23

FROZEN, MICROWAVE, AND REFRIGERATED FOODS

		CALORIES		
FOOD	AMOUNT	TOTAL	FAT	SAT-FAT
Yu Sing (Michelina's) (cont.)				
Shrimp Fried Rice	1 pkg (227 g)	360	50	5
Shrimp Lo Mein	1 pkg (227 g)	220	15	0
Sweet & Sour Chicken	1 pkg (241 g)	340	35	9
PIZZAS, FROZEN				
Amy's Pizza				
Cheese	⅓ pizza (123 g)	310	100	36
Spinach	⅓ pizza (132 g)	320	100	36
Vegetable, no cheese	⅓ pizza (113 g)	270	70	9
Celeste Pizza-for-One				
Cheese	1 pizza (170 g)	420	180	90
Deluxe	1 pizza (202 g)	470	220	81
Four Cheese				
Original	1 pizza (174 g)	480	240	99
Zesty	1 pizza (174 g)	470	210	108
Pepperoni	1 pizza (170 g)	470	240	81
Suprema	1 pizza (221 g)	530	260	90
Vegetable	1 pizza (187 g)	420	180	63
Di Giorno				
Four Cheese				
small	⅓ pizza (114 g)	280	90	45
large	⅙ pizza (139 g)	330	100	54
Pepperoni				
small	⅓ pizza (120 g)	320	120	54
large	⅙ pizza (148 g)	390	150	63
Spinach, Mushroom & Garlic	⅓ pizza (125 g)	270	80	36
Supreme	⅙ pizza (165 g)	400	150	63
Fox De Luxe				
Sausage & Pepperoni	1 pizza (184 g)	460	160	45
Healthy Choice French Bread Pizza				
Cheese	1 pizza (170 g)	340	45	14
Pepperoni	1 pizza (170 g)	340	45	14
Supreme	1 pizza (180 g)	330	45	14
Vegetable	1 pizza (170 g)	280	35	14
Hot Pockets				
Pizza Mini's				
Double Cheese	6 pieces (85 g)	240	80	36
Pepperoni	6 pieces (85 g)	250	100	36
Sausage & Pepperoni	6 pieces (85 g)	230	80	27
Pizza snacks				
Pepperoni	6 pieces (85 g)	220	70	31
Toaster Breaks Pizza				
Double Cheese	1 piece (60 g)	190	80	27
Pepperoni	1 piece (60 g)	200	90	31
Jeno's Crisp 'n Tasty Pizza				
Chompin' Cheese	1 pizza (195 g)	460	170	54

FROZEN, MICROWAVE, AND REFRIGERATED FOODS

FOOD	AMOUNT	CALORIES		
		TOTAL	FAT	SAT-FAT
Jeno's Crisp 'n Tasty Pizza (cont.)				
Crazy Combination (Sausage				
& Pepperoni)	1 pizza (198 g)	520	250	63
Power Pepperoni	1 pizza (192 g)	510	240	54
Lean Cuisine French Bread Pizza				
Deluxe	1 pkg (173 g)	300	50	23
Pepperoni	1 pkg (148 g)	310	60	27
Mama Celeste				
Four Cheese	⅙ pizza (140 g)	340	90	41
Pepperoni	⅙ pizza (142 g)	380	140	63
Supreme	⅙ pizza (157 g)	380	150	63
McCain Ellio's				
Cheese	1 slice (75 g)	160	45	18
Ore Ida Bagel Bites				
Cheese & Pepperoni	4 pieces (88 g)	200	60	31
Cheese, Sausage & Pep-				
peroni	4 pieces (88 g)	190	60	32
Three Cheese	4 pieces (88 g)	190	50	31
Red Baron Deep Dish Singles Pizzas				
Cheese	1 pizza (168 g)	500	230	90
Pepperoni	1 pizza (168 g)	540	280	99
Supreme	1 pizza (168 g)	490	240	90
Safeway Select Gourmet Club				
French Bread Pepperoni Pizza	1 pizza (85 g)	230	90	36
Stouffer's French Bread Pizza				
Cheese	1 pizza (147 g)	370	150	54
Deluxe	1 pizza (175 g)	420	160	63
Extra Cheese	1 pizza (167 g)	400	140	63
Five Cheese	1 pizza (147 g)	370	150	54
Grilled Vegetable	1 pizza (165 g)	350	100	45
Pepperoni	1 pizza (159 g)	390	140	54
Pepperoni & Mushroom	1 pizza (174 g)	440	170	63
Sausage & Pepperoni	1 pizza (177 g)	470	200	72
Three Meat (sausage, pep-				
peroni, bacon)	1 pizza (177 g)	470	200	72
Tombstone				
Light				
Vegetable	⅕ pizza (131 g)	240	60	23
Original				
Pepperoni	¼ pizza (152 g)	400	190	81
Supreme	⅕ pizza (130 g)	320	140	63
Thin Crust				
Four Meat Combination	¼ pizza (143 g)	380	200	90
Pepperoni	¼ pizza (138 g)	400	230	99
Tombstone for One Deep Dish Pizza				
Cheese	1 pizza (177 g)	470	190	108
Pepperoni	1 pizza (177 g)	510	240	117

FROZEN, MICROWAVE, AND REFRIGERATED FOODS

		CALORIES		
FOOD	AMOUNT	TOTAL	FAT	SAT-FAT
Totino's Party Pizza				
Pepperoni	½ pizza (145 g)	380	**190**	45
Supreme	½ pizza (155 g)	390	**190**	41
Totino's Pizza Rolls				
Cheese	6 rolls (85 g)	210	**70**	27
Combination (Sausage & Pepperoni)	6 rolls (85 g)	220	**100**	27
Pepperoni	6 rolls (85 g)	240	**110**	27
Pepperoni Supreme	6 rolls (85 g)	230	**100**	23
Supreme	6 rolls (85 g)	220	**90**	18
Wolfgang Puck's Pizza				
Artichoke Heart	½ pizza (140 g)	340	**150**	54
Barbecue Chicken	½ pizza (150 g)	340	**100**	45
Four Cheese	½ pizza (130 g)	360	**130**	54
Pepperoni Mushroom	½ pizza (155 g)	390	**130**	54
Zucchini & Tomato	½ pizza (146 g)	290	**100**	45
POULTRY				
Perdue				
Breaded Chicken Breast Cutlets				
Homestyle	84 g	120	**15**	0
Italian Style	84 g	130	**25**	9
Breaded Chicken Breast Nuggets	5 pieces (93 g)	200	**110**	27
Breaded Chicken Breast Tenderloins	84 g	160	**60**	23
Swift Premium Turkey Roast				
Boneless White Turkey	5 oz (40 g)	160	**80**	27
White & Dark Turkey	5 oz (40 g)	190	**110**	41
Tyson				
Barbecue Style Chicken Wings	3 pieces (91 g)	200	**110**	31
Breaded Chicken Breast Fillets	2 fillets (81 g)	180	**70**	14
Breaded Chicken Breast Patties	1 patty (73 g)	190	**110**	27
fat free	1 patty (74 g)	80	**0**	0
Breaded Chicken Breast Tenders	3 tenders (92 g)	100	**0**	0
Chicken Fajitas	3½ fajitas (374 g)	460	**100**	27
Hot 'n Spicy Chicken Wings	4 pcs (96 g)	220	**130**	31
Mandarin Sesame Wraps	1½ wraps (416 g)	630	**140**	31
Wamplers				
100% Pure Ground Chicken	4 oz (112 g)	220	**120**	36
100% Pure Ground Turkey	4 oz (112 g)	210	**130**	27
100% Pure Turkey Burgers	1 burger (112 g)	210	**130**	27
Turkey Mignons	1 mignon (142 g)	230	**110**	45

FROZEN, MICROWAVE, AND REFRIGERATED FOODS

FOOD	AMOUNT	CALORIES TOTAL	FAT	SAT-FAT
SANDWICHES				
Amy's in a Pocket Sandwich				
Spinach Feta	1 (128 g)	200	**60**	27
Vegetable·Pie	1 (142 g)	230	**60**	5
Banquet Hot Sandwich Toppers				
Creamed Chipped Beef	1 bag (113 g)	120	**50**	23
Gravy & Salisbury Steak	1 bag (141 g)	210	**140**	63
Gravy & Sliced Beef	1 bag (113 g)	70	**20**	9
Gravy & Sliced Turkey	1 bag (141 g)	160	**100**	36
Bob Evans Farms				
Sausage & Biscuit	2 sandwiches (112 g)	370	**210**	63
Chef America				
Croissant Pockets				
Chicken, Broccoli & Cheddar	1 piece (128 g)	290	**80**	36
Egg, Sausage & Cheese	1 piece (128 g)	340	**130**	54
Ham & Cheese	1 piece (128 g)	320	**110**	54
Pepperoni Pizza	1 piece (128 g)	360	**140**	63
Turkey & Ham with Swiss	1 piece (128 g)	290	**90**	36
Hot Pockets				
Beef & Cheddar	1 piece (128 g)	350	**150**	81
Beef with Barbecue	1 piece (128 g)	340	**110**	45
Chicken & Cheddar with Broccoli	1 piece (128 g)	300	**90**	45
Meatballs with Mozzarella	1 piece (128 g)	320	**100**	54
Pepperoni & Sausage Pizza	1 piece (128 g)	330	**120**	54
Pepperoni Pizza	1 piece (128 g)	360	**140**	63
Lean Pockets				
Chicken Broccoli Supreme	1 piece (128 g)	260	**60**	27
Chicken Fajita	1 piece (128 g)	270	**60**	23
Chicken Parmesan	1 piece (128 g)	280	**60**	23
Ham & Cheddar	1 piece (128 g)	280	**70**	27
Pepperoni Pizza Deluxe (reduced fat)	1 piece (128 g)	270	**60**	23
Philly Steak & Cheese	1 piece (128 g)	260	**60**	27
Turkey, Broccoli & Cheese	1 piece (128 g)	250	**60**	27
Toaster Breaks Melts				
Ham & Cheese	1 piece (61 g)	180	**80**	23
Veggie Pockets				
Bar-B-Q Style	1 pocket (127 g)	290	**80**	5
Broccoli & Cheddar Style	1 pocket (127 g)	290	**80**	5
Greek Style	1 pocket (127 g)	250	**80**	5
Indian Style	1 pocket (127 g)	260	**80**	5
Oriental Style	1 pocket (127 g)	250	**80**	5
Pizza Style	1 pocket (127 g)	270	**80**	5
Tex-Mex Style	1 pocket (127 g)	280	**80**	5
Veggie Burger	1 sandwich (71 g)	130	**10**	0

FROZEN, MICROWAVE, AND REFRIGERATED FOODS

		CALORIES		
FOOD	AMOUNT	TOTAL	FAT	SAT-FAT
Gardenburger Veggie Patties				
Fire Roasted Vegetable	1 patty (71 g)	120	25	14
Gardenburger with cheese	1 patty (71 g)	110	25	14
Savory Mushroom	1 patty (71 g)	120	25	14
The Original	1 patty (71 g)	130	25	9
Veggie Medley	1 patty (71 g)	100	0	0
Green Giant Harvest Burgers				
Original flavor	1 patty (90 g)	140	35	14
Healthy Choice Hearty Handfuls				
Chicken & Broccoli	1 hearty handful (173 g)	320	50	14
Chicken & Mushrooms	1 hearty handful (173 g)	310	45	14
Garlic Chicken	1 hearty handful (173 g)	330	45	14
Ham & Cheese	1 hearty handful (173 g)	320	45	14
Italian Style Meatball	1 hearty handful (173 g)	320	45	14
Philly Beef Steak	1 hearty handful (173 g)	290	45	14
Jimmie Dean				
Bacon, Egg, & Cheese on a Biscuit	1 sandwich (102 g)	300	150	54
Sausage, Egg, & Cheese on a Biscuit	1 sandwich (128 g)	390	240	90
Sausage Biscuits	2 sandwiches (113 g)	390	220	72
Morningstar Farms				
Better 'n Burgers	1 patty (78 g)	70	0	0
Chik Nuggets	4 nuggets (86 g)	160	40	5
Chik Patties	1 patty (71 g)	150	50	9
Garden Veggie Patties	1 patty (67 g)	100	25	5
Spicy Black Bean	1 patty (78 g)	110	10	0
Veggie Dogs	1 link (57 g)	80	5	0
Quaker Maid				
Italian Meatball Sandwich	1 (170 g)	460	220	90
Philly Cheese Steak	1 sandwich (170 g)	400	80	36
Pure Beef Sandwich Steak	1 steak (56 g)	170	130	54
Safeway Stuffed Sandwiches				
Barbecue Beef	1 piece (127 g)	310	120	23
Ham & Cheese	1 piece (128 g)	320	140	54
Lean Turkey, Broccoli & Cheddar	1 piece (128 g)	240	60	18
Pepperoni Pizza	1 piece (128 g)	370	170	63
Steak-umm				
100% All Beef Sandwich Steaks	1 steak, raw (57 g)	190	150	63

FROZEN, MICROWAVE, AND REFRIGERATED FOODS

FOOD	AMOUNT	CALORIES		
		TOTAL	FAT	SAT-FAT
Steak-umm (cont.)				
Reduced Fat Real Beef				
Sandwich Steaks	1 steak, raw (57 g)	110	**63**	18,
Sandwich to Go Cheese Steak	1 sandwich (133 g)	290	**120**	54
Tennessee Pride				
Sausage & Buttermilk Biscuit	2 sandwiches (91 g)	320	**180**	63
Sausage & Egg with Cheese				
Biscuit	2 sandwiches (125 g)	400	**230**	81
Weight Watchers Sandwiches				
English Muffin with Ham &				
Cheese	1 sandwich (113 g)	210	**50**	27
White Castle				
Cheeseburger	2 sandwiches (104 g)	310	**160**	81
Hamburger	2 sandwiches (90 g)	270	**130**	54
VEGETABLES AND SIDE DISHES (*see also* **VEGETABLES**)				
Birds Eye Side Orders				
Bavarian Style Vegetables	1 cup (156 g)	150	**70**	36
French Green Beans with				
Toasted Almonds	¾ cup (116 g)	80	**35**	0
New England Style Vegetables	1 pkg (255 g)	260	**130**	45
Peas & Pearl Onions	⅔ cup (121 g)	90	**5**	0
Budget Gourmet				
Cheddared Potatoes &				
Broccoli	1 pkg (141 g)	160	**70**	54
Oriental Rice with Vegetables	1 pkg (148 g)	200	**100**	41
Rice Pilaf with Green Beans	1 pkg (141 g)	220	**90**	27
Spinach au Gratin	1 pkg (141 g)	160	**110**	63
Green Giant				
Alfredo Vegetables	¾ cup (109 g)	80	**25**	14
Broccoli & Cheese	⅔ cup (112 g)	70	**25**	9
Cheesy Rice & Broccoli	1 pkg (283 g)	300	**45**	14
Creamed Spinach	½ cup (109 g)	80	**25**	14
Cut Leaf Spinach in Butter				
Sauce	½ cup (98 g)	40	**15**	9
Green Bean Casserole	⅔ cup (109 g)	90	**45**	9
Rice Pilaf	1 pkg (283 g)	260	**25**	14
Shoepeg White Corn & Butter	¾ cup (112 g)	120	**25**	14
Southwestern Style Corn &				
Roasted Red Peppers	¾ cup (99 g)	90	**10**	0
Teriyaki Vegetables	1¼ cup (110 g)	100	**60**	9
Vegetable Medley & Butter	¾ cup (103 g)	60	**20**	14
White & Wild Rice	1 pkg (283 g)	280	**50**	9
Ore Ida				
Country Style Hash Browns	1¼ cup (91 g)	80	**0**	0
Country Style Potato Wedges	13 pieces (84 g)	120	**40**	5

FROZEN, MICROWAVE, AND REFRIGERATED FOODS

		CALORIES		
FOOD	AMOUNT	TOTAL	FAT	SAT-FAT
Ore Ida (cont.)				
Country Style Steak Fries	8 pieces (84 g)	110	30	0
Crispers	17 fries (84 g)	220	110	18
Golden Crinkles	14 pieces (84 g)	120	30	9
Golden Fries	16 pieces (84 g)	120	35	5
Golden Patties Shredded				
Potatoes	1 patty (71 g)	140	70	14
Mashed Potatoes	⅔ cup (69 g)	90	20	0
Mini Tater Tots	19 pieces (84 g)	180	90	18
Onion Ringers	6 rings (88 g)	210	100	14
Onion Rings	4 pieces (84 g)	220	100	18
Oven Chips	7 pieces (84 g)	180	70	9
Potato Wedges with skins	8 pieces (84 g)	110	25	5
Shoestrings	44 pieces (84 g)	150	50	9
Tater Tots	9 pieces (86 g)	150	60	14
Toaster Hash Browns	2 patties (99 g)	190	90	18
Topped Baked Potatoes,				
Broccoli & Cheese	½ baker (159 g)	160	35	18
Twice Baked Potatoes				
Cheddar cheese	1 piece (141 g)	190	70	18
Sour cream & chives	1 piece (141 g)	190	60	14
Safeway Select Side Dish				
BBQ Beans	½ cup	200	15	5
Cheddar Cheese & Bacon				
Mashed Potatoes	⅔ cup	190	90	54
Creamed Spinach	½ cup	130	90	54
Roasted Garlic Mashed				
Potatoes	⅔ cup	110	40	27
Stouffer's				
Creamed Spinach	½ cup (125 g)	180	100	63
Corn Souffle	½ cup (125 g)	170	60	18
Spinach Soufflé	½ cup (118 g)	140	80	18

FRUITS AND FRUIT JUICES

		CALORIES		
FOOD	AMOUNT	TOTAL	FAT	SAT-FAT
Apple				
fresh	1	81	0	0
cooked, boiled	½ cup slices	46	0	0
canned, sweetened	½ cup slices	68	0	0
Apple butter	1 tbsp	35	0	0
Apple juice	1 cup	116	0	0

FRUITS AND FRUIT JUICES

FOOD	AMOUNT	CALORIES		
		TOTAL	FAT	SAT-FAT
Applesauce				
unsweetened	½ cup	53	0	0
sweetened	½ cup	97	0	0
Apricot	3	51	0	0
dried, uncooked	10 halves	83	0	0
	1 cup halves	310	0	0
dried, cooked	1 cup halves	211	0	0
Avocado, fresh				
California	1	306	270	41
Florida	1	339	243	48
Banana, fresh	1	105	5	2
Blackberries, fresh	½ cup	37	0	0
Blueberries, fresh	1 cup	82	0	0
Boysenberries, canned, heavy syrup	½ cup	113	0	0
Cantaloupe, fresh	½ fruit	94	0	0
	1 cup cubes	57	0	0
Cherries, sour, red, fresh	1 cup with pits	51	0	0
canned, light syrup	½ cup	94	0	0
canned, heavy syrup	½ cup	116	0	0
Cherries, sweet, fresh	10	49	0	0
	1 cup	104	0	0
canned, light syrup	½ cup	85	0	0
canned, heavy syrup	½ cup	107	0	0
Cranberries, fresh	1 cup whole	46	0	0
dried cranberries	⅓ cup	130	0	0
Cranberry juice cocktail	1 cup	147	0	0
Cranberry sauce	½ cup	209	0	0
Dates	5–6 pitted dates	120	0	0
	1 cup chopped	489	7	3
Figs, fresh	1 medium	37	0	0
	1 large	47	0	0
dried, uncooked	2	150	0	0
	1 cup	508	21	4
dried, cooked	1 cup	279	11	2
Fruit cocktail, canned				
juice pack	1 cup	113	0	0
light syrup pack	1 cup	110	0	0
heavy syrup pack	1 cup	186	0	0
Grapefruit, fresh	½ fruit	38	0	0
	1 cup sections	74	0	0
Grapefruit juice				
fresh	4 oz	47	0	0
canned, unsweetened	4 oz	47	0	0
canned, sweetened	4 oz	57	0	0
Grapes, fresh	10	15	0	0
	1 cup	58	0	0

FRUITS AND FRUIT JUICES

| FOOD | AMOUNT | CALORIES | | |
		TOTAL	FAT	SAT-FAT
Grape juice, canned or bottled	1 cup	155	0	0
Guava, fresh	1	45	0	0
Honeydew melon	⅟₁₀ melon	46	0	0
	1 cup cubes	60	0	0
Kiwi, fresh	1 medium	46	0	0
	1 large	55	0	0
Kumquat, fresh	1	12	0	0
Lemon, fresh	1 medium	17	0	0
	1 large	25	0	0
Lemon juice	1 tbsp	4	0	0
	1 cup	60	0	0
Lime, fresh	1	20	0	0
Lime juice	1 tbsp	4	0	0
	1 cup	66	0	0
Mango, fresh	1	135	0	0
	1 cup slices	108	0	0
Mixed fruit, dried	11 oz package	712	13	0
Mulberries, fresh	10	7	0	0
	1 cup	61	0	0
Nectarine, fresh	1	67	0	0
	1 cup slices	68	0	0
Orange, fresh	1	60	0	0
Orange juice	juice from 1 fruit	39	0	0
	1 cup	111	0	0
Papaya, fresh	1	117	0	0
	1 cup cubes	54	0	0
Peaches, fresh	1	37	0	0
canned in juice	1 cup halves	109	0	0
canned in light syrup	1 cup halves	136	0	0
canned in heavy syrup	1 cup halves	190	0	0
dried, uncooked	10 halves	311	9	1
	1 cup halves	383	11	1
dried, cooked	1 cup halves	198	6	1
Pears, fresh	1	98	0	0
canned in juice	1 cup halves	123	0	0
canned in light syrup	1 cup halves	144	0	0
canned in heavy syrup	1 cup halves	188	0	0
dried, uncooked	10 halves	459	10	1
	1 cup halves	472	10	1
dried, cooked	1 cup halves	325	7	0
Pineapple, fresh	1 slice (¾" thick)	42	0	0
	1 cup diced pieces	77	0	0
canned in juice	1 cup chunks	150	0	0
canned in light syrup	1 cup	131	0	0
canned in heavy syrup	1 cup	199	0	0

FRUITS AND FRUIT JUICES

| FOOD | AMOUNT | CALORIES | | |
		TOTAL	FAT	SAT-FAT
Pineapple juice	1 cup	139	0	0
Plantain, fresh	1	218	6	0
cooked	1 cup slices	179	3	0
Plums, fresh	1	36	0	0
	1 cup slices	91	0	0
Prunes				
canned in heavy syrup	5 fruits	90	0	0
	1 cup	245	0	0
dried, uncooked	10 fruits	201	0	0
	1 cup	385	7	0
dried, cooked	1 cup	227	4	0
Prune juice	1 cup	181	0	0
Raisins, seedless	1 cup packed	494	7	0
Raspberries, fresh	1 cup	61	0	0
Rhubarb, fresh	1 cup diced pieces	26	0	0
Strawberries, fresh	1 cup	45	0	0
canned in heavy syrup	1 cup	234	0	0
Tangerine, fresh	1	37	0	0
	1 cup sections	86	0	0
Watermelon, fresh	1 cup diced pieces	50	0	0

GRAINS AND PASTA

| FOOD | AMOUNT | CALORIES | | |
		TOTAL	FAT	SAT-FAT
BREAD				
Bagels				
Freshly baked, grocery				
Blueberry	1 (114 g)	280	10	0
Bran	1 (114 g)	260	10	0
Cinnamon Raisin	1 (114 g)	280	10	0
Combination	1 (114 g)	280	15	0
Garlic	1 (114 g)	270	10	0
Honey Wheat	1 (114 g)	260	10	0
Oat Bran	1 (114 g)	270	10	0
Onion	1 (114 g)	270	10	0
Plain	1 (114 g)	270	10	0
Poppy Seed	1 (114 g)	280	20	0
Pumpernickel	1 (114 g)	260	10	0
Raisin Bran	1 (114 g)	260	10	0
Rye	1 (114 g)	270	10	0
Sesame Seed	1 (114 g)	280	20	0
Sourdough	1 (114 g)	280	10	0

GRAINS AND PASTA

		CALORIES		
FOOD	**AMOUNT**	**TOTAL**	**FAT**	**SAT-FAT**
Bagels (cont.)				
Frozen				
Lenders				
Bagelettes	2 (25 g)	140	10	0
Big 'n Crusty				
Cinnamon Raisin	1 (85 g)	230	15	0
Plain or Onion	1 (85 g)	230	10	0
Blueberry Swirl or	1 (57 g)			
Cinnamon Swirl		160	5	0
Onion or Egg	1 (57 g)	160	15	0
Plain	1 (57 g)	150	5	0
Soft	1 (71 g)	210	30	0
Sara Lee				
Cinnamon & Raisin	1 (79 g)	220	5	0
Oat bran or poppy seed	1 (79 g)	210	10	0
Plain	1 (79 g)	210	0	0
Bialy	1 (110 g)	270	15	0
Biscuits (*see also* **FAST FOODS**)				
Beaten Biscuits	2" biscuit	98	60	24
Pillsbury Ready-to-Bake				
Big Country				
Butter Tastin'	1 biscuit (34 g)	100	35	9
Buttermilk	1 biscuit (34 g)	100	35	9
Grands!				
Golden Wheat	1 biscuit (61 g)	200	70	18
Butter Tastin' Biscuits	1 biscuit (61 g)	200	90	23
Buttermilk Biscuits	1 biscuit (61 g)	200	90	27
Golden Corn	1 biscuit (61 g)	210	90	23
Flaky Biscuits	1 biscuit (61 g)	200	80	18
Southern Style Biscuits	1 biscuit (61 g)	200	90	23
Biscuit Baking Mix (Jiffy)	¼ cup mix (32 g)	130	40	9
	baked	190	60	20
Bisquick All-Purpose Baking Mix (Betty Crocker)				
Biscuits, Pancakes	⅓ cup mix (40 g)	170	50	14
reduced fat	⅓ cup mix (40 g)	150	25	5
Buttermilk Biscuit Mix				
(Washington)	5 tbsp mix (40 g)	160	45	14
Hungry Jack				
Butter Tastin' or				
Buttermilk	1 biscuit (34 g)	100	40	9
Bran'nola	1 slice (38 g)	100	15	0
Country Oat	1 slice (38 g)	90	25	5
Bread Crumbs				
Cracker Meal (OTC)	¼ cup (28 g)	110	0	0
Italian Style	¼ cup (28 g)	110	15	0
Plain	¼ cup (28 g)	100	15	0

GRAINS AND PASTA

FOOD	AMOUNT	CALORIES		
		TOTAL	FAT	SAT-FAT
Bread Crumbs (cont.)				
Kellogg's Corn Flake Crumbs	2 tbsp (11 g)	40	0	0
Oven Fry				
Extra Crispy Chicken	⅛ packet (15 g) (coats 1 piece)	60	10	0
Extra Crispy Pork	⅛ pkt (15 g) (coats 1 chop)	60	10	0
Shake 'n Bake				
Barbecue Chicken Glaze	⅛ packet (12 g) (coats 1–2 pieces)	45	10	0
Buffalo Wings	¹⁄₁₀ pkg (10 g) (coats 2 pieces)	40	5	0
Honey Mustard Chicken Glaze	¼ packet (25 g) (coats 2 pieces)	100	20	9
Hot & Spicy Chicken or Pork coating	⅛ pkg (10 g) (coats 1 piece)	40	10	0
Pork Original Recipe	⅛ packet (11 g) (coats 1 chop)	40	0	0
Tangy Honey Glaze	¼ packet (25 g) (coats 2 pieces)	90	15	5
Bread Mixes				
Bread Machine				
Dromedary				
Country White	½ inch (50 g)	140	10	5
Italian Herb	½ inch (50 g)	140	20	14
Sourdough	½ inch (50 g)	140	15	9
Stoneground Wheat	½ inch (50 g)	140	15	9
Pillsbury				
Cracked Wheat	¹⁄₁₂ pkg (36 g)	130	20	0
Crusty White	¹⁄₁₂ pkg (36 g)	130	15	0
Brown Bread Raisin, New England Style (B & M)	½" slice (56 g)	130	5	0
	baked with water & 2 eggs	70	35	14
Hot Roll Mix (Pillsbury)	1 pan roll (28 g)	100	10	0
Quick Mix (Pillsbury)				
Apple Cinnamon	¹⁄₁₂ loaf (37 g mix)	140	10	0
Banana	¹⁄₁₂ loaf (33 g mix)	120	10	0
Spoon Bread Mix (Washington)	2 tbsp mix (13 g)	60	30	9
Bread Sticks				
(Stella D'Oro)	1 stick (9 g)	40	10	0
Grissini-Style fat free (Stella D'Oro)	3 sticks (15 g)	60	0	0
Italian (Angonoa's)	3 sticks (15 g)	60	10	0
Mini Sesame (Angonoa's)	24 sticks (28 g)	130	35	5
Sesame (Stella D'Oro)	1 stick (11 g)	50	20	0

GRAINS AND PASTA

FOOD	AMOUNT	CALORIES TOTAL	FAT	SAT-FAT
Bread Sticks (cont.)				
Sesame	4 sticks (28 g)	130	35	5
Soft (Bread Du Jour)	1 stick (53 g)	130	10	0
Soft (Pillsbury)	1 stick (39 g)	110	25	5
Soft, Cheese	1 stick (28 g)	80	20	9
Bread Stick Mixes				
Pillsbury				
Breadsticks	1 stick (39 g)	110	20	0
Garlic Breadsticks	2 sticks (60 g)	180	60	14
Bread Stuffing				
Arnold				
Cornbread	2 cups (67 g)	250	35	9
Seasoned	2 cups (67 g)	250	30	5
Pepperidge Farm Top of Stove Stuffing Mix				
Apple & Raisin	½ cup (36 g)	140	15	0
Corn Bread	¾ cup (43 g)	170	20	0
Country Garden Herb	½ cup (34 g)	150	45	9
Herb Seasoned Stuffing	¾ cup (43 g)	170	15	0
Cubed	¾ cup (37 g)	140	15	0
Honey Pecan	½ cup (34 g)	140	45	5
Pepperidge Farm Crunchy Croutons				
Cheese & Garlic	9 croutons (7 g)	35	15	0
Onion & Garlic	9 croutons (7 g)	30	15	0
Seasoned	9 croutons (7 g)	35	15	0
Ritz Stuffing Mix	⅔ cup (38 g)	200	80	18
Stove Top Stuffing Mix (Kraft)				
Cornbread	⅙ box (28 g)	110	5	0
	½ cup prep.	170	80	18
for Chicken	½ cup dry (28 g)	120	25	0
	½ cup prep.	170	80	14
lower sodium	⅙ box (28 g)	110	10	0
	½ cup prep.	180	80	14
for Pork	⅙ box (28 g)	110	10	0
	½ cup prep.	170	80	18
for Turkey	⅙ box (28 g)	110	10	0
	½ cup prep.	170	80	18
Savory Herbs	⅙ box (28 g)	110	10	0
	½ cup prep.	170	80	14
Wild Rice & Mushroom	⅔ cup (37 g)	170	50	14
Challah	1" slice (50 g)	160	35	9
Cocktail				
Rye or pumpernickel	3 slices (31 g)	80	10	0
Corn Bread	⅛ of 8" diameter	225	77	22
	3" x 4.5"	325	100	35
	2" x 2"	104	57	28
Crackling Corn Bread	⅛ of 8" diameter	263	150	55

GRAINS AND PASTA

FOOD	AMOUNT	CALORIES		
		TOTAL	FAT	SAT-FAT
Corn Bread Mixes				
Buttermilk Corn Bread Mix				
(Washington)	3 tbsp (25 g)	90	15	5
	baked with whole			
	milk & 1 egg	110	30	14
Corn Bread mix (Aunt				
Jemima)	⅓ cup mix (35 g)	140	35	9
	as prepared	160	45	11
Corn Bread Mix (Marie				
Callender's)	¼ cup mix (66 g)	150	30	0
Cornbread Twists (Pillsbury)	1 twist (41 g)	130	50	14
Cracked Wheat Bread				
Pepperidge Farm	1 slice (25 g)	70	10	0
Croissant				
Almond Filled	1 (98 g)	430	280	36
Apple Filled	1 (110 g)	290	150	27
Butter	1 (55 g)	200	100	63
Butter (Vie-de-France)	1 (56 g)	230	110	72
Cheese Filled	1 (104 g)	380	250	81
Cherry Filled	1 (110 g)	330	140	27
Chocolate Filled	1 (91 g)	350	180	36
Margarine	1 (70 g)	260	140	27
Croissant Mixes				
Pillsbury				
Original Crescent	1 roll (28 g)	110	50	14
reduced fat	1 roll (28 g)	100	40	9
Croutons				
Pepperidge Farm	2 tbsp (7 g)	30	10	0
English Muffins				
Thomas	1 (57 g)	120	10	0
Bran'nola (Arnolds)	1 (66 g)	130	15	0
Raisin	1 (61 g)	140	10	0
Raisin (Sun Maid)	1 (68 g)	160	10	0
Flatbread (New York)				
low fat				
all flavors	1 piece (11 g)	50	15	5
fat free				
Roasted Garlic	1 piece (11 g)	40	0	0
Mini's				
Low fat	3 pieces (13 g)	58	17	0
Fat free	3 pieces (13 g)	45	0	0
French Bread	1 slice (2")	130	0	0
French Loaf (Bread Du Jour)	3" slice (56 g)	130	10	0
Crusty French Loaf				
(Pillsbury)	⅕ loaf (62 g)	150	10	0
French Loaf Mix (Pillsbury)	⅕ pkg (62 g)	150	20	9

GRAINS AND PASTA

| FOOD | AMOUNT | CALORIES | | |
		TOTAL	FAT	SAT-FAT
French Toast (see also **FROZEN, MICROWAVE, AND REFRIGERATED FOODS**)				
Garlic Bread	3½" slice (56 g)	190	80	14
with cheese	3½" slice (56 g)	180	60	14
Italian Bread	1¼" slice (46 g)	130	10	0
Pepperidge Farm	2" slice (57 g)	150	20	9
Italian Bread Shell (Boboli)	⅕ shell (57 g)	150	30	9
Italian Olive Bread	2 slices (50 g)	150	30	5
Multi-grain Bread	1" slice (50 g)	160	20	NA
Oatmeal (Pepperidge Farm)	1 slice (25 g)	60	10	0
Soft (Pepperidge Farm)	1 slice (25 g)	60	5	NA
Pita				
White	1 (45 g)	110	5	0
Whole-wheat	1 (45 g)	110	5	0
Pizza Crusts				
Boboli				
Thin Pizza Crust	⅕ crust (57 g)	160	35	14
2 Pizza Crusts	½ crust (57 g)	150	30	9
Popover Mix, New England				
Style (Washington)	¼ cup mix (27 g)	110	25	9
	baked with water			
	& 2 eggs	140	40	14
Pumpernickel Bread	1 slice (32 g)	80	10	0
Raisin Bread (Pepperidge Farm)	1 slice (28 g)	80	10	0
Rolls				
Cinnamon rolls (Pillsbury)	1 roll (40 g)	140	45	14
Club (Pepperidge Farm)	1 (47 g)	120	10	5
Cornbread Twists (Pillsbury)	1 twist (41 g)	130	50	14
Dinner rolls				
Arnold	2 (38 g)	110	25	5
Country Style (Pepperidge Farm)	3 (57 g)	150	30	9
Crescent (Pillsbury)	2 (57 g)	200	100	23
Parker House (Pepperidge Farm)	3 (53 g)	150	40	14
Party (Pepperidge Farm)	5 (53 g)	170	40	14
Egg Twist	1 (47 g)	180	35	14
French (Pepperidge Farm)	½ roll (71 g)	180	20	5
Seven Grain (Pepperidge Farm)	1 (38 g)	80	20	0
Hamburger	1 (43 g)	130	20	9
Potato roll (Martins)	1 (53 g)	150	20	0
Hard rolls	1 (57 g)	160	10	5
Hoagie with sesame seeds (Pepperidge Farm)	1 (69 g)	200	40	23
Hot dog	1 (39 g)	110	20	5
Italian rolls (Bread Du Jour)	1 (35 g)	80	5	0

GRAINS AND PASTA

FOOD	AMOUNT	CALORIES		
		TOTAL	FAT	SAT-FAT
Rolls (cont.)				
Oat Bran	1 roll (52 g)	140	20	5
Pumpernickel	1 roll (57 g)	160	20	0
Sub rolls (8") (La Parisienne)	⅖ roll (50 g)	130	0	0
Wheat	1 roll (57 g)	190	25	5
White	1 (6" in diam)	150	10	0
Whole-wheat	1 (6" in diam)	180	10	0
Roll Mixes (refrigerated)				
Pillsbury				
Cinnamon Raisin Rolls with Icing	1 roll (49 g)	170	50	14
Cinnamon Rolls with Icing	1 roll (41 g)	150	45	14
reduced fat	1 roll (44 g)	140	30	9
Dinner Rolls	1 roll (40 g)	110	20	0
Grands!				
Cinnamon rolls with cream cheese icing	1 roll (99 g)	330	100	27
Cinnamon rolls with icing	1 roll (99 g)	320	90	23
reduced fat	1 roll (99 g)	300	60	18
Orange Sweet Rolls with Icing	1 roll (49 g)	170	60	14
Rye Bread				
Jewish	1 slice (32 g)	80	10	0
Seeded	1 slice (22 g)	55	9	5
Onion	1 slice (32 g)	80	10	0
Sunflower seed	1 slice (50 g)	120	7	0
Seven Grain Bread	1 slice (50 g)	120	18	0
Sicilian Bread	¼ loaf (57 g)	150	15	0
Sourdough Bread	1" slice (50 g)	130	10	0
Sourdough Boule (La Parisienne)	1 slice (57 g)	120	10	0
Spoon Bread	1 slice	325	185	100
Tortillas				
Corn	1 tortilla (28 g)	60	0	0
Flour	1 tortilla (35 g)	110	25	0
White Bread	1 slice (25-27 g)	65-80	8-15	0
Light White	1 slice (22 g)	40	5	0
Very Thin White (Pepperidge Farm)	1 slice (15 g)	37	5	0
Whole-wheat Bread				
Pepperidge Farm	1 slice (25 g)	60	10	0
Pepperidge Farm Soft	1 slice (25 g)	60	5	0
Stroehmann	1 slice (36 g)	80	15	0
Wonder	1 slice (34 g)	80	15	0
BREAKFAST CEREALS, COLD				
100% Bran	⅓ cup (29 g)	80	5	0
All-Bran, original	½ cup (31 g)	80	10	0

GRAINS AND PASTA

FOOD	AMOUNT	CALORIES		
		TOTAL	FAT	SAT-FAT
All-Bran, Extra Fiber	½ cup (26 g)	50	10	0
Alpha-Bits				
Frosted	1 cup (32 g)	130	10	0
Marshmallow	1 cup (29 g)	120	10	0
Apple Jacks	1 cup (33 g)	120	0	0
Amaranth	¾ cup (28 g)	100	0	0
Banana Nut Crunch	1 cup (59 g)	250	50	9
Basic 4	1 cup (55 g)	200	25	0
Berry Berry Kix	¾ cup (30 g)	120	10	0
Blueberry Morning	1¼ cups (55 g)	210	20	5
Bran, 100% Natural	¾ cup (49 g)	160	0	0
Bran, Health Fiber	¾ cup (28 g)	100	0	0
Cap'n Crunch	¾ cup (27 g)	110	15	5
Crunch Berries	¾ cup (26 g)	100	15	5
Peanut Butter Crunch	¾ cup (27 g)	110	25	5
Cheerios	1 cup (30 g)	110	15	0
Apple Cinnamon	¾ cup (30 g)	120	15	0
Frosted	1 cup (30 g)	120	0	0
Honey Nut	1 cup (30 g)	120	10	0
Multi-grain Plus	1 cup (30 g)	110	10	0
Cinnamon Grahams	¾ cup (30 g)	120	10	0
Cinnamon Toast Crunch	¾ cup (30 g)	130	30	5
Cocoa Frosted Flakes	¾ cup (31 g)	120	0	0
Cocoa Krispies	¾ cup (30 g)	120	10	5
Cocoa Pebbles	¾ cup (29 g)	120	10	9
Cocoa Puffs	1 cup (30 g)	120	10	0
Complete Bran Flakes	¾ cup (29 g)	90	5	0
Complete Oat Bran Flakes	¾ cup (30 g)	110	10	0
Complete Wheat Bran Flakes	¾ cup (29 g)	90	5	0
Cookie Crisp Chocolate Chip	1 cup (30 g)	120	10	0
Corn Chex	1 cup (30 g)	110	0	0
Corn Flakes	1 cup (28 g)	100	0	0
Corn Flakes Honey Crunch	¾ cup (30 g)	110	10	0
Corn Pops	1 cup (31 g)	120	0	0
Count Chocula	1 cup (30 g)	120	10	0
Cracklin' Oat Bran	¾ cup (49 g)	190	50	0
Crispix	1 cup (29 g)	110	0	0
Crispy Wheaties 'n Raisins	1 cup (55 g)	190	5	0
Crunchy Corn Bran	¾ cup (27 g)	90	10	0
Double Chex	1¼ cups (30 g)	120	0	0
Fiber One	½ cup (30 g)	60	10	0
French Toast Crunch	¾ cup (30 g)	120	10	0
Froot Loops	1 cup (32 g)	120	10	5
Frosted Flakes	¾ cup (31 g)	120	0	0
Frosted Mini-Wheats	5 biscuits (51 g)	180	10	0
Bite-size	1 cup (59 g)	200	10	0

GRAINS AND PASTA

FOOD	AMOUNT	CALORIES		
		TOTAL	FAT	SAT-FAT
Fruit & Fiber Peaches, Raisins & Almonds	1 cup (55 g)	210	25	5
Fruity Pebbles	¾ cup (27 g)	110	10	0
Golden Crisp	¾ cup (27 g)	110	0	0
Golden Grahams	¾ cup (30 g)	120	10	0
Granola, low-fat (Kellogg's)				
with raisins	⅔ cup (60 g)	220	30	9
without raisins	½ cup (49 g)	190	25	5
98% Fat Free	⅔ cup (55 g)	180	10	0
Grape Nuts	½ cup (58 g)	200	10	0
Grape Nuts Flakes	¾ cup (29 g)	100	10	0
Great Grains				
Crunchy Pecan	⅔ cup (53 g)	220	60	9
Raisin, Date, Pecan	⅔ cup (54 g)	210	45	5
Healthy Choice				
Almond Crunch with Raisins	1 cup (58 g)	210	20	0
Multigrain Raisins, Crunchy Oat Clusters & Almonds	1 cup (54 g)	210	20	0
Multigrain Squares	1 cup (54 g)	190	10	0
Toasted Brown Sugar Squares	1 cup (54 g)	190	10	0
Honey Bunches of Oats				
Honey Roasted	¾ cup (30 g)	120	15	5
with Almonds	¾ cup (31 g)	130	30	5
Honeycomb	1⅓ cups (29 g)	110	5	0
Honey Nut Clusters	1 cup (55 g)	210	20	0
Just Right				
Crunchy Nugget	1 cup (55 g)	210	15	0
Fruit & Nut	1 cup (60 g)	220	20	0
Kix	1⅓ cups (30 g)	120	5	0
Life	¾ cup (32 g)	120	15	0
Cinnamon	¾ cup (32 g)	120	10	0
Lucky Charms	1 cup (30 g)	120	10	0
Muesli				
Cranberry with almonds or walnuts	¾ cup (58 g)	220	25	0
Raspberry with almonds	¾ cup (58 g)	220	25	0
Swiss (Familia)				
Granola No Added Sugar	½ cup (57 g)	200	30	5
Granola Original Recipe	½ cup (60 g)	210	30	5
Granola Original Recipe Lowfat	⅔ cup (55 g)	180	15	0
Puffed Wheat	½ cup (47 g)	170	45	9
Müeslix				
Apple & Almond Crunch	¾ cup (57 g)	200	45	9
Raisin & Almond Crunch	⅔ cup (55 g)	200	25	0

GRAINS AND PASTA

FOOD	AMOUNT	TOTAL	FAT	SAT-FAT
		CALORIES		
Multi Bran Chex	1 cup (58 g)	200	15	0
Natural Bran Flakes	⅔ cup (28 g)	90	5	0
100% Natural				
Oats, Honey & Raisins	½ cup (51 g)	230	80	32
Low fat	⅔ cup (55 g)	210	27	9
Nutri-Grain Almond Raisin	1¼ cups (49 g)	180	25	0
Oatmeal Crisp				
with Almonds	1 cup (55 g)	220	45	5
with Raisins	1 cup (55 g)	210	25	0
Oatmeal Squares	1 cup (56 g)	220	25	5
Oat Bran O's	1¼ cup (28 g)	100	0	0
Oat Bran Flakes	1¼ cup (28 g)	100	0	0
Product 19	1 cup (30 g)	100	0	0
Puffed Rice	1 cup (14 g)	50	0	0
Puffed Wheat	1¼ cups (15 g)	50	0	0
Puffins	¾ cup (27 g)	90	10	0
Raisin Bran	1 cup (61 g)	200	15	0
Raisin Bran Flakes	1¼ cup (55 g)	190	0	0
Raisin Nut Bran	¾ cup (55 g)	200	35	5
Raisin Squares	¾ cup (53 g)	180	14	0
Reese's Peanut Butter Puffs	¾ cup (30 g)	130	25	5
Rice Chex	1¼ cups (31 g)	120	0	0
Rice Krispies	1¼ cups (33 g)	120	0	0
Razzle-Dazzle	¾ cup (28 g)	110	0	0
Shredded Wheat (Barbara's)	2 biscuits (40 g)	140	10	0
Shredded Wheat (Post)	2 biscuits (46 g)	160	5	0
Frosted Shredded Wheat	1 cup (52 g)	190	10	0
Honey Nut Shredded Wheat	1 cup (52 g)	200	15	0
Spoon Size Shredded Wheat	1 cup (49 g)	170	5	0
Wheat 'N Bran Shredded				
Wheat	1¼ cups (59 g)	200	5	0
Smacks	¾ cup (27 g)	10	5	0
Smart Starts	1 cup (50 g)	180	5	0
Special K	1 cup (31 g)	110	0	0
10 Bran Cereal	¾ cup (27 g)	100	0	0
Toasted Oatmeal				
Honey Nut	1 cup (49 g)	190	25	5
With Clusters	1 cup (49 g)	190	25	5
Total	¾ cup (30 g)	110	10	0
Corn Flakes	1⅓ cups (30 g)	110	0	0
Raisin Bran	1 cup (55 g)	180	10	0
Whole Grain	¾ cup (30 g)	110	10	0
Triples	1 cup (30 g)	120	10	0
Trix	1 cup (30 g)	120	15	0
Waffle Crisp	1 cup (30 g)	130	25	0
Wheat Chex	1 cup (50 g)	180	10	0

GRAINS AND PASTA

| FOOD | AMOUNT | CALORIES | | |
		TOTAL	FAT	SAT-FAT
Wheaties	1 cup (30 g)	110	10	0
Honey Gold	¾ cup (30 g)	110	0	0

BREAKFAST CEREALS, HOT (Dry unless otherwise noted)

FOOD	AMOUNT	TOTAL	FAT	SAT-FAT
Alpen	⅔ cup (55 g)	200	25	0
Cream of Rice	1 oz	100	0	0
Cream of Wheat	1 pkt (35 g)	100	0	0
	1 cup cooked	120	0	0
Flavored	1 pkt (35 g)	130	0	0
regular, quick, instant, cooked	3 tbsp (33 g)	120	0	0
Farina (Pillsbury)	3 tbsp (28 g)	100	0	0
Grits (Quaker)	¼ cup (41 g)	140	5	0
Instant (Quaker)				
Country bacon	1 pkt (28 g)	100	5	0
Original	1 pkt (28 g)	100	0	0
Real butter	1 pkt (28 g)	100	15	5
Real cheddar cheese	1 pkt (28 g)	100	15	5
Red Eye Gravy & Country Ham	1 pkt (28 g)	10	5	0
Malt-O-Meal	1 cup, cooked	110	0	0
Maypo	1 oz	100	9	0
Oatmeal				
Quaker	½ cup (40 g)	150	25	5
	1 cup cooked	150	25	5
Instant	½ cup (40 g)	150	25	5
Irish (John McCann's)	⅓ cup (60 g)	230	40	9
Oat Bran				
Quaker	½ cup (40 g)	150	30	5
Mother's Oat Bran	½ cup (40 g)	150	25	9
Quinoa	¼ cup	159	22	2
Ralston 100% Wheat	½ cup (38 g)	130	10	0
Wheatena	⅓ cup (41 g)	150	5	0
Whole Wheat (Mother's)	½ cup (40 g)	130	5	0

CEREAL GRAINS (*see also* **FLOUR**)

FOOD	AMOUNT	TOTAL	FAT	SAT-FAT
Barley, pearled				
uncooked	½ cup	352	10	0
cooked	½ cup	97	3	0
Buckwheat	½ cup	292	26	6
Buckwheat groats, roasted				
uncooked	½ cup	283	20	4
cooked	½ cup	91	5	0
Kasha	¼ cup (45 g)	170	15	NA
Bulgur				
uncooked	½ cup	239	8	0
cooked	½ cup	76	2	0

GRAINS AND PASTA

		CALORIES		
FOOD	**AMOUNT**	**TOTAL**	**FAT**	**SAT-FAT**
Corn Grits				
uncooked	½ cup	290	8	0
cooked	1 cup	146	5	0
Couscous				
uncooked	½ cup	346	5	0
cooked (no added fat)	½ cup	101	1	0
Farina				
uncooked	½ cup	325	4	0
cooked	1 cup	116	2	0
Hominy, canned	½ cup	57	6	0
Millet				
uncooked	½ cup	378	38	7
cooked	½ cup	143	11	2
Oat bran				
uncooked	½ cup	116	30	6
cooked	1 cup	87	17	3
Oatmeal				
uncooked	⅓ cup	104	15	3
cooked	1 cup	145	22	4
Quinoa	¼ cup (42 g)	159	18	0
Rice				
Brown				
uncooked	1 cup	684	49	10
cooked	½ cup	109	8	0
White, long-grain				
uncooked	1 cup	676	11	3
cooked	½ cup	131	3	0
White, long-grain, parboiled				
uncooked	1 cup	686	9	2
cooked	½ cup	100	2	0
White, glutinous				
uncooked	1 cup	685	9	2
cooked	½ cup	116	2	0
White, Instant				
uncooked	1 cup	360	2	0
cooked	½ cup	80	1	0
Wild				
uncooked	1 cup	571	16	2
cooked	½ cup	83	3	0
Rice bran, crude	⅓ cup	88	53	10
Rye	½ cup	282	18	2
Wheat bran	½ cup	65	12	2
	1 tbsp	8	1	0
Wheat germ, toasted	1 tbsp	27	7	0
	½ cup	216	54	9

GRAINS AND PASTA

| FOOD | AMOUNT | CALORIES | | |
		TOTAL	FAT	SAT-FAT
FLOUR				
Arrowroot flour	1 tbsp	29	0	0
Bisquick, original (Betty Crocker)	⅓ cup (40 g)	170	50	14
reduced fat	⅓ cup (40 g)	140	25	5
Buckwheat flour	½ cup	201	17	5
Cake flour	½ cup	195	4	0
Corn flour				
whole grain	½ cup	209	20	3
masa	⅓ cup	139	13	2
Cornmeal, yellow	½ cup	210	10	1
Cornstarch	1 tbsp	31	0	0
Pastry flour	⅓ cup (30 g)	100	5	0
Potato starch	1 tbsp (10 g)	30	0	0
Rice flour				
brown	½ cup	287	20	4
white	½ cup	289	10	3
Rye flour				
dark	½ cup	207	15	2
medium	½ cup	181	8	1
Semolina	½ cup	303	8	1
Soy flour	½ cup	179	78	12
White flour	½ cup	200	0	0
All-purpose flour	½ cup	226	5	0
Bread flour	½ cup	249	10	0
Whole-wheat flour	½ cup	203	10	2

PASTAS (*see also* **FROZEN, MICROWAVE, AND REFRIGERATED FOODS**)
All dry types, cooked

FOOD	AMOUNT	TOTAL	FAT	SAT-FAT
Macaroni, noodles,				
spaghetti, shells, etc.	2 oz dry	211	8	0
	1 cup cooked	197	8	0
Barley egg	¼ cup (55 g)	220	25	NA
Cellophane (Chinese)	1 cup dry	174	7	0
Chinese Style Noodles	57 g dry	200	5	0
Egg noodles	2 oz dry	217	22	5
	1 cup cooked	212	21	5
Whole-wheat	2 oz dry	198	7	0
	1 cup cooked	174	7	0
Chow Mein noodles				
Goodman's	⅔ cup (26 g)	120	40	NA
La Choy	½ cup (28 g)	140	60	9
Chung King	⅓ cup (28 g)	140	65	NA
Soba noodles (Japanese)	2 oz dry	192	4	0
	1 cup cooked	113	0	0
Somen noodles (Japanese)	2 oz dry	203	4	0
	1 cup cooked	230	3	0

GRAINS AND PASTA

		CALORIES		
FOOD	AMOUNT	TOTAL	FAT	SAT-FAT
Oriental noodles, miscellaneous				
Chinese Style	57 g	200	**5**	0
Japanese Style	55 g	200	**15**	0
Oriental Style	55 g	195	**1**	0
Rice Stick	¼ cup (55 g)	200	**5**	0
Refrigerated pasta				
Celentano				
Broccoli Stuffed Shells	3 shells (280 g)	190	**35**	NA
Contadina				
Angel hair	1¼ cup (80 g)	230	**20**	9
Fettuccine	1¼ cup (83 g)	240	**20**	9
Linguine	1¼ cup (85 g)	240	**20**	9
Ravioli				
Chicken & Herb	1¼ cups (113 g)	370	**120**	36
Four Cheese	1 cup (88 g)	230	**35**	18
Garden Vegetable	1 cup (90 g)	250	**45**	18
Spinach Fettuccine	1¼ cups (89 g)	250	**30**	14
Tortelloni				
Cheese & Herb	1 cup (111 g)	320	**80**	45
Chicken & Prosciutto	1 cup (109 g)	360	**110**	41
Garlic & Cheese	1 cup (104 g)	280	**40**	23
Mushroom & Cheese	1 cup (104 g)	290	**50**	18
Sausage & Bell Pepper	1 cup	330	**90**	NA
Sun-dried Tomato	1 cup (100 g)	320	**90**	23
Sweet Italian Sausage	1 cup (107 g)	320	**70**	27
3 Cheese	¾ cup (85 g)	250	**45**	27
DiGiorno				
Angel hair	⅕ pkg (56 g)	160	**10**	0
Fettuccine	¼ pkg (70 g)	200	**15**	0
Four Cheese Ravioli	1 cup (110 g)	350	**140**	81
Linguine	¼ pkg (70 g)	200	**15**	0
Mozzarella Garlic Tortelloni	1 cup (99 g)	300	**80**	45
Three Cheese Tortellini	¾ cup (81 g)	250	**60**	31
Refrigerated Pasta Sauces: *see* **SAUCES, GRAVIES, AND DIPS**				
Mixed Pasta Dishes				
Fettuccine Alfredo	1 cup	880	**610**	377
Chef Boyardee				
Beef Ravioli	1 cup (253 g)	240	**50**	23
Beefaroni	1 cup (249 g)	260	**60**	27
Cheese Ravioli	1 cup (246 g)	220	**30**	14
Lasagna	1 cup (249 g)	270	**70**	27
Mini Ravioli	1 cup (252 g)	240	**60**	27
Spaghetti & Meatballs	1 cup (257 g)	270	**90**	45
Tortellini	1 cup (258 g)	230	**210**	0

GRAINS AND PASTA

		CALORIES		
FOOD	AMOUNT	TOTAL	FAT	SAT-FAT
Chef Boyardee 99% Fat Free				
Beef Ravioli	1 cup (244 g)	210	**10**	0
Cheese Ravioli	1 cup (251 g)	240	**25**	9
Franco-American				
Garfield				
Beef Ravioli	1 cup (252 g)	300	**90**	36
Life with Louie				
Pasta with Meatballs	1 cup (252 g)	260	**100**	45
Pasta with Tomato &				
Cheese Sauce	1 cup (252 g)	190	**20**	5
RavioliOs				
Beef Ravioli	1 cup (252 g)	230	**30**	14
Sonic the Hedgehog				
Pasta with Meatballs	1 cup (252 g)	280	**100**	36
Spaghetti in Tomato Sauce	1 cup (252 g)	210	**20**	9
SpaghettiOs				
Pasta with Meatballs	1 cup (252 g)	260	**100**	45
Pasta with Sliced Franks	1 cup (252 g)	250	**100**	45
Pasta with Tomato &				
Cheese Sauce	1 cup (252 g)	190	**20**	5
Superiore				
Beef Ravioli	1 cup (259 g)	280	**80**	36
Spaghetti & Meatballs	1 cup (252 g)	270	**90**	45
TeddyOs				
Pasta with Tomato &				
Cheese Sauce	1 cup (252 g)	190	**20**	5
Where's Waldo				
Pasta in Tomato Sauce	1 cup (252 g)	190	**20**	5
Pasta with Meatballs	1 cup (252 g)	260	**100**	45
Hamburger Helper (Betty Crocker)				
Cheddar Cheese Melt	¾ cup mix (42 g)	150	**15**	5
	1 cup prepared	310	**100**	36
Cheeseburger Macaroni	⅓ cup mix (45 g)	180	**40**	14
	1 cup prepared	360	**140**	54
Chili Macaroni	⅓ cup mix (41 g)	140	**10**	0
	1 cup prepared	290	**90**	36
Italian Herb	½ cup mix (40 g)	130	**10**	0
	1 cup prepared	270	**90**	36
Lasagne	⅔ cup mix (41 g)	140	**5**	0
	1 cup prepared	280	**90**	36
Ravioli	½ cup mix (41 g)	140	**5**	0
	1 cup prepared	280	**90**	36
Southwestern Beef	⅓ cup mix (44 g)	150	**10**	0
	1 cup prepared	300	**90**	36
Stroganoff	⅔ cup mix (41 g)	160	**25**	9
	1 cup prepared	320	**110**	45

GRAINS AND PASTA

FOOD	AMOUNT	CALORIES TOTAL	FAT	SAT-FAT
Hamburger Helper (Betty Crocker) (cont.)				
Supreme Topping				
Italian Parmesan	⅓ cup mix (44 g)	160	**15**	0
	1 cup prepared	300	**100**	36
Cheesy Hashbrowns	½ cup mix (48 g)	170	**15**	5
	1 cup prepared	400	**170**	54
Hormel				
Italian Style Lasagna	1 bowl (284 g)	350	**72**	NA
Macaroni & Cheese	1 cup (213 g)	270	**100**	NA
Noodles & Chicken (Hearty				
Helpings)	1 cup (298 g)	250	**100**	NA
Spaghetti	1 bowl (284 g)	240	**23**	NA
Kid's Kitchen (Hormel)				
Beefy Mac	1 cup (213 g)	190	**50**	23
Cheezy Mac 'n Beef	1 cup (213 g)	260	**60**	27
Cheezy Mac 'n Cheese	1 cup (213 g)	260	**100**	54
Mini Beef Ravioli	1 cup (213 g)	240	**60**	27
Noodle Rings & Chicken	1 cup (213 g)	150	**35**	14
Spaghetti & Mini Meatballs	1 cup (213 g)	220	**60**	36
Spaghetti Rings & Franks	1 cup (213 g)	240	**80**	31
Spaghetti Rings with Meatballs	1 cup (213 g)	230	**60**	27
Kraft				
Deluxe Macaroni & Cheese Dinner				
Four Cheese	98 g mix	320	**90**	63
Light	98 g mix	290	**40**	23
Original	98 g mix	320	**90**	54
Macaroni & Cheese Dinner				
The Cheesiest, Cheesy				
Alfredo, Spirals, Super				
Heroes, Rugrats, Bugs				
Bunny, ABC's, 123	70 g mix	260	**25**	9
	1 cup prepared	410	**170**	41
Thick 'n Creamy	70 g mix	260	**25**	9
	1 cup prepared	420	**170**	45
Three Cheese	70 g mix	260	**25**	9
	1 cup prepared	410	**160**	41
White Cheddar	70 g mix	260	**25**	9
	1 cup prepared	410	**160**	41
Velveeta Shells & Cheese	112 g mix	360	**120**	72
Lipton				
Noodles & Sauce				
Alfredo	⅔ cup (62 g)	250	**60**	36
	1 cup prepared	330	**130**	54
Beef Flavor	⅔ cup (60 g)	230	**30**	9
	1 cup prepared	280	**90**	23

GRAINS AND PASTA

FOOD	AMOUNT	CALORIES		
		TOTAL	FAT	SAT-FAT
Lipton (cont.)				
Butter & Herb	⅔ cup (62 g)	250	60	31
	1 cup prepared	300	110	41
Chicken Broccoli	⅔ cup (59 g)	230	35	14
	1 cup prepared	310	100	27
Chicken Flavor	⅔ cup (60 g)	240	40	18
	1 cup prepared	290	100	27
Creamy Chicken	⅔ cup (59 g)	240	50	27
	1 cup prepared	320	110	43
Parmesan	⅔ cup (60 g)	250	70	36
	1 cup prepared	330	140	54
Stroganoff	⅔ cup (56 g)	220	35	18
	1 cup prepared	300	100	36
Pasta & Sauce				
Cheddar Broccoli	⅔ cup (68 g)	260	35	14
	1 cup prepared	340	100	30
Creamy Garlic	⅔ cup (69 g)	270	50	23
	1 cup prepared	350	120	40
Mild Cheddar Cheese	¾ cup (59 g)	210	25	14
	1 cup prepared	290	90	28
Roasted Garlic & Olive Oil with Tomatoes	¾ cup (60 g)	220	25	5
	1 cup prepared	270	80	18
Roasted Garlic Chicken Flavor	¾ cup (56 g)	210	20	9
	1 cup prepared	290	90	23
Rice-A-Roni				
Pasta Roni				
Angel Hair Pasta with Herbs	56 g mix	200	25	5
	1 cup prepared	320	120	30
Angel Hair Pasta with Lemon & Butter	70 g mix	250	30	9
	1 cup prepared	360	140	30
Angel Hair Pasta with Parmesan Cheese	56 g mix	210	40	9
	1 cup prepared	320	130	31
Broccoli	56 g mix	200	30	5
	1 cup prepared	340	140	36
Fettuccine Alfredo	70 g mix	270	60	18
	1 cup prepared	470	230	54
Garlic & Olive Oil with Vermicelli	70 g mix	250	30	5
	1 cup prepared	360	140	27
Herb & Butter	56 g mix	200	25	5
	1 cup prepared	380	170	40

GRAINS AND PASTA

		CALORIES		
FOOD	**AMOUNT**	**TOTAL**	**FAT**	**SAT-FAT**
Rice-A-Roni (cont.)				
Homestyle Chicken	56 g mix	190	**15**	0
	1 cup prepared	230	**50**	45
Parmesano	70 g mix	260	**35**	9
	1 cup prepared	390	**150**	36
Shells & White Cheddar	70 g mix	270	**50**	23
	1 cup prepared	380	**210**	45
White Cheddar & Broccoli	70 g mix	270	**50**	18
	1 cup prepared	400	**170**	43
Tuna Helper (Betty Crocker)				
Cheesy Pasta	¾ cup mix (44 g)	170	**25**	9
	1 cup prepared	280	**100**	23
Creamy Broccoli	⅔ cup mix (50 g)	190	**40**	14
	1 cup prepared	310	**110**	27
Creamy Pasta	¾ cup mix (46 g)	190	**50**	14
	1 cup prepared	300	**120**	30
Pancakes and Waffles: *see* **FAST FOODS; FROZEN, MICROWAVE, AND REFRIGERATED FOODS; RESTAURANT FOODS**				
Pancake Mix				
Buttermilk (Flap-Stax)	½ cup mix (63 g)	240	**35**	9

MEATS (BEEF, GAME, LAMB, PORK, AND VEAL)

The following cuts of meat are braised, roasted, or broiled, unless otherwise noted. *See also* **SAUSAGES AND LUNCHEON MEATS** for cold cuts made from beef and pork products and **FROZEN, MICROWAVE, AND REFRIGERATED FOODS.**

		CALORIES		
FOOD	**AMOUNT**	**TOTAL**	**FAT**	**SAT-FAT**
BEEF				
*Remember that most of the following calorie figures are for **only 1 ounce** of beef!*				
Arm pot roast, braised				
lean and fat	1 oz	99	**66**	27
lean only	1 oz	68	**25**	11
Backribs	2 ribs (140 g)	360	**220**	90
Bottom round steak, braised				
lean and fat	1 oz	74	**38**	14
lean only	1 oz	67	**25**	9
Brisket flat half, braised				
lean and fat	1 oz	116	**89**	37
lean only	1 oz	74	**40**	17
Chuck steak, braised				
lean and fat	1 oz	108	**78**	32
lean only	1 oz	77	**39**	18

MEATS (BEEF, GAME, LAMB, PORK, AND VEAL)

		CALORIES		
FOOD	AMOUNT	TOTAL	FAT	SAT-FAT
Club steak, broiled				
lean and fat	1 oz	129	104	50
lean only	1 oz	69	33	16
Flank steak, braised				
lean and fat	1 oz	73	39	18
lean only	1 oz	69	35	16
Ground beef, raw				
extra lean	1 oz	66	44	17
lean	1 oz	75	53	21
regular	1 oz	88	68	28
Ground beef, broiled, medium				
extra lean	1 oz	72	42	16
lean	1 oz	77	47	18
regular	1 oz	82	53	21
Ground beef, pan-fried, medium				
extra lean	1 oz	72	42	16
lean	1 oz	78	49	19
regular	1 oz	87	58	23
Porterhouse steak, broiled				
lean and fat	1 oz	85	54	22
lean only	1 oz	62	28	13
Rib roast				
lean and fat	1 oz	108	81	34
lean only	1 oz	68	35	17
Round, broiled				
lean and fat	1 oz	78	47	19
lean only	1 oz	55	20	7
Rump roast				
lean and fat	1 oz	98	70	33
lean only	1 oz	59	24	7
Shortribs, braised				
lean and fat	1 oz	133	107	45
lean only	1 oz	84	46	20
Sirloin steak, broiled				
lean and fat	1 oz	79	46	19
lean only	1 oz	59	22	12
T-bone steak, broiled				
lean and fat	1 oz	92	63	26
lean only	1 oz	61	26	11
Tenderloin steak, broiled				
lean and fat	1 oz	75	44	18
lean only	1 oz	58	24	9
Top round, broiled				
lean and fat	1 oz	60	22	8
lean only	1 oz	54	16	6

MEATS (BEEF, GAME, LAMB, PORK, AND VEAL)

FOOD	AMOUNT	CALORIES TOTAL	FAT	SAT-FAT
MIXED BEEF DISHES				
Beef Barbecue (Brookwood Farms)	¼ cup (63 g)	350	**220**	90
Beef and vegetable stew	1 cup	220	**99**	40
Chili con carne, canned	1 cup	340	**144**	52
Lasagne	¹⁄₁₂ casserole	570	**210**	142
Spaghetti w/meatballs and tomato				
sauce, canned	1 cup	260	**90**	22
VARIETY MEATS AND BY-PRODUCTS				
Brain, simmered	1 oz	45	**32**	7
Liver, braised	1 oz	46	**12**	5
Liver Paté	½ cup	289	**204**	104
	1 tbsp	36	**26**	13
Tripe	1 oz	28	**10**	5
Tongue, simmered	1 oz	81	**53**	23
GAME MEATS				
*Remember that the following calorie figures are for **only 1 ounce** of game!*				
Antelope, roasted	1 oz	42	**7**	2
Bear, simmered	1 oz	73	**34**	NA
Beefalo, composite of cuts, roasted	1 oz	53	**16**	7
Bison, roasted	1 oz	41	**6**	2
Boar, wild, roasted	1 oz	45	**11**	3
Buffalo, water, roasted	1 oz	37	**5**	2
Caribou, roasted	1 oz	47	**11**	4
Deer, roasted	1 oz	45	**8**	3
Elk, roasted	1 oz	41	**5**	2
Goat, roasted	1 oz	41	**8**	2
Horse, roasted	1 oz	50	**15**	5
Moose, roasted	1 oz	38	**2**	1
Muskrat, roasted	1 oz	52	**23**	NA
Opossum, roasted	1 oz	63	**26**	NA
Rabbit				
domesticated, composite of cuts				
roasted	1 oz	44	**16**	5
stewed	1 oz	58	**21**	6
wild, stewed	1 oz	49	**9**	3
Raccoon, roasted	1 oz	72	**37**	NA
Squirrel, roasted	1 oz	39	**9**	1
LAMB				
*Remember that most of the following calorie figures are for **only 1 ounce** of lamb!*				
Foreshank, braised				
lean and fat	1 oz	69	**34**	14
lean only	1 oz	53	**15**	6
Leg, whole (shank and sirloin), roasted				
lean and fat	1 oz	73	**42**	18
lean only	1 oz	54	**20**	7

MEATS (BEEF, GAME, LAMB, PORK, AND VEAL)

FOOD	AMOUNT	CALORIES		
		TOTAL	FAT	SAT-FAT
Leg, shank half, roasted				
lean and fat	1 oz	64	**32**	13
lean only	1 oz	51	**17**	6
Leg, sirloin half, roasted				
lean and fat	1 oz	83	**53**	23
lean only	1 oz	58	**23**	8
Loin, roasted				
lean and fat	1 oz	88	**60**	25
lean only	1 oz	57	**25**	9
Chop, with bone, broiled				
lean and fat	1 chop (3.5 oz)	357	**265**	145
lean only	1 chop (3.5 oz)	189	**74**	37
Rib, broiled or roasted				
lean and fat	1 oz	102	**76**	33
lean only	1 oz	67	**34**	12
Chop, with bone, broiled				
lean and fat	1 chop (3.5 oz)	398	**315**	148
lean only	1 chop (3.5 oz)	212	**105**	40
Shoulder, whole (arm and blade) braised				
lean and fat	1 oz	97	**63**	27
lean only	1 oz	80	**40**	16
Cubed lamb for stew or kabob (leg and shoulder), lean only				
braised	1 oz	63	**22**	8
broiled	1 oz	53	**19**	7
Ground lamb				
broiled	1 oz	81	**50**	26

PORK

*Remember that many of the following calorie figures are for **only 1 ounce** of pork!*

Loin				
whole, broiled				
lean and fat, without bone	1 oz	98	**69**	25
	1 chop (104 g)	284	**202**	73
lean only	1 oz	73	**39**	13
	1 chop (104 g)	169	**91**	31
blade, pan-fried				
lean and fat	1 oz	117	**94**	34
	1 chop (104 g)	368	**296**	107
lean only	1 oz	85	**51**	19
	1 chop (89 g)	177	**111**	39
center loin, pan fried				
lean and fat	1 oz	106	**78**	28
	1 chop (112 g)	333	**244**	88
lean only	1 oz	75	**41**	14
	1 chop (112 g)	178	**96**	33

MEATS (BEEF, GAME, LAMB, PORK, AND VEAL)

		CALORIES		
FOOD	**AMOUNT**	**TOTAL**	**FAT**	**SAT-FAT**
Loin (cont.)				
center rib, broiled				
lean and fat	1 oz	97	**67**	24
	1 chop (104 g)	264	**183**	66
lean only	1 oz	73	**38**	13
	1 chop (104 g)	162	**85**	29
sirloin, broiled				
lean and fat	1 oz	94	**64**	23
	1 chop (106 g)	278	**191**	69
lean only	1 oz	69	**35**	12
	1 chop (106 g)	165	**83**	29
tenderloin, roasted				
lean only	1 oz	47	**12**	4
top loin, broiled				
lean and fat	1 oz	102	**85**	26
	1 chop (104 g)	295	**211**	76
lean only	1 oz	73	**39**	13
	1 chop (104 g)	165	**86**	30
Shoulder cut				
whole, roasted				
lean and fat	1 oz	92	**65**	24
lean only	1 oz	69	**38**	13
arm picnic, roasted				
lean and fat	1 oz	94	**67**	24
lean only	1 oz	65	**32**	11
blade, Boston, roasted				
lean and fat	1 oz	91	**64**	23
lean only	1 oz	73	**43**	15
Spareribs, cooked				
lean and fat	1 oz	113	**77**	30
Pork Ribs (Spare the Ribs)	5 oz (140 g)	380	**260**	72
Pork Baby Back Ribs (Lloyd's)	3 ribs (140 g)	330	**190**	72
PORK PRODUCTS, CURED (*see also* **SAUSAGES AND LUNCHEON MEATS**)				
Bacon, cooked	1 strip	36	**28**	10
Breakfast strips, cooked	1 strip	52	**37**	13
Canadian bacon, grilled	1 slice	43	**18**	6
Ham, boneless				
Extra lean (5% fat)	1 slice (28 g)	41	**14**	5
Regular (11% fat)	1 slice (28 g)	52	**27**	9
Ham, canned				
Extra lean (4% fat)	1 slice (28 g)	39	**12**	4
Regular (13% fat)	1 slice (28 g)	64	**39**	13

MEATS (BEEF, GAME, LAMB, PORK, AND VEAL)

		CALORIES		
FOOD	**AMOUNT**	**TOTAL**	**FAT**	**SAT-FAT**
Ham, center slice				
Country-style				
Lean and fat	1 oz	57	**33**	12
Lean	1 oz	55	**21**	1
Salt pork, raw	1 oz	212	**205**	75
PORK DISHES, MIXED				
Barbecue Pork	½ cup	320	**220**	72
Hash	1 cup	410	**250**	117
VARIETY MEATS & BY-PRODUCTS				
Backfat, raw	1 oz	230	**226**	226
Chitterlings, simmered	1 oz	86	**73**	37
Feet				
pickled	1 oz	58	**41**	14
simmered, without bone	1 oz	55	**32**	11
Liver paté	2 oz (56 g)	200	**160**	54

For cold cuts made from pork products, *see* **SAUSAGES AND LUNCHEON MEATS.**

VEAL

*Remember that the following calorie figures are for **only 1 ounce** of veal!*

Breast, lean and fat, braised	1 oz	86	**54**	26
Cutlet, lean and fat, braised	1 oz	62	**27**	12
Ground, broiled	1 oz	49	**19**	8
Leg				
top round, lean and fat, braised	1 oz	60	**16**	6
top round, lean, braised	1 oz	57	**13**	5
Loin				
lean and fat, braised	1 oz	81	**44**	16
lean only, braised	1 oz	64	**23**	7
lean and fat, roasted	1 oz	61	**31**	16
lean only, roasted	1 oz	50	**18**	7
Rib				
lean and fat, braised	1 oz	71	**32**	13
lean only, braised	1 oz	62	**20**	7
lean and fat, roasted	1 oz	65	**36**	14
lean only, roasted	1 oz	50	**19**	6
Shoulder				
arm, lean and fat, braised	1 oz	67	**26**	10
arm, lean only, braised	1 oz	57	**14**	4
blade, lean and fat, braised	1 oz	64	**26**	9
blade, lean, braised	1 oz	56	**17**	5
Sirloin				
lean and fat, braised	1 oz	72	**34**	13
lean only, braised	1 oz	58	**17**	5
Veal cubed for stew (leg and shoulder)				
lean only braised	1 oz	53	**11**	3

NUTS AND SEEDS

		CALORIES		
FOOD	AMOUNT	TOTAL	FAT	SAT-FAT
NUTS				
Almonds				
slivered or sliced	½ cup	400	**315**	30
whole, dry-roasted	1 oz (24 nuts)	167	**132**	13
	½ cup	405	**320**	30
Almond butter				
plain	1 tbsp	101	**85**	8
honey-cinnamon	1 tbsp	96	**75**	7
Almond paste	1 oz	127	**69**	7
	1 cup	1012	**556**	53
Beechnuts, dried	1 oz	164	**128**	15
Brazil nuts, shelled, dried	1 oz (8 med. nuts)	186	**169**	41
Butternuts, dried	1 oz	174	**146**	3
Cashew nuts				
dry-roasted	1 oz (18 med. nuts)	163	**118**	23
	1 cup	787	**572**	113
oil-roasted	1 oz (18 med. nuts)	163	**123**	24
	1 cup	748	**564**	112
jumbo	12 nuts (30 g)	190	**130**	27
Cashew butter, plain	1 oz	167	**126**	25
	1 tbsp	94	**71**	14
Chestnuts, Chinese				
raw	1 oz	64	**3**	0
dried	1 oz	103	**5**	1
boiled and steamed	1 oz	44	**2**	0
roasted	1 oz	68	**3**	0
Chestnuts, European				
raw, unpeeled	1 oz	60	**6**	1
raw, peeled	1 oz	56	**3**	1
dried, unpeeled	1 oz	106	**11**	2
dried, peeled	1 oz	105	**10**	2
boiled and steamed	1 oz	37	**4**	1
roasted	1 oz (3 nuts)	70	**6**	1
	1 cup	350	**28**	5
Chestnuts, Japanese				
raw	1 oz	44	**1**	0
dried	1 oz	102	**3**	0
boiled and steamed	1 oz	16	**1**	0
roasted	1 oz	57	**2**	0
Coconut meat				
dried, creamed	1 oz	194	**177**	157
dried, sweetened, flaked	1 oz	135	**82**	73
	1 cup	351	**214**	190
dried, toasted	1 oz	168	**120**	107
fresh frozen with sugar	2 tbsp (13 g)	45	**25**	18

NUTS AND SEEDS

| FOOD | AMOUNT | CALORIES | | |
		TOTAL	FAT	SAT-FAT
Coconut meat (cont.)				
fresh, shredded or grated	1 oz	101	**86**	76
	1 cup	283	**241**	214
Coconut cream				
fresh	1 tbsp	49	**47**	42
	1 cup	792	**749**	664
canned	1 tbsp	36	**30**	27
	1 cup	568	**472**	419
Coconut milk				
fresh	1 tbsp	35	**32**	29
	1 cup	552	**515**	457
canned	1 tbsp	30	**29**	26
	1 cup	445	**434**	385
frozen	1 tbsp	30	**28**	25
	1 cup	486	**449**	398
Filberts (hazelnuts)				
dried	1 oz	179	**160**	12
	1 cup, chopped	727	**648**	48
dry-roasted	1 oz	188	**169**	12
oil-roasted	1 oz	187	**163**	12
Hickory nuts, dried	1 oz	187	**165**	18
Macadamia nuts				
dried	1 oz	199	**188**	28
oil-roasted	1 oz (24 halves)	204	**196**	29
	1 cup	962	**923**	139
Mixed nuts				
dry-roasted, with peanuts	1 oz	169	**131**	18
	1 cup	814	**634**	85
oil-roasted, with peanuts	1 oz	175	**144**	22
	1 cup	876	**720**	112
oil-roasted, without peanuts	1 oz	175	**144**	23
	1 cup	886	**728**	118
Peanuts, shelled				
dry-roasted	1 oz (35 kernels)	161	**126**	17
	1 cup	827	**646**	90
	1 tbsp	50	**35**	9
oil-roasted	1 oz (35 kernels)	165	**126**	18
	1 cup	841	**642**	89
Planters Peanuts				
Hot Spicy Peanuts (to heat)	37 pieces (28 g)	160	**120**	18
Snack Mix (to heat)	¼ cup (28 g)	140	**70**	9
Sweet 'N Crunchy	18 pieces (28 g)	140	**60**	9
Peanut butter	2 tbsp	190	**148**	24
Jif				
Extra Crunchy	2 tbsp (32 g)	190	**130**	27
Simply Creamy	2 tbsp (31 g)	190	**130**	27
reduced fat	2 tbsp (36 g)	190	**110**	23

NUTS AND SEEDS

		CALORIES		
FOOD	AMOUNT	TOTAL	FAT	SAT-FAT
Peanut butter (cont.)				
Peter Pan				
Creamy	2 tbsp (32 g)	190	**140**	31
reduced fat	2 tbsp (36 g)	180	**90**	23
Crunchy	2 tbsp (32 g)	190	**130**	27
Reese's Creamy	2 tbsp (32 g)	200	**140**	27
Skippy				
Creamy	2 tbsp (32 g)	190	**140**	31
reduced fat	2 tbsp (36 g)	190	**100**	23
Super Chunk	2 tbsp (32 g)	190	**140**	31
reduced fat	2 tbsp (35 g)	190	**100**	23
Pecans				
dried	1 oz	190	**173**	14
dry-roasted	1 oz (14 halves)	187	**165**	13
	⅓ cup	230	**210**	18
oil-roasted	1 oz	195	**182**	15
Pine nuts	¼ cup	190	**140**	32
Pistachio nuts				
dried	1 oz	164	**124**	16
dry-roasted	1 oz (47 kernels)	172	**135**	17
Walnuts	¼ cup (32 g)	210	**180**	14
walnut halves	⅓ cup (33 g)	210	**190**	18
walnut pieces	¼ cup (30 g)	190	**170**	18
black walnuts	¼ cup (30 g)	200	**150**	9
English, dried	1 oz (14 halves)	182	**158**	14
	1 cup	770	**668**	60
SEEDS				
Poppy	1 tsp	15	**11**	NA
	1 tbsp	66	**51**	NA
Pumpkin and squash				
whole, roasted	1 oz	127	**50**	9
kernels, dried	1 oz	154	**117**	22
kernels, roasted	1 oz	148	**108**	20
Sesame seed kernels, dried	1 tbsp	47	**39**	6
	1 cup	882	**739**	104
Sunflower				
whole	1 oz	80	**59**	8
kernels				
dried	1 oz	162	**127**	13
dry-roasted	1 oz	165	**127**	13
	1 tbsp	48	**34**	7
	1 cup	745	**574**	60
oil-roasted	1 oz	175	**147**	15
	1 tbsp	47	**44**	5

NUTS AND SEEDS

| FOOD | AMOUNT | CALORIES | | |
		TOTAL	FAT	SAT-FAT
Sunflower (cont.)				
toasted	1 oz	176	**145**	15
	1 tbsp	51	**43**	5
Tahini	1 tbsp	90	**72**	10
Watermelon, dried	1 oz	158	**121**	25

POULTRY

See also **SAUSAGES AND LUNCHEON MEATS** for cold cuts made from poultry products and **FROZEN, MICROWAVE, AND REFRIGERATED FOODS.**

*Remember that many of the following calorie figures are for **only 1 ounce** of poultry!*

| FOOD | AMOUNT | CALORIES | | |
		TOTAL	FAT	SAT-FAT
CHICKEN				
Back				
meat and skin				
raw	½ back (99 g)	316	**256**	74
	1 oz	90	**73**	21
fried, batter-dipped	½ back (120 g)	397	**237**	63
	1 oz	94	**56**	15
fried, flour-coated	½ back (72 g)	238	**134**	36
	1 oz	94	**53**	14
roasted	½ back (53 g)	159	**100**	28
	1 oz	85	**54**	15
meat only				
raw	½ back (51 g)	70	**27**	7
	1 oz	39	**15**	4
fried	½ back (58 g)	167	**80**	22
	1 oz	82	**39**	10
roasted	½ back (51 g)	70	**27**	7
	1 oz	39	**15**	4
Breast				
meat and skin				
raw	1 breast (145 g)	250	**121**	35
	1 oz	49	**24**	7
fried, batter-dipped	1 breast (140 g)	364	**166**	44
	1 oz	74	**34**	9
fried, flour-coated	1 breast (98 g)	218	**78**	22
	1 oz	63	**23**	6
roasted	1 breast (98 g)	193	**69**	19
	1 oz	56	**20**	6

POULTRY

		CALORIES		
FOOD	AMOUNT	TOTAL	FAT	SAT-FAT
Chicken, Breast (cont.)				
meat only				
raw	1 breast (118 g)	129	**13**	3.5
	1 oz	31	**3**	1
fried	1 breast (86 g)	161	**36**	10
	1 oz	53	**12**	3
roasted	1 breast (86 g)	129	**13**	3.5
	1 oz	31	**3**	1
Drumstick				
meat and skin				
raw	1 drumstick (73 g)	117	**57**	16
	1 oz	46	**22**	6
fried, batter-dipped	1 drumstick (72 g)	193	**102**	27
	1 oz	76	**40**	10
fried, flour-coated	1 drumstick (49 g)	120	**60**	16
	1 oz	69	**35**	9
roasted	1 drumstick (52 g)	112	**52**	14
	1 oz	61	**28**	8
meat only				
raw	1 drumstick (62 g)	74	**19**	5
	1 oz	34	**9**	2
fried	1 drumstick (42 g)	82	**31**	8
	1 oz	55	**21**	5
roasted	1 drumstick (44 g)	74	**19**	5
	1 oz	34	**9**	2
Gizzard				
raw	1 gizzard (37 g)	44	**14**	4
	1 oz	33	**11**	3
simmered	1 cup	222	**48**	14
	1 oz	43	**9**	3
Ground Chicken				
Fresh (Perdue)	1 oz	48	**30**	9
Frozen (Longacre)	1 oz	55	**30**	9
Leg				
meat and skin				
raw	1 leg (167 g)	312	**182**	51
	1 oz	53	**31**	9
fried, batter-dipped	1 leg (158 g)	431	**230**	61
	1 oz	77	**41**	11
fried, flour-coated	1 leg (112 g)	285	**145**	39
	1 oz	72	**37**	10
roasted	1 leg (114 g)	265	**138**	38
	1 oz	66	**34**	9
meat only				
raw	1 leg (130 g)	156	**45**	11
	1 oz	34	**10**	2

POULTRY

FOOD	AMOUNT	CALORIES		
		TOTAL	FAT	SAT-FAT
Leg (cont.)				
fried	1 leg (94 g)	195	**79**	21
	1 oz	59	**24**	6
roasted	1 leg (95 g)	156	**45**	11
	1 oz	34	**10**	2
Liver				
raw	1 liver (32 g)	40	**11**	4
	1 oz	35	**10**	3
simmered	1 cup	219	**69**	23
	1 oz	44	**14**	5
Neck				
meat and skin				
raw	1 neck (50 g)	148	**118**	33
	1 oz	84	**67**	18
fried, batter dipped	1 neck (52 g)	172	**110**	29
	1 oz	94	**60**	16
fried, flour coated	1 neck (36 g)	119	**76**	21
	1 oz	94	**60**	16
simmered	1 neck (38 g)	94	**62**	17
	1 oz	70	**46**	13
meat only				
raw	1 neck (20 g)	31	**16**	4
	1 oz	44	**22**	6
fried	1 neck (22 g)	50	**23**	6
	1 oz	65	**30**	8
simmered	1 neck (18 g)	32	**13**	3
	1 oz	44	**21**	5
Thigh				
meat and skin				
raw	1 thigh (94 g)	199	**129**	36
	1 oz	60	**39**	11
fried, batter-dipped	1 thigh (86 g)	238	**128**	34
	1 oz	78	**42**	11
fried, flour-coated	1 thigh (62 g)	162	**84**	23
	1 oz	74	**38**	11
roasted	1 thigh (62 g)	153	**86**	24
	1 oz	70	**40**	11
meat only				
raw	1 thigh (69 g)	82	**24**	6
	1 oz	34	**10**	3
fried	1 thigh (52 g)	113	**48**	13
	1 oz	62	**26**	7
roasted	1 thigh (52 g)	82	**24**	6
	1 oz	34	**10**	3

POULTRY

| FOOD | AMOUNT | CALORIES | | |
		TOTAL	FAT	SAT-FAT
Wing				
meat and skin				
raw	1 wing (49 g)	109	**70**	20
	1 oz	63	**41**	11
fried, batter-dipped	1 wing (49 g)	159	**96**	26
	1 oz	92	**56**	15
fried, flour-coated	1 wing (32 g)	103	**64**	17
	1 oz	91	**57**	15
roasted	1 wing (34 g)	99	**60**	17
	1 oz	82	**50**	14
meat only				
raw	1 wing (29 g)	36	**9**	2
	1 oz	36	**9**	2
fried	1 wing (20 g)	42	**16**	5
	1 oz	60	**23**	6
roasted	1 wing (21 g)	36	**9**	2
	1 oz	36	**9**	2
MIXED CHICKEN DISHES (*see also* **FROZEN, MICROWAVE, AND REFRIGERATED FOODS**)				
Chicken à la king	1 cup	470	**306**	116
Chicken and noodles	1 cup	365	**162**	46
Chicken potpie	⅓ pie	545	**279**	93
DUCK, DOMESTICATED				
meat and skin				
raw	½ duck (634 g)	2561	**2245**	754
	1 oz	115	**100**	33
roasted	½ duck (382 g)	1287	**975**	332
	1 oz	96	**72**	25
meat only				
raw	½ duck (303 g)	399	**162**	63
	1 oz	37	**15**	6
roasted	½ duck (221 g)	445	**223**	83
	1 oz	57	**29**	11
liver, raw	1 liver (44 g)	60	**18**	6
	1 oz	39	**12**	4
DUCK, WILD				
meat and skin, raw	½ duck (270 g)	571	**369**	125
	1 oz	60	**39**	13
breast meat only, raw	1 breast (83 g)	102	**32**	10
	1 oz	35	**11**	3
GOOSE, DOMESTICATED				
meat and skin				
raw	½ goose (1319 g)	4893	**3991**	1161
	1 oz	105	**86**	25

POULTRY

| FOOD | AMOUNT | CALORIES | | |
		TOTAL	FAT	SAT-FAT
meat and skin (cont.)				
roasted	½ goose (774 g)	2362	**1527**	479
	1 oz	86	**56**	18
meat only				
raw	½ goose (766 g)	1237	**492**	192
	1 oz	46	**18**	7
roasted	½ goose (591 g)	1406	**674**	242
	1 oz	67	**32**	12
liver, raw	1 liver (94 g)	125	**36**	14
	1 oz	38	**11**	4
PHEASANT				
meat and skin, raw	½ pheasant (400 g)	723	**335**	97
	1 oz	51	**24**	7
meat only, raw	½ pheasant (352 g)	470	**115**	39
	1 oz	38	**9**	3
breast meat only, raw	1 breast (182 g)	243	**53**	18
	1 oz	38	**8**	3
leg meat only, raw	1 leg (107 g)	143	**41**	14
	1 oz	38	**11**	4
QUAIL				
meat and skin, raw	1 quail (109 g)	210	**118**	33
	1 oz	54	**31**	9
meat only, raw	1 quail (92 g)	123	**38**	11
	1 oz	38	**12**	3
breast meat only, raw	1 breast (56 g)	69	**15**	4
	1 oz	35	**8**	2
SQUAB (PIGEON)				
meat and skin, raw	1 squab (199 g)	584	**426**	151
	1 oz	83	**61**	21
meat only, raw	1 squab (168 g)	239	**113**	30
	1 oz	40	**19**	5
breast meat only, raw	1 breast (101 g)	135	**41**	11
	1 oz	38	**12**	3
TURKEY				
Dark meat, roasted				
meat and skin	1 oz	52	**18**	5
meat only	1 oz	46	**11**	4
Light meat, roasted				
meat and skin	1 oz	46	**12**	3
meat only	1 oz	40	**3**	1
Back				
meat and skin				
raw	½ back (183 g)	275	**120**	35
	1 oz	43	**18**	5

POULTRY

FOOD	AMOUNT	CALORIES TOTAL	FAT	SAT-FAT
Turkey, Back (cont.)				
roasted	½ back (130 g)	265	120	35
	1 oz	58	26	8
meat only				
raw	½ back (150 g)	180	47	16
	1 oz	34	9	3
roasted	½ back (96 g)	180	47	16
	1 oz	34	9	3
Breast				
meat and skin				
raw	1 oz	35	7	2
roasted	1 oz	43	8	2
meat only				
raw	1 oz	31	2	1
roasted	1 oz	31	2	1
Cutlet, braised	1 oz	31	2	1
Ground Turkey				
Fresh				
Breast, 99% fat free (Shady Brook Farm)	112 g (4 oz)	120	5	0
Perdue	1 oz	40	18	6
lean (Shady Brook Farm)	112 g (4 oz)	160	70	18
Frozen (Longacre)	1 oz	53	33	7
Turkey Meatballs (Shady Brook Farms)	3 meatballs (85 g)	130	60	23
Leg				
meat and skin				
raw	1 leg (349 g)	412	112	34
	1 oz	33	9	3
roasted	1 leg (245 g)	418	119	37
	1 oz	48	14	4
meat only				
raw	1 leg (329 g)	356	70	24
	1 oz	31	6	2
roasted	1 leg (224 g)	355	76	24
	1 oz	45	10	3
Wing				
meat and skin				
raw	1 wing (128 g)	203	89	24
	1 oz	45	20	5
roasted	1 wing (90 g)	186	80	22
	1 oz	59	25	7
meat only				
raw	1 wing (90 g)	96	9	3
	1 oz	30	3	1

POULTRY

FOOD	AMOUNT	CALORIES		
		TOTAL	FAT	SAT-FAT
Wing (cont.)				
roasted	1 wing (60 g)	96	9	3
	1 oz	30	3	1

RESTAURANT FOODS

FOOD	AMOUNT	CALORIES		
		TOTAL	FAT	SAT-FAT
AU BON PAIN				
Breads				
Bagels				
Cinnamon Raisin	1	280	9	5
Plain, Onion, or Sesame	1	270	9	5
Loaf				
Baguette	1 loaf	810	18	5
Cheese	1 loaf	1670	261	81
Four Grain	1 loaf	1420	99	5
Onion Herb	1 loaf	1430	117	5
Parisienne	1 loaf	1490	36	5
Muffins				
Blueberry	1	390	99	36
Bran	1	390	99	27
Carrot	1	450	198	45
Corn	1	460	153	27
Cranberry Walnut	1	350	117	18
Oat Bran Apple	1	400	90	18
Pumpkin	1	410	144	18
Whole Grain	1	440	144	18
Rolls				
Alpine	1	220	27	5
Country Seed	1	220	36	5
Hearth	1	250	18	5
Petit Pain	1	220	9	5
Pumpernickel	1	210	18	5
Rye	1	230	18	5
3 Seed Raisin	1	250	36	5
Vegetable	1	230	45	5
Sandwich				
Braided Roll	1 roll	387	99	27
Croissant	1 roll	300	126	72
French Sandwich	1 roll	320	9	5
Hearth Sandwich	1 roll	370	27	5
Multigrain Slice	2 slices	391	27	9
Pita Pocket	1 pocket	80	9	5
Rye Slice	2 slices	374	36	9

RESTAURANT FOODS

		CALORIES		
FOOD	AMOUNT	TOTAL	FAT	SAT-FAT
Cookies				
Chocolate Chip	1 serving	280	135	81
Chocolate Chunk Pecan	1 serving	290	153	54
Oatmeal Raisin	1 serving	250	81	27
Peanut Butter	1 serving	290	135	54
White Chocolate Chunk Pecan	1 serving	300	153	54
Croissants				
Dessert				
Almond	1	420	225	108
Apple	1	250	90	54
Blueberry Cheese	1	380	180	108
Chocolate	1	400	216	126
Cinnamon Raisin	1	390	117	72
Coconut Pecan	1	440	207	108
Hazelnut Chocolate	1	480	252	126
Plain	1	220	90	54
Strawberry or Raspberry Cheese	1	400	180	108
Sweet Cheese	1	420	207	126
Hot Filled				
Ham & Cheese	1	370	180	108
Spinach & Cheese	1	290	144	90
Turkey & Cheddar	1	410	198	117
Turkey & Havarti	1	410	189	117
Salads				
Chicken Tarragon Garden	1	310	135	18
Cracked Pepper Chicken Garden	1	100	18	5
Grilled Chicken Garden	1	110	18	5
Large Garden	1	40	9	5
Shrimp Garden	1	102	18	5
Small Garden	1	20	9	5
Tuna Garden	1	350	225	36
Salad Dressings				
Balsamic Vinaigrette	2.25 oz	311	297	45
Champagne Vinaigrette	2.25 oz	251	234	36
County Blue Cheese	2.25 oz	325	279	54
Honey with Poppy Seed	2.25 oz	351	315	54
Low Cal Italian	2.25 oz	68	54	5
Olive Oil Caesar	2.25 oz	255	144	NA
Parmesan & Pepper	2.25 oz	235	189	45
Sesame French	2.25 oz	339	243	36
Tomato Basil	2.25 oz	66	9	0
Sandwich Fillings				
Cheese				
Brie Cheese	1 serving	300	216	135

RESTAURANT FOODS

FOOD	AMOUNT	CALORIES		
		TOTAL	**FAT**	**SAT-FAT**
Sandwich Fillings (cont.)				
Cheddar Cheese	1 serving	110	**81**	45
Herb Cheese	1 serving	290	**261**	162
Provolone Cheese	1 serving	155	**113**	66
Swiss Cheese	1 serving	330	**216**	135
Meats				
Albacore Tuna Salad	1 serving	310	**216**	36
Bacon	1 serving	140	**108**	36
Chicken Tarragon	1 serving	270	**135**	18
Country Ham	1 serving	150	**63**	27
Cracked Pepper Chicken	1 serving	120	**18**	5
Grilled Chicken	1 serving	130	**36**	5
Roast Beef	1 serving	180	**72**	36
Smoked Turkey	1 serving	100	**9**	5
Soups				
Beef Barley	1 cup	75	**18**	5
	1 bowl	112	**23**	9
Chicken Noodle	1 cup	79	**9**	5
	1 bowl	119	**15**	5
Clam Chowder	1 cup	289	**162**	81
	1 bowl	433	**243**	126
Cream of Broccoli	1 cup	201	**153**	72
	1 bowl	302	**234**	108
Garden Vegetarian	1 cup	29	**9**	5
	1 bowl	44	**9**	5
Minestrone	1 cup	105	**9**	5
	1 bowl	158	**15**	5
Split Pea	1 cup	176	**9**	5
	1 bowl	264	**15**	5
Tomato Florentine	1 cup	61	**9**	5
	1 bowl	92	**15**	5
Vegetarian Chili	1 cup	139	**27**	5
	1 bowl	208	**36**	5
BOSTON MARKET				
¼ white meat chicken				
without skin & wing	140 g	170	**35**	9
with skin & wing	152 g	280	**110**	32
¼ dark meat chicken				
without skin	95 g	190	**90**	27
with skin	125 g	320	**190**	54
½ chicken with skin	277 g	590	**300**	90
Baked Italian pasta	¾ cup (170 g)	190	**80**	32
BBQ baked beans	¾ cup (201 g)	270	**45**	18
Brownie	1 piece (95 g)	450	**240**	63
Butternut squash	¾ cup (193 g)	160	**60**	36

RESTAURANT FOODS

		CALORIES		
FOOD	AMOUNT	TOTAL	FAT	SAT-FAT
Caesar salad				
entree	1 (283 g)	510	**380**	99
without dressing	1 (225 g)	230	**110**	54
side	1 (113 g)	200	**159**	41
Chicken Caesar salad	1 (369 g)	650	**410**	108
Chicken gravy	28 g	15	**10**	0
Chicken noodle soup	1 cup (257 g)	130	**40**	9
Chicken potpie	1 pie (425 g)	780	**410**	117
Chicken salad sandwich	1 (327 g)	680	**270**	45
Chicken sandwich				
with cheese & sauce	1 (352 g)	750	**300**	108
without cheese & sauce	1 (281 g)	430	**40**	9
Chicken tortilla soup	1 cup (238 g)	220	**100**	36
Chocolate chip cookie	1 (79 g)	340	**150**	54
Chunky chicken salad	1¾ cup (58 g)	370	**240**	41
Cinnamon apple pie	⅕ pie (136 g)	390	**200**	36
Corn bread	1 loaf (68 g)	200	**50**	14
Creamed spinach	¾ cup (181 g)	260	**180**	117
Fruit salad	¾ cup (156 g)	70	**5**	0
Green bean casserole	¾ cup (170 g)	130	**80**	41
Ham & turkey club				
with cheese & sauce	1 (379 g)	890	**390**	180
without cheese & sauce	1 (266 g)	420	**50**	14
Ham sandwich				
with cheese & sauce	1 (337 g)	750	**310**	108
without cheese & sauce	1 (266 g)	440	**70**	23
Hearth honey ham	142 g	210	**80**	32
Homestyle mashed potatoes	⅔ cup (161 g)	190	**80**	54
with gravy	¾ cup (189 g)	210	**90**	54
Hot cinnamon apples	¾ cup (181 g)	250	**40**	5
Macaroni & cheese	¾ cup (192 g)	280	**100**	54
Meat loaf & chunky tomato sauce	227 g	370	**160**	72
Meat loaf & brown gravy	198 g	390	**200**	72
Meat loaf sandwich				
with cheese	1 (383 g)	860	**290**	144
without cheese	1 (351 g)	690	**190**	63
New potatoes	¾ cup (131 g)	130	**20**	0
Old fashioned potato salad	¾ cup (176 g)	340	**210**	36
Rice Pilaf	⅔ cup (145 g)	180	**45**	9
Savory stuffing	¾ cup (174 g)	310	**110**	18
Skinless rotisserie turkey breast	142 g	170	**10**	5
Steamed vegetables	⅔ cup (105 g)	35	**5**	0
Turkey sandwich				
with cheese & sauce	1 (337 g)	710	**260**	90
without cheese & sauce	1 (266 g)	400	**30**	9
Whole kernel corn	¾ cup (146 g)	180	**40**	5

RESTAURANT FOODS

		CALORIES		
FOOD	AMOUNT	TOTAL	FAT	SAT-FAT

CHAIN FAMILY-STYLE RESTAURANTS, such as Applebee's, Bennigans, Chili's, TGI Friday's, Grady's American Grill, Hard Rock Cafe, Houlihan's, Houston's, and Ruby Tuesday*

Appetizers				
Buffalo Wings	12 wings	700	**432**	144
Chili	1½ cups	350	**144**	72
Fried Mozzarella Sticks	9 sticks	830	**459**	252
Stuffed Potato Skins	8 skins	1120	**711**	360
Entrees				
Beef				
BBQ Baby Back Ribs	14 ribs	770	**486**	189
Hamburger	1	660	**324**	153
Mushroom Cheeseburger	1	900	**513**	252
Sirloin Steak	7 oz	410	**180**	90
Steak Fajitas with Tortillas	1 order	860	**279**	108
with guacamole, sour				
cream, & cheese		1190	**567**	252
Chicken				
Bacon & Cheese Grilled				
Chicken Sandwich	1	650	**270**	108
Chicken Caesar Salad with				
dressing	4 cups	660	**414**	99
Chicken Fajitas with Tortillas	1 order	840	**216**	54
with guacamole, sour				
cream, & cheese		1170	**504**	198
Chicken Fingers	5 pieces	620	**306**	117
Grilled Chicken	6 oz	270	**72**	27
with loaded baked				
potato & vegetables		950	**378**	207
Oriental Chicken Salad				
with dressing	4 cups	750	**441**	108
Side Orders				
Cole Slaw	1 cup	170	**126**	18
French Fries	2 cups	590	**279**	108
Loaded Baked Potato	1	620	**279**	171
Onion Rings	11	900	**576**	207
Vegetable of the Day	1 cup	60	**27**	9
Dessert				
Fudge Brownie Sundae	10 oz	1130	**513**	270

CHILI'S				
Chicken fajitas	1 order	870	**306**	NA
Chicken sandwich	1	1082	**450**	NA

*Adapted from *Nutrition Action Health Letter,* October 1996.

RESTAURANT FOODS

FOOD	AMOUNT	CALORIES TOTAL	FAT	SAT-FAT
Diet by Chocolate cake with				
hot fudge sauce	1 slice	370	**18**	5
Grilled chicken platter	1	757	**189**	NA
Guiltless Grill				
chicken fajitas	1 order	690	**54**	18
chicken platter	1	450	**32**	9
chicken salad	1	254	**30**	10
chicken sandwich	1	485	**47**	14
Tuna sandwich	1	950	**342**	NA

CHINESE RESTAURANT

FOOD	AMOUNT	CALORIES TOTAL	FAT	SAT-FAT
Barbecued pork (not fried)	1 whole dish	1374	**986**	355
Barbecued spareribs	1 whole dish	1863	**1232**	480
Beef with vegetables	1 whole dish	1572	**1068**	263
Chicken with cashews	1 whole dish	1765	**1075**	186
Chicken with vegetables	1 whole dish	1224	**652**	102
Chinese Noodle Soup	1 serving	265	**81**	NA
Egg rolls	1	152	**103**	30
Hot and sour soup	1 serving	165	**72**	NA
Hunan shrimp (not fried)	1 whole dish	1068	**755**	100
Kung Pao beef	1 whole dish	2458	**1706**	444
Kung Pao chicken	1 whole dish	1806	**1134**	158
Kung Pao shrimp	1 whole dish	1068	**755**	115
Moo shu pork	1 whole dish	1383	**1053**	258
Orange beef	1 whole dish	1710	**1216**	342
Pork with vegetables	1 whole dish	1574	**1219**	338
Sweet and sour pork	1 whole dish	1845	**1509**	389
Sweet and sour shrimp	1 whole dish	1069	**805**	130
Szechuan pork	1 whole dish	1694	**1339**	356
Velvet corn soup	1 serving	115	**27**	NA
Wonton soup	1 serving	283	**108**	NA

COFFEE BAR COFFEES

If whipped cream is added to your coffee, add 60 total calories and 45 fat calories.

COFFEE BEANERY

FOOD	AMOUNT	CALORIES TOTAL	FAT	SAT-FAT
Cafe Mocha				
with whole milk	8 fl oz	94	**45**	NA
with 2% milk	8 fl oz	76	**27**	NA
with nonfat milk	8 fl oz	54	**0**	NA
Cappuccino				
with whole milk	12 fl oz	296	**81**	NA
with 2% milk	12 fl oz	267	**54**	NA
with nonfat milk	12 fl oz	232	**9**	NA
Espresso	2.4 fl oz	0	**0**	NA
Latte				
with whipped cream and				
grated chocolate	16 fl oz	350	**180**	NA
with whole milk	16 fl oz	263	**126**	NA

RESTAURANT FOODS

FOOD	AMOUNT	CALORIES		
		TOTAL	FAT	SAT-FAT
Latte (cont.)				
with 2% milk	16 fl oz	211	**72**	NA
with nonfat milk	16 fl oz	151	**9**	NA
GLORIA JEAN'S (only made with 2% milk)				
Cafe Mocha	8 fl oz	222	**36**	NA
Grande	16 fl oz	312	**63**	NA
Iced	12 fl oz	282	**54**	NA
Espresso	2.7 fl oz	0	**0**	NA
Latte	8 fl oz	76	**27**	NA
Grande	16 fl oz	166	**54**	NA
STARBUCKS				
Coffee Drinks				
Caffe Latte				
Short				
with whole milk	8 fl oz	140	**60**	41
with lowfat milk	8 fl oz	110	**35**	23
with nonfat milk	8 fl oz	80	**0**	0
with soy milk	8 fl oz	70	**35**	0
Tall				
with whole milk	12 fl oz	210	**100**	63
with lowfat milk	12 fl oz	170	**50**	36
with nonfat milk	12 fl oz	120	**5**	0
with soy milk	12 fl oz	110	**60**	5
Grande				
with whole milk	16 fl oz	270	**130**	81
with lowfat milk	16 fl oz	220	**70**	45
with nonfat milk	16 fl oz	160	**10**	5
with soy milk	16 fl oz	150	**70**	0
Venti				
with whole milk	20 fl oz	350	**160**	108
with lowfat milk	20 fl oz	270	**90**	54
with nonfat milk	20 fl oz	200	**10**	5
with soy milk	20 fl oz	190	**90**	9
Caffe Mocha with whipping cream				
Short				
with whole milk	8 fl oz	250	**150**	90
with lowfat milk	8 fl oz	220	**120**	72
with nonfat milk	8 fl oz	200	**100**	63
Tall				
with whole milk	12 fl oz	340	**190**	117
with lowfat milk	12 fl oz	300	**150**	90
with nonfat milk	12 fl oz	260	**100**	63
Grande				
with whole milk	16 fl oz	410	**220**	135
with lowfat milk	16 fl oz	370	**160**	99
with nonfat milk	16 fl oz	320	**110**	72
Venti				
with whole milk	20 fl oz	500	**250**	162

RESTAURANT FOODS

FOOD	AMOUNT	CALORIES		
		TOTAL	FAT	SAT-FAT
Starbucks, Coffee Drinks (cont.)				
with lowfat milk	20 fl oz	440	**190**	117
with nonfat milk	20 fl oz	380	**120**	72
Caffe Mocha (iced) with whipping cream				
Short				
with whole milk	8 fl oz	180	**110**	72
with lowfat milk	8 fl oz	170	**90**	54
with nonfat milk	8 fl oz	150	**80**	45
Tall				
with whole milk	12 fl oz	290	**160**	99
with lowfat milk	12 fl oz	260	**130**	81
with nonfat milk	12 fl oz	230	**100**	63
Grande				
with whole milk	16 fl oz	390	**220**	135
with lowfat milk	16 fl oz	350	**180**	108
with nonfat milk	16 fl oz	310	**130**	81
Caffe Rhumba				
Tall				
with lowfat milk	12 fl oz	250	**45**	36
Grande				
with lowfat milk	16 fl oz	330	**60**	45
Venti				
with lowfat milk	20 fl oz	410	**70**	63
Cappuccino				
Short				
with whole milk	8 fl oz	100	**45**	31
with lowfat milk	8 fl oz	80	**25**	14
with nonfat milk	8 fl oz	60	**0**	0
with soy milk	8 fl oz	50	**25**	0
Tall				
with whole milk	12 fl oz	140	**60**	41
with lowfat milk	12 fl oz	110	**35**	23
with nonfat milk	12 fl oz	80	**0**	0
with soy milk	12 fl oz	70	**35**	0
Grande				
with whole milk	16 fl oz	180	**80**	54
with lowfat milk	16 fl oz	140	**45**	27
with nonfat milk	16 fl oz	110	**5**	0
with soy milk	16 fl oz	100	**50**	5
Venti				
with whole milk	20 fl oz	200	**90**	63
with lowfat milk	20 fl oz	160	**50**	32
with nonfat milk	20 fl oz	120	**5**	0
with soy milk	20 fl oz	110	**50**	5
Espresso				
Solo	1 fl oz	5	**0**	0
Doppio	2 fl oz	10	**0**	0

RESTAURANT FOODS

FOOD	AMOUNT	CALORIES		
		TOTAL	FAT	SAT-FAT
Coffee Drinks (cont.)				
Con Panna				
Solo	1 fl oz	30	**25**	18
Doppio	2 fl oz	35	**25**	18
Macchiato				
Solo				
with whole milk	1 fl oz	15	**5**	0
with lowfat milk	1 fl oz	10	**0**	0
with nonfat milk	1 fl oz	10	**0**	0
Doppio				
with whole milk	2 fl oz	20	**5**	0
with lowfat milk	2 fl oz	15	**0**	0
with nonfat milk	2 fl oz	15	**0**	0
Frappuccino				
Tall				
with lowfat milk	12 fl oz	200	**25**	14
Grande				
with lowfat milk	16 fl oz	270	**35**	23
Venti				
with lowfat milk	20 fl oz	340	**45**	27
Power Frappuccino				
Tall	12 fl oz	290	**20**	9
Grande	16 fl oz	350	**25**	14
Venti	20 fl oz	410	**25**	18
Power Mocha Frappuccino				
Tall	12 fl oz	320	**25**	14
Grande	16 fl oz	390	**25**	18
Venti	20 fl oz	460	**30**	23
Cocoa Drinks				
Cocoa with whipping cream				
Short				
with whole milk	8 fl oz	260	**160**	99
with lowfat milk	8 fl oz	230	**130**	81
with nonfat milk	8 fl oz	210	**100**	63
Tall				
with whole milk	12 fl oz	350	**190**	126
with lowfat milk	12 fl oz	310	**150**	90
with nonfat milk	12 fl oz	270	**100**	63
Grande				
with whole milk	16 fl oz	440	**230**	144
with lowfat milk	16 fl oz	390	**170**	108
with nonfat milk	16 fl oz	330	**110**	72
Venti				
with whole milk	20 fl oz	530	**270**	171
with lowfat milk	20 fl oz	460	**200**	126
with nonfat milk	20 fl oz	390	**120**	72

RESTAURANT FOODS

FOOD	AMOUNT	CALORIES		
		TOTAL	FAT	SAT-FAT
Tea Drinks				
Chai Tea Latte hot				
Short				
with whole milk	8 fl oz	160	**60**	36
with lowfat milk	8 fl oz	130	**30**	18
with nonfat milk	8 fl oz	110	**0**	0
Tall				
with whole milk	12 fl oz	220	**80**	54
with lowfat milk	12 fl oz	190	**45**	27
with nonfat milk	12 fl oz	150	**0**	0
Grande				
with whole milk	16 fl oz	310	**120**	72
with lowfat milk	16 fl oz	260	**60**	41
with nonfat milk	16 fl oz	210	**5**	0
Venti				
with whole milk	20 fl oz	400	**150**	99
with lowfat milk	20 fl oz	330	**80**	54
with nonfat milk	20 fl oz	270	**10**	5
Cakes, Cookies, and Pastries				
Biscotti				
Chocolate Hazelnut				
standard size	1 (29 g)	110	**45**	18
mini size	1 (12 g)	50	**20**	9
Vanilla Almond				
standard size	1 (28 g)	110	**40**	14
mini size	1 (14 g)	50	**20**	9
Brownies & Bars				
Blondies	1 (76 g)	350	**170**	81
Fantasy Bar	⅓ bar (35 g)	180	**80**	41
Raspberry Crumb Bar	⅓ bar (35 g)	160	**70**	27
Ultra Chocolate Brownie	1 bar (98 g)	418	**146**	75
Ultra Hazelnut Brownie	1 bar (35 g)	433	**174**	72
Walnut Brownie	1 brownie (98 g)	450	**240**	99
Cookie				
Oatmeal Raisin	1 (85 g)	400	**130**	45
Croissants				
Almond	1 (74 g)	320	**150**	81
Butter	1 (99 g)	410	**210**	144
Chocolate	1 (99 g)	400	**200**	136
Cupcakes				
Carrot Cake	1 (114 g)	440	**210**	81
Chocolate Chocolate	1 (113 g)	380	**140**	63
Focaccia				
Tomato & Cheese	1 (170 g)	640	**385**	90
Muffins				
Chocolate Chunk	1 muffin (145 g)	580	**280**	81

RESTAURANT FOODS

FOOD	AMOUNT	CALORIES		
		TOTAL	FAT	SAT-FAT
Cakes, Cookies, and Pastries (cont.)				
Cranberry Orange	1 muffin (145 g)	520	300	36
Lemon Poppyseed	1 muffin (145 g)	540	210	45
Blueberry	1 muffin (145 g)	490	230	63
Blueberry, lowfat	1 muffin (113 g)	250	10	0
Pecan Rolls	1 (145 g)	450	150	54
Rugelach				
Cinnamon Raisin (traditional)	3 dolcini (64 g)	380	270	108
Scones				
Apricot reduced fat	1 (128 g)	320	50	41
Blueberry (no cholesterol)	1 (128 g)	380	100	54
Chocolate	1 (1298 g)	420	140	81
Cinnamon	1 (128 g)	420	130	63
Maple Oat Nut	1 (124 g)	540	250	126
Multigrain (50% reduced fat)	1 (128 g)	320	50	41
Very Blueberry	1 (124 g)	530	210	126
DELI SANDWICH SHOPS				
Bacon, lettuce, and tomato	8 oz	599	333	108
Chicken salad (plain bread)	10 oz	537	288	54
with mayo	10 oz	655	414	72
Corned beef with mustard	9 oz	497	180	72
Egg salad (plain bread)	10 oz	546	279	90
with mayo	10 oz	664	396	108
Grilled cheese (plain bread)	5 oz	511	297	153
Ham with mustard	9 oz	563	243	90
with mayo	9 oz	666	360	108
Reuben	14 oz	916	450	180
Roast beef with mustard	9 oz	462	108	36
with mayo	9 oz	565	216	54
Tuna salad (plain bread)	11 oz	716	387	72
with mayo	11 oz	833	504	90
Turkey Club	13 oz	737	306	90
Turkey with mustard	9 oz	370	54	18
with mayo	9 oz	473	171	36
Vegetarian	12 oz	753	360	126
DENNY'S				
Baked potato	1	180	0	0
Banana/Strawberry Medley	½ cup	170	9	0
Biscuit	1	217	63	NA
BLT Sandwich	1	492	306	NA
Blueberry Muffin	1	309	126	NA
Catfish	1 entree	576	432	NA
Buttermilk Pancakes, plain	3	410	54	18
Chicken Strips	4 oz	240	90	NA
Chili	8 oz	238	135	NA

RESTAURANT FOODS

		CALORIES		
FOOD	AMOUNT	TOTAL	FAT	SAT-FAT
Cinnamon Roll	1	450	126	NA
Club Sandwich	1	590	180	NA
Coleslaw	1 cup	119	86	NA
Country Gravy	1 oz	140	72	NA
Eggs Benedict	1	658	320	NA
French Fries	1 order	303	142	NA
French Toast	2 slices	729	504	NA
Fried Chicken, entree only	4 pieces	463	270	NA
Fried Shrimp, entree only	1	230	135	NA
Grilled Cheese Sandwich	1	454	261	NA
Grilled Chicken, entree only	1	130	36	9
Grilled Chicken Sandwich	1	439	108	NA
Guacamole	1 oz	60	55	NA
Hamburger				
Bacon Swiss burger	1	819	468	NA
Denny burger	1	629	340	NA
San Fran burger	1	872	432	NA
Works burger	1	944	549	NA
Hashed Browns	4 oz	164	18	NA
Liver with Bacon and Onions, entree only	2 slices	334	130	NA
Mozzarella Sticks	1 piece	88	60	NA
Omelet				
Denver	1	567	243	NA
Ultimate	1	577	369	NA
Veggie Cheese	1	350	180	NA
Onion Rings	3 rings	258	135	NA
Patty Melt	1	761	423	NA
Rice Pilaf	⅓ cup	89	21	NA
Salads				
California Grilled Chicken, no dressing	1	280	90	9
Chef	1	492	180	NA
Chicken salad, no shell	1	207	36	NA
Garden, no dressing	1	115	36	9
Taco, no shell	1	514	180	NA
Tuna salad	1	340	162	NA
Sausage	1 link	113	90	NA
Senior Grilled Chicken, entree only	1	130	36	9
Soups				
Cheese	1 bowl	309	198	NA
Chicken Noodle	1 bowl	45	9	0
Clam Chowder	1 bowl	235	126	NA
Cream of Potato	1 bowl	175	81	63
Split Pea	1 bowl	231	45	NA
Spaghetti with Tomato Sauce	1 order	600	72	0

RESTAURANT FOODS

FOOD	AMOUNT	CALORIES		
		TOTAL	FAT	SAT-FAT
Stir-fry, entree only	1	328	**99**	NA
Stuffing	½ cup	180	**81**	NA
Super Bird Sandwich	1	625	**216**	NA
Steak				
Chicken Fried Steak, entree				
only, no gravy	2 pieces	252	**131**	NA
Hamburger Steak	1 entree	669	**484**	NA
New York Steak, entree only	1	582	**324**	NA
Top Sirloin Steak, entree only	1	223	**57**	NA
Tortilla Shell, fried	1	439	**270**	NA
Turkey, no gravy, entree only	1	505	**130**	NA
Waffle	1	261	**94**	NA

INTERNATIONAL HOUSE OF PANCAKES

FOOD	AMOUNT	CALORIES		
Pancakes				
Buttermilk	1 pancake (56 g)	108	**28**	6
Buckwheat	1 pancake (63 g)	134	**45**	11
Country Griddle	1 pancake (63 g)	134	**34**	9
Egg	1 pancake (56 g)	102	**45**	11
Harvest Grain 'N Nut	1 pancake (63 g)	160	**74**	12
Foods prepared with Eggstro'dnaire				
Broccoli & Mushroom				
Omelette	1 omelette	310	**62**	NA
Breakfast Burrito	1 burrito	456	**109**	NA
Chicken Fajita Burrito	1 burrito	523	**89**	NA
French Toast	1 piece	99	**18**	NA
Waffles				
Regular	1 waffle (112 g)	305	**133**	30
Belgian				
Regular	1 waffle (168 g)	408	**177**	100
Harvest Grain 'N Nut	1 waffle (168 g)	445	**251**	107

ITALIAN RESTAURANT

FOOD	AMOUNT	CALORIES		
Appetizers				
Antipasto	1.5 lbs	629	**423**	132
Entrees				
Eggplant Parmigiana with				
spaghetti	2.5 cups	1208	**558**	145
Fettuccine Alfredo	2.5 cups	1498	**873**	434
Lasagna	2 cups	958	**477**	192
Linguine with red clam sauce	3 cups	892	**207**	36
Linguine with white clam sauce	3 cups	907	**261**	45
Spaghetti with meat sauce	3 cups	918	**225**	92
Spaghetti with meatballs	3.5 cups	1155	**351**	94
Spaghetti with sausage	2.5 cups	1043	**351**	92
Spaghetti with tomato sauce	3.5 cups	849	**153**	34
Veal Parmigiana with spaghetti	1.5 cups	1064	**396**	128

RESTAURANT FOODS

FOOD	AMOUNT	CALORIES		
		TOTAL	FAT	SAT-FAT
Side Dishes				
Fried calamari	3 cups	1037	**630**	83
Garlic bread	8 oz	822	**360**	90
Spaghetti with tomato sauce	1.5 cups	409	**72**	16
MEXICAN RESTAURANT				
Appetizers				
Beef and cheese nachos				
with sour cream and				
guacamole	1 serving	1362	**801**	250
Cheese quesadilla				
with sour cream and				
guacamole	1 serving	900	**531**	220
Cheese Nachos	1 serving	807	**500**	225
Entrees				
Beef Burrito	1 serving	833	**360**	121
with beans, rice, sour				
cream, and guacamole	1 serving	1639	**711**	248
Beef Chimichanga	1 serving	802	**423**	113
with beans, rice, sour				
cream, and guacamole	1 serving	1607	**774**	241
Beef Enchilada	1 serving	324	**171**	67
two enchiladas with beans				
and rice	1 serving	1253	**522**	140
Chicken Fajitas and Flour				
Tortillas	1 serving	839	**216**	54
with beans, rice, sour				
cream, and guacamole	1 serving	1661	**567**	173
Chile Rellenos	1 serving	487	**342**	45
two chile rellenos with				
beans and rice	1 serving	1578	**864**	173
Chicken Enchilada	1 serving	329	**162**	103
two enchiladas with beans				
and rice	1 serving	1264	**513**	270
Crispy Chicken Taco	1 serving	219	**99**	27
two tacos with beans and rice	1 serving	1042	**378**	119
Taco Salad				
with sour cream and				
guacamole	1 serving	1099	**639**	177
Side Dishes				
Rice	¾ cup	229	**34**	5
Refried beans	¾ cup	375	**146**	60
Tortilla chips	50 chips	645	**432**	81
OLIVE GARDEN				
Breadsticks				
garlic	1 stick	160	**32**	14
plain	1 stick	140	**14**	0

RESTAURANT FOODS

		CALORIES		
FOOD	AMOUNT	TOTAL	FAT	SAT-FAT
Capellini pomodoro	1 dinner	520	144	32
	1 lunch	340	72	18
Capellini primavera	1 dinner	380	63	27
	1 lunch	270	45	18
Garden salad, no dressing	1 order	70	9	0
Grilled chicken with peppers	1 dinner	470	81	32
Julius				
banana	16 oz	210	9	5
banana Julius Smoothy	16 oz	270	54	45
Cool Cappuccino Julius Java	16 oz	390	63	63
Cool Mocha Julius Java	16 oz	460	90	72
lemon, orange, peach, pineapple, or strawberry Julius	16 oz	190-220	5	0
pinata colada Julius Smoothy	16 oz	330	54	45
strawberry Julius Smoothy	16 oz	330	54	45
tropical Julius Smoothy	16 oz	330	54	45
Minestrone soup	6 oz	80	9	0
Pasta e fagioli soup	6 oz	140	45	14
Raspberry sorbetto	170 g	110	0	0
Shrimp primavera	1 dinner	420	108	27
	1 lunch	320	90	18
Spaghetti				
with marinara sauce	1 dinner	500	81	14
	1 lunch	340	54	9
with Sicilian sauce	1 dinner	530	108	14
	1 lunch	370	72	9
with tomato sauce	1 dinner	550	90	14
	1 lunch	390	63	9
Venetian grilled chicken	1 dinner	240	45	14
RAX				
Baked Potato				
Barbecue with 2 oz cheese	1 serving	730	216	NA
Chili with 2 oz cheese	1 serving	700	207	NA
Plain	1 serving	270	0	0
with margarine	1 serving	370	99	NA
with sour cream topping	1 serving	400	99	NA
with 3 oz cheese & bacon	1 serving	780	252	NA
with 3 oz cheese & broccoli	1 serving	760	234	NA
Barbecue Sandwich	1	420	126	NA
Beans				
Garbanzo	½ cup	360	45	NA
Kidney	1 cup	220	9	NA
Breadstick, sesame	28 g	150	90	NA
Chili Topping	84 g	80	18	NA
Coleslaw	98 g	70	36	NA
Chocolate Chip Cookie	1	130	54	NA

RESTAURANT FOODS

FOOD	AMOUNT	CALORIES TOTAL	FAT	SAT-FAT
French Fries				
large	1 order	390	**180**	NA
regular	1 order	260	**117**	NA
Hot Chocolate	1 serving	110	**99**	NA
Milkshakes, without whipped topping				
Chocolate	1 serving	560	**117**	NA
Strawberry	1 serving	560	**117**	NA
Vanilla	1 serving	500	**126**	NA
Pasta & Noodles				
Pasta Shells	98 g	170	**36**	NA
Pasta/Vegetable Blend	98 g	100	**36**	NA
Rainbow Rotini	98 g	180	**36**	NA
Potato Salad	1 cup	260	**153**	NA
Pudding, all flavors	98 g	140	**54**	NA
Refried Beans	84 g	120	**36**	NA
Roast Beef	1 serving	140	**54**	NA
Salads				
Chef, no dressing	1 serving	230	**126**	NA
Garden, no dressing	1 serving	160	**99**	NA
Garden, Lighterside	1 serving	134	**54**	NA
Macaroni	98 g	160	**63**	NA
Pasta	98 g	80	**9**	NA
Potato	1 cup	260	**63**	NA
Three Bean	½ cup	100	**9**	NA
Salad dressing (see **FATS AND OILS**)				
Sandwiches				
Beef				
BBQ Beef, Bacon, Chicken	1 serving	720	**441**	NA
Philly Beef & Cheese	1 serving	480	**198**	NA
Fish	1 serving	460	**153**	NA
Ham & Cheese	1	430	**207**	NA
Roast Beef				
large	1 serving	570	**315**	NA
regular	1 serving	320	**99**	NA
small	1 serving	260	**126**	NA
Turkey Bacon Club	1 serving	670	**387**	NA
Sauces				
Cheese				
Nacho	98 g	470	**198**	NA
Regular	98 g	420	**153**	NA
Spaghetti				
Regular	98 g	80	**9**	NA
With Meat	98 g	150	**72**	NA
Spicy Meat	98 g	80	**36**	NA
Taco	98 g	30	**9**	NA

RESTAURANT FOODS

FOOD	AMOUNT	CALORIES		
		TOTAL	FAT	SAT-FAT
Soups				
Chicken Noodle	98 g	40	9	NA
Cream of Broccoli	98 g	50	18	NA
Soy Nuts	28 g	120	63	NA
Spaghetti	98 g	140	36	NA
Taco Shell	1 shell	40	18	NA
Tortilla	1 tortilla	110	18	NA
Turkey Bits	56 g	70	27	NA
Whipped Topping	1 dollop	50	36	NA
RED LOBSTER				
Alaskan snow crab legs	1 order (454 g)	200	99	54
Bay platter	1	680	243	81
Bayou-style seafood gumbo	170 g	180	45	9
Broiled fish fillet sandwich	1	230	86	5
Broiled flounder fillets	1 order (142 g)	150	54	27
Broiled rock lobster	1 order (369 g)	250	45	18
Fish fillet sandwich	1	230	85	9
Grilled chicken breast				
dinner menu	228 g	340	108	36
lunch menu	114 g	170	54	18
Grilled chicken (114 g) and 10				
shrimp	1 order	490	180	54
Grilled Chicken sandwich	1	340	90	36
Grilled shrimp salad, lite dressing	1 order	170	72	9
Grilled shrimp skewers	120 shrimp	290	81	36
Ice cream	1 order (128 g)	260	126	81
Live Maine lobster	1 order (511 g)	200	45	18
Rice pilaf	114 g	140	27	4
Seafood Lover's platter	1	650	243	108
Sherbet	1 order (128 g)	180	27	18
Shrimp				
cocktail	6 shrimp	90	18	4
in the shell	170 g	130	18	5
scampi	11 shrimp	310	207	126
Today's fresh catch *(for lunch portions, halve the total calories, fat calories, and sat-fat calories)*				
Atlantic cod	1 dinner (10 oz)	300	108	54
Atlantic salmon	1 dinner (10 oz)	460	306	108
Catfish	1 dinner (10 oz)	440	270	108
Coho salmon	1 dinner (10 oz)	480	252	90
Grouper	1 dinner (10 oz)	300	108	54
Haddock	1 dinner (10 oz)	320	108	54
King salmon	1 dinner (10 oz)	580	360	72
Mahi mahi	1 dinner (10 oz)	320	108	54
Ocean perch	1 dinner (10 oz)	360	162	90
Orange roughy	1 dinner (10 oz)	440	270	54

RESTAURANT FOODS

		CALORIES		
FOOD	AMOUNT	TOTAL	FAT	SAT-FAT
Red Lobster, Today's fresh catch (cont.)				
Rainbow trout	1 dinner (10 oz)	440	252	72
Red rockfish	1 dinner (10 oz)	280	108	54
Sea bass	1 dinner (10 oz)	360	144	72
Snapper	1 dinner (10 oz)	320	108	54
Sole	1 dinner (10 oz)	320	108	54
Swordfish	1 dinner (10 oz)	300	162	108
Walleye pike	1 dinner (10 oz)	340	108	54
Yellow lake perch	1 dinner (10 oz)	340	108	54
SWISS CHALET				
Apple Pie	1 serving	413	171	36
Back Rib	full rib	810	468	162
Caesar Salad Entrée	1 serving	454	342	36
Caesar Salad Appetizer	1 serving	345	171	36
Chicken				
White (with skin)	¼ chicken	381	198	36
White (skinless)	¼ chicken	225	72	18
Dark (with skin)	¼ chicken	313	153	45
Dark (skinless)	¼ chicken	232	90	27
Chicken (with skin)	½ chicken	694	351	81
Chicken Pot Pie	1 pie	494	216	45
Chicken Salad & Roll	1 serving	466	198	36
Roll	1 roll	116	9	0
MISCELLANEOUS RESTAURANT FOODS				
Beef Gyro	1 sandwich (122 g)	340	190	99
Caesar salad*	1 salad	660	414	NA
Fettuccine with creamed spinach*	1 serving	1050	738	NA
Focaccia club sandwich*	1 sandwich	1222	585	NA
Gnocchi*	1 serving	700	423	NA
Lasagna*	1 serving	960	477	NA
Omelet	for 1	337	250	110
Cheese	for 1	377	276	126
Denver	for 1	425	290	125
Porterhouse steak dinner*	1 dinner	1860	1125	NA
Risotto	1 serving	1280	990	NA
Tuna salad sandwich*	1 sandwich	720	387	NA

*Source: Marion Burrows, *New York Times*

SALAD BAR FOODS

		CALORIES		
FOOD	AMOUNT	TOTAL	FAT	SAT-FAT
Bacon bits	1 tbsp (7 g)	30	10	0
Baked beans	½ cup	160	36	5

SALAD BAR FOODS

FOOD	AMOUNT	CALORIES		
		TOTAL	FAT	SAT-FAT
Breadsticks, mini, sesame	2 (7 g)	35	10	0
Sauces				
nacho cheese	¼ cup	120	90	54
Cheese, shredded				
cheddar	⅓ cup	110	80	45
mozzarella	¼ cup	80	45	27
Chow mein noodles	½ cup	140	60	NA
Cottage cheese (4% fat)	½ cup	120	45	27
Crackers				
Oyster	1 pkg (14 g)	60	25	5
Saltine	2 crackers (14 g)	25	5	0
Croutons	2 tbsp (7 g)	35	20	0
Eggs, chopped, hard boiled	28 g	45	25	9
Olives, green or ripe	2 tbsp (16 g)	30	25	0
Puddings & Desserts				
Bread pudding	½ cup	170	36	NA
Chocolate mousse	½ cup	160	45	NA
Chocolate pudding	½ cup	110	18	9
Lemon mousse	½ cup	160	45	NA
Rice pudding	½ cup	120	15	9
Strawberry Creme dessert	1 container (99 g)	100	10	9
Strawberry Fruit dessert	1 container (113 g)	90	0	0
Tapioca Pudding	1 container (113 g)	120	15	9
Salads				
Carrot Waldorf	½ cup	190	108	18
Creamy coleslaw	½ cup	220	60	18
Pasta				
Chicken	¾ cup	320	225	27
Fiesta	⅔ cup	240	80	18
Macaroni	½ cup	370	220	27
Penne mozzarella	¾ cup	190	70	18
Rigati Garden	½ cup	170	80	9
Seafood	¾ cup	290	190	23
Sicilian Tortellini	1 cup	280	50	18
Spaghetti	¾ cup	310	160	36
Tuna supreme	½ cup	240	160	18
Vegetable Pasta (cholesterol				
free)	⅔ cup	170	15	5
with broccoli	⅔ cup	190	50	5
Polynesian	½ cup	160	45	14
Potato	½ cup	210	80	9
Red skin potato	⅔ cup	260	155	45
Three bean	⅓ cup	90	5	0
Waldorf	½ cup	250	225	30
Salad dressings (see **FATS AND OILS**)				
Sauces				
Salsa	2 tbsp	10	0	0

SALAD BAR FOODS

		CALORIES		
FOOD	AMOUNT	TOTAL	FAT	SAT-FAT
Soup bar				
Bean and ham	1 cup	180	25	9
Beef barley	1 cup	127	24	NA
Beef stew	1 cup	270	130	45
Chicken corn noodle	1 cup	150	20	5
Chicken noodle	1 cup	170	30	14
Chicken rice	1 cup	50	10	0
Chili con carne with beans	1 cup	320	100	45
Clam chowder New England style	1 cup	130	35	18
Crab	1 cup	73	24	NA
Cream of broccoli	1 cup	140	60	36
Cream of potato with bacon	1 cup	130	30	14
Vegetable beef	1 cup	190	25	9
Vegetable crab	1 cup	80	20	14
Sunflower seeds	¼ cup (30 g)	160	110	14
Suremi (imitation crabmeat)	½ cup (85 g)	80	0	0
Tofu	½ cup (85 g)	90	45	5
Tortilla chips, regular & blue corn	8 chips (28 g)	140	60	9
Turkey, diced	56 g	115	80	23
SALAD TOPPINGS				
Bac-o's, bits or chips (Betty Crocker)	1½ tbsp (7 g)	30	10	0
Bac'n Pieces (McCormick)	1½ tbsp (7 g)	30	15	0
Croutons				
Pepperidge Farm				
Cheese & Garlic	9 croutons (7 g)	35	15	0
Cracked Pepper & Parmesan	6 croutons (7 g)	35	10	0
Seasoned	9 croutons (7 g)	35	15	0
Zesty Italian	6 croutons (7 g)	35	15	0
Real Bacon Bits (Hormel)	1 tbsp (7 g)	30	15	9
Salad Crispins, Mini Croutons (Hidden Valley)				
Italian Parmesan	1 tbsp (7 g)	35	10	0
Original Ranch	1 tbsp (7 g)	35	10	0

SAUCES, GRAVIES, AND DIPS

		CALORIES		
FOOD	AMOUNT	TOTAL	FAT	SAT-FAT
SAUCES				
Barbecue				
Chinese	2 tbsp	45	2	0
Masterpiece	2 tbsp	40–60	0	0

SAUCES, GRAVIES, AND DIPS

FOOD	AMOUNT	CALORIES		
		TOTAL	**FAT**	**SAT-FAT**
Barbecue (cont.)				
Kraft	2 tbsp	40	0	0
Open Pit	2 tbsp	50	5	0
Bean Sauce	1 tbsp	23	8	0
Black Bean Garlic Sauce	1 tbsp	25	0	0
Bearnaise	1 tbsp	53	48	29
	½ cup	423	383	232
Browning & Seasoning (Kitchen Bouquet)	1 tsp	15	0	0
Cheese Sauce	1 tbsp	31	21	14
	½ cup	250	170	110
Chili Paste with Garlic	1 Tbsp	10	9	0
Clam Sauce, White	½ cup	120	80	14
Cream	1 tbsp	28	22	14
	½ cup	225	175	110
Curry Cream	1 tbsp	40	31	20
	½ cup	317	250	160
Fish Sauce	1 Tbsp	0	0	0
Hoisin Sauce	2 Tbsp	60	10	0
Hollandaise	1 tbsp	82	80	47
	½ cup	660	627	377
Horseradish (Kraft)	1 tbsp	20	15	0
Hunan Sauce	4 tsp	25	10	0
Korean Bulkogi Marinade Sauce	30 g	54	1	0
Kung Pao Sauce	4 tsp	35	15	0
Louis	1 tbsp	63	60	14
	½ cup	504	480	112
Nacho Cheese Sauce (Kaukauna)	2 tbsp	90	60	18
Nacho Topping (Tostitos)				
Beef Fiesta	¼ cup	120	70	27
Chicken Quesadilla	¼ cup	90	50	18
Pasta & Spaghetti Sauces				
Contadina				
Alfredo	¼ cup	180	140	90
Light	¼ cup	80	45	27
Garden Vegetable	½ cup	40	0	0
Marinara	½ cup	80	35	9
Mushroom Alfredo	¼ cup	100	60	45
Pesto with Basil	¼ cup	290	220	63
reduced fat	¼ cup	230	170	36
Roasted Garlic Marinara	½ cup	60	15	5
DiGiorno				
Alfredo	¼ cup	180	160	63
Marinara	¼ cup	180	160	63
Healthy Choice				
all flavors	½ cup	50	0	0

SAUCES, GRAVIES, AND DIPS

		CALORIES		
FOOD	AMOUNT	TOTAL	FAT	SAT-FAT
Pasta & Spaghetti Sauces (cont.)				
Prego				
Diced Onion & Garlic	½ cup	110	45	5
Flavored with meat	½ cup	140	50	14
Fresh Mushrooms	½ cup	150	45	14
Garden combination	½ cup	90	15	5
Mushroom Parmesan	½ cup	120	30	9
Mushroom Supreme	½ cup	130	40	5
Roasted Garlic & Herb	½ cup	110	30	5
Three cheese	½ cup	100	20	9
Tomato & Basil	½ cup	110	30	5
Tomato Parmesan	½ cup	120	25	9
Tomato, onion, & garlic	½ cup	110	30	9
Traditional	½ cup	140	40	14
Ragú				
Cheese Creations				
Double Cheese	¼ cup	110	90	36
Roasted Garlic Parmesan	¼ cup	120	100	36
Spicy Cheddar & Tomato	¼ cup	50	20	14
Chunky Garden Style				
Mushroom & Green Pepper	½ cup	110	30	5
Roasted Red Pepper & Onion	½ cup	110	30	5
Super Chunky Mushroom	½ cup	120	30	5
Super Garlic	½ cup	100	20	0
Super Vegetable Primavera	½ cup	110	30	5
Tomato, Basil & Italian Cheese	½ cup	110	25	9
Tomato, Garlic & Onion	½ cup	120	30	5
Robust Blend, Hearty				
Parmesan & Romano	½ cup	120	30	9
Red Wine & Herbs	½ cup	100	25	0
Sauteed Onion & Garlic	½ cup	120	35	5
Spicy Red Pepper	½ cup	110	15	0
Old World Style				
flavored with meat	½ cup	80	30	9
Mushroom	½ cup	80	25	5
Traditional	½ cup	80	25	5
Light				
Chunky Mushroom & Garlic	½ cup	70	0	0
Tomato & Basil	½ cup	50	0	0
Safeway Select Verdi				
Alfredo	½ cup	120	100	63
Light	½ cup	160	100	63
Creamy Sundried Tomato Pesto	½ cup	210	150	90
Pizza Sauce				
Boboli	½ pouch	40	0	0

SAUCES, GRAVIES, AND DIPS

FOOD	AMOUNT	CALORIES TOTAL	FAT	SAT-FAT
Plum Sauce	2 Tbsp	90	0	0
Soy	1 tbsp	11	0	0
Double Black Soy	1 tbsp	15	0	0
Stir Fry Sauce	4 tsp	40	0	0
Tartar				
Fat-free (Kraft)	2 tbsp	25	0	0
Regular (Hellman's)	1 tbsp	70	70	9
Thai Peanut Stir-Fry & Dipping Sauce	2 tbsp	70	25	5
Tomato (*see under* Pasta & Spaghetti Sauces above)				
White	1 tbsp	24	17	11
	½ cup	195	138	88
Worcestershire	1 tbsp	0	0	0

GRAVIES

FOOD	AMOUNT	TOTAL	FAT	SAT-FAT
Gravies by type				
Beef, canned	½ cup	62	25	13
Gravies by brand name				
Franco-American				
Beef	¼ cup	30	15	5
Chicken	¼ cup	40	25	9
Fat free				
all flavors	¼ cup	15	0	0
Mushroom	¼ cup	20	10	0
Turkey	¼ cup	25	10	0
Heinz				
Classic chicken	¼ cup	25	10	0
Fat-free, all	¼ cup	15	0	0
Rich mushroom	¼ cup	20	5	0
Roasted turkey	¼ cup	30	15	0
Savory beef	¼ cup	25	10	0
Zesty onion	¼ cup	25	10	0

DIPS

FOOD	AMOUNT	TOTAL	FAT	SAT-FAT
Bacon Horseradish				
Heluva Good	2 tbsp	60	45	27
Bean Dip (Frito-Lay)	2 tbsp	40	10	0
Cheddar Cheese, mild (Utz)	2 tbsp	45	25	14
Jalapeño (Frito-Lay)	2 tbsp	50	30	9
Jalapeño & Cheddar (Utz)	2 tbsp	30	25	9
Chesapeake Clam Dip				
Breakstone's	2 tbsp	50	40	27
Chili Cheese Flavor (Fritos)	2 tbsp	45	30	9
French Onion				
Frito-Lay's	2 tbsp	60	45	27

SAUCES, GRAVIES, AND DIPS

FOOD	AMOUNT	CALORIES		
		TOTAL	FAT	SAT-FAT
French Onion (cont.)				
Heluva Good	2 tbsp	60	45	27
Fat Free	2 tbsp	25	0	0
French Onion Dip				
Kraft	2 tbsp	45	35	23
Lucerne	2 tbsp	70	60	27
Green Onion (Lucerne)	2 tbsp	50	45	27
Guacamole				
Calavo (all flavors)	2 tbsp	60	45	9
Lucerne	2 tbsp	90	80	23
Hummus	2 tbsp	57	30	27
Jalapeño				
Frito-Lay	2 tbsp	50	30	9
Jalapeño & Cheddar				
Utz	2 tbsp	30	25	9
Jalapeño Cheese Sauce				
Pablo's	2 tbsp	150	90	32
Nacho Cheese Dip (Snyder's of				
Hanover)	2 tbsp	30	25	9
New England Clam				
Heluva Good	2 tbsp	50	40	27
Ranch				
Heluva Good	2 tbsp	60	45	27
Hidden Valley	28 g prepared	70	50	36
Lucerne	2 tbsp	110	100	18
Salsa				
Chunky (Herr's)	2 tbsp	12	0	0
Chunky (Utz)	2 tbsp	60	0	0
Dip (Pace)	2 tbsp	10	0	0
Dip (Tostitos)	2 tbsp	15	0	0
Mexican (Kaukauna)	2 tbsp	15	0	0
Mild (Rojo's)	2 tbsp	10	0	0
Salsa and Cream Cheese				
(Kaukauna)	2 tbsp	70	50	NA
Salsa Con Queso (Kaukauna)	2 tbsp	70	40	27
Salsa con Queso (Tostitos)	2 tbsp .	40	20	5
Southwest, mild (Safeway)	2 tbsp	10	0	0
Sour Cream & Onion Dip				
Herr's	2 tbsp	60	45	27
Utz	2 tbsp	60	45	27
Vegetable Dip				
Heluva Good	2 tbsp	60	45	27

SAUSAGES AND LUNCHEON MEATS

FOOD	AMOUNT	CALORIES		
		TOTAL	FAT	SAT-FAT
Bacon	2 slices (11 g)	60	45	18
Hickory Smoked (Smithfield)	2 slices (15 g)	90	70	27
Thick Sliced (Gwaltney)	1 slice (8 g)	45	35	9
Turkey (Louis Rich)	1 slice (14 g)	30	20	5
Barbecue loaf, pork, beef	28 g	49	23	8
	1 slice (22 g)	40	18	7
Beer 'n Bratwurst (Johnsonville)	1 grilled link (85 g)	290	230	81
Beerwurst, beer salami				
beef	28 g	92	75	31
	1 slice (22 g)	75	61	25
pork	28 g	67	48	16
	1 slice (22 g)	55	39	13
Berliner, pork, beef	28 g	65	44	15
	1 slice (22 g)	53	36	13
Bockwurst, raw	28 g	87	70	26
	1 link (64 g)	200	161	59
Bologna				
Beef (Hebrew National)	56 g	180	150	54
Beef (Oscar Mayer)	1 slice (28 g)	90	70	36
Chicken (Gwaltney)	1 slice (32 g)	80	50	18
Chicken, Pork, & Beef (Thorn Apple)	1 slice (37 g)	120	90	18
Pork	1 slice (28 g)	70	51	18
Pork & Beef (Oscar Mayer)	1 slice (28 g)	90	70	27
Pork, Chicken, & Beef (Oscar Mayer)	1 slice (28 g)	90	70	27
Light	1 slice (28 g)	60	35	14
Pork & Turkey (Gwaltney)	1 slice (38 g)	120	100	36
Turkey (Louis Rich)	1 slice (28 g)	50	35	9
Bratwurst, pork, beef	28 g	92	71	25
	1 link (70 g)	226	175	63
Bratwurst, pork, cooked	28 g	85	66	24
	1 link (84 g)	256	198	71
Braunschweiger, pork				
Jones	56 g	150	110	36
Jones Sandwich slices	1 slice (34 g)	110	90	27
Kahn's	56 g	180	140	81
Oscar Mayer	1 slice (56 g)	190	150	54
Breakfast strips, beef, cured cooked	1 slice (11 g)	51	35	15
Canadian bacon, grilled	1 slice	43	18	6
Cheese Dog (Oscar Mayer)	1 frank (45 g)	140	120	45
Chicken breast				
Deli Thin				
Fat Free (Oscar Mayer)	4 slices (52 g)	40	0	0
Oven roasted (Louis Rich)	5 slices (55 g)	60	15	5

SAUSAGES AND LUNCHEON MEATS

		CALORIES		
FOOD	AMOUNT	TOTAL	FAT	SAT-FAT
Chicken roll, white meat				
(Tysons)	3 slices (55 g)	90	50	18
Chipped Beef	28 g	50	20	9
Corned Beef				
Hormel	56 g	130	60	27
thin sliced (Hebrew National)	4 slices (56 g)	90	40	18
Corned beef brisket				
Cooked	28 g	71	48	16
Loaf, jellied	1 slice (28 g)	43	16	7
Thorn Apple Valley	84 g	190	150	63
Corned Beef Hash				
Libby's	1 cup (252 g)	420	220	99
Cured Beef				
Oven Roasted (Hillshire				
Farms)	6 slices (57 g)	50	5	0
Dried beef, cured (beef jerky)	28 g	47	10	4
Dutch brand loaf, pork, beef	1 slice (28 g)	68	45	16
Frankfurter				
Beef	1 frank (57g)	190	150	63
Beef Franks (Hebrew				
National)	1 frank (48 g)	150	120	45
Big 8's Jumbo Beef Hot				
Dogs (Gwaltney)	1 frank (56 g)	190	150	63
Esskay Beef Franks	1 frank (56 g)	170	130	36
Oscar Mayer Beef Franks	1 frank (45 g)	150	120	54
Quarter pound (Hebrew				
National)	1 frank (114 g)	350	300	108
Safeway Jumbo Beef Franks	1 frank (57 g)	170	140	63
Smithfield Jumbo Beef Hot				
Dogs	1 frank (56 g)	190	150	63
Chicken				
Gwaltney Great Dogs	1 frank (56 g)	140	90	27
Wampler-LongAcre	1 frank (56 g)	120	100	27
Chicken, Pork & Beef				
Safeway Jumbo Franks	1 frank (57 g)	180	150	54
Corn Dogs (Ball Park)	1 corn dog (75 g)	220	110	27
Turkey				
Louis Rich	1 frank (57 g)	110	70	23
Safeway Jumbo Turkey				
Franks	1 frank (57 g)	120	80	23
Turkey & Chicken				
Louis Rich Bun-Length	1 frank (57 g)	110	70	23
Turkey & Pork Wiener (Oscar				
Mayer)	1 frank (45 g)	150	120	41
Jumbo Wiener	1 frank (57 g)	180	150	54

SAUSAGES AND LUNCHEON MEATS

FOOD	AMOUNT	CALORIES		
		TOTAL	FAT	SAT-FAT
Low-fat and Fat-free Franks				
Ball Park				
Fat Free Beef Franks	1 frank (50 g)	45	0	0
Lite Franks	1 frank (50 g)	100	70	18
Healthy Choice				
Beef Franks	1 frank (50 g)	60	15	5
Turkey, Pork, Beef Franks	1 frank (40 g)	50	10	5
Oscar Mayer				
Fat Free Hot Dogs	1 frank (50 g)	40	0	0
Light Beef Franks	1 frank (57 g)	110	70	31
Ham				
Baked (Oscar Mayer)	3 slices (63 g)	60	10	5
Boiled (Oscar Mayer)	3 slices (63 g)	70	15	5
Chopped	1 slice (28 g)	50	30	14
	1 slice (21 g)	50	36	12
Cured (Hormel)	85 g	100	45	14
Danish (Plumrose)	2 slices (56 g)	65	25	9
Deli Thins				
Baked Ham	4 slices (52 g)	50	10	0
Honey Ham	4 slices (52 g)	50	15	5
Minced	28 g	75	53	18
	1 slice (21 g)	55	39	14
Salad spread	28 g	61	40	13
	1 tbsp	32	21	7
Smoked				
Esskay	85 g	120	50	18
Hickory Smoked	3 slices (89 g)	160	100	36
Oscar Mayer	3 slices (63 g)	60	20	9
Smok-a-Roma	57 g	120	70	27
Turkey Ham (*see* Turkey, below)				
Ham and cheese loaf or roll				
Oscar Mayer	1 slice (28 g)	60	40	23
Ham and cheese spread	28 g	69	47	22
	1 tbsp	37	25	12
Headcheese, pork	1 slice (28 g)	60	40	13
Honey loaf, pork, beef	1 slice (28 g)	36	11	4
Honey roll sausage, beef	28 g	52	27	10
	1 slice (22 g)	42	22	8
Kielbasa				
pork, beef (Eckrich)	56 g	180	140	63
	1 slice (25 g)	81	64	23
beef polska (Hillshire Farm)	2 oz (56 g)	190	150	72
Healthy Choice	2 oz (56 g)	70	15	5
turkey (Mr. Turkey & Hillshire Farm)	56 g	90	45	23

SAUSAGES AND LUNCHEON MEATS

		CALORIES		
FOOD	AMOUNT	TOTAL	FAT	SAT-FAT
Knockwurst, beef (Hebrew National)	1 link (85 g)	260	**210**	81
Lebanon bologna, beef	28 g	64	**38**	16
	1 slice (22 g)	52	**31**	13
Liver cheese, pork	28 g	86	**65**	23
Liver pudding, pork	45 g	170	**110**	9
Liverwurst (see Braunschweiger)				
Luncheon meat				
beef, loaved	1 slice (28 g)	87	**67**	29
beef, thin sliced	28 g	35	**8**	3
	5 slices (21 g)	26	**6**	2
pork, beef	1 slice (28 g)	100	**82**	30
pork, canned	28 g	95	**77**	28
	1 slice (21 g)	70	**57**	20
Luxury loaf, pork	1 slice (28 g)	40	**12**	4
Mortadella, beef, pork	28 g	88	**65**	24
	1 slice (14 g)	47	**34**	13
Mother's loaf, pork	28 g	80	**57**	20
	1 slice (21 g)	59	**42**	15
Safeway	1 slice (35 g)	100	**70**	23
Olive loaf	1 slice (28 g)	70	**45**	15
Pastrami				
beef	1 slice (28 g)	99	**74**	27
turkey	1 slice (28 g)	40	**16**	9
Paté				
Chicken liver	1 tbsp	26	**15**	4
Goose liver	28 g	131	**112**	NA
	1 tbsp	60	**51**	NA
Pork	28 g	100	**80**	27
Peppered Beef (Carl Buddig)	71 g	100	**45**	18
Peppered loaf, pork, beef	1 slice (28 g)	42	**16**	6
Pepperoni				
Hormel	15 slices (28 g)	140	**120**	54
	1 sausage (252 g)	1248	**993**	364
Bridgford	1 oz (28 g)	130	**110**	36
Pickle and pimento loaf (Oscar Mayer)	1 slice (28 g)	70	**50**	18
Picnic loaf, pork, beef	1 slice (28 g)	66	**42**	15
Pork Cracklins (fried pork fat with skin)	½ oz (14 g)	80	**50**	9
Potted Meat Food Product	¼ cup (58 g)	110	**80**	27
Prosciutto				
Citterio	2 slices (30 g)	70	**40**	14
Salami				
Beef (Hebrew National)	56 g	170	**130**	54
Cotto (Oscar Mayer)	1 slice (28 g)	60	**40**	18

SAUSAGES AND LUNCHEON MEATS

| FOOD | AMOUNT | CALORIES | | |
		TOTAL	FAT	SAT-FAT
Salami (cont.)				
Hard, pork & beef (Oscar Mayer)	3 slices (27 g)	100	**70**	27
Genoa salami	3 slices (30 g)	100	**70**	27
Sandwich spread, pork, beef	28 g	67	**44**	15
	1 tbsp	35	**23**	8
Sausage				
Beef sausage (Jones Dairy Farm)	2 links (45 g)	170	**140**	NA
Beerwurst Sausage	2 oz (56 g)	160	**130**	45
Biscuits (Jimmy Dean)	2 (96 g)	330	**190**	63
Blood sausage	28 g	107	**88**	34
	1 slice (25 g)	95	**78**	30
Cajun Brand Andouille Sausage (Aidells Sausage Company)	1 link (90 g)	200	**140**	63
Farmer Summer Sausage	2 oz (56 g)	200	**160**	63
Ham sausage (Smithfield)	48 g	180	**140**	54
Italian sausage, cooked, pork	28 g	92	**66**	23
	1 link (5/lb)	216	**155**	55
	1 link (4/lb)	268	**192**	68
Johnsonville	1 grilled link (85 g)	290	**230**	81
Usinger's	1 (84 g)	270	**230**	90
Italian Turkey Sausage (Shady Brook Farms)	1 link (64 g)	100	**45**	14
Liver sausage, liverwurst, pork	28 g	93	**73**	27
	1 slice (17 g)	59	**46**	17
Luncheon sausage, pork and beef	28 g	74	**53**	19
	1 slice (22 g)	60	**43**	16
New England brand sausage, pork, beef	28 g	46	**19**	6
	1 slice (22 g)	37	**16**	5
New Mexico Brand Smoked Turkey & Chicken Sausage (Aidells Sausage Company)	1 link (90 g)	190	**130**	41
Polish sausage, beef (Hebrew National)	1 link (85 g)	240	**190**	90
Polish sausage, pork	28 g	92	**73**	26
	1 sausage (8 oz)	739	**587**	211
Pork Sausage				
Bob Evans	2 patties pan-fried (53 g)	230	**180**	63
Country	28 g	120	**100**	36
Hot				
Gwaltney	39 g	150	**130**	45
Jamestown	36 g	170	**140**	45

SAUSAGES AND LUNCHEON MEATS

FOOD	AMOUNT	CALORIES		
		TOTAL	FAT	SAT-FAT
Sausage (cont.)				
Links (Parks)	2 links (42 g)	170	150	54
Smoked	1 link (85 g)	290	230	81
Pork and beef sausage, cooked	1 patty (28 g)	112	92	33
	1 link (13 g)	52	33	15
Smoked link sausage				
Hot Links	1 (76 g)	250	200	99
Lite (Hillshire Farms)	2 oz (56 g)	110	70	32
pork	28 g	110	81	29
	1 link (67 g)	265	194	69
	1 link (16 g)	62	46	16
pork and beef	28 g	95	77	27
	1 link (67 g)	229	186	65
	1 link (16 g)	54	44	15
Summer sausage, beef	3 slices (57 g)	180	140	63
Vienna sausage (Hormel)	28 g	70	60	36
Scrapple				
Parks	2 oz (56 g)	90	45	14
Rapa	2 oz (56 g)	120	70	27
Spam	56 g	170	140	54
Lite	56 g	110	70	27
Tongue, beef				
raw	28 g	63	41	18
cook, simmered	28 g	80	53	23
Tripe, beef, raw	28 g	28	10	5
Turkey breast, processed				
Oven Roasted (Oscar Mayer)	3 slices (63 g)	70	15	0
Fat Free Deli Thin (Oscar Mayer)	4 slices (52 g)	40	0	0
Smoked white (Louis Rich)	1 slice (28 g)	30	10	0
Turkey Cold Cuts				
bacon (Louis Rich)	1 slice (14 g)	30	20	5
bologna (Louis Rich)	1 slice (28 g)	50	35	9
ham				
Chopped	1 slice (28 g)	40	20	9
Jennie-O	56 g	80	40	7
Louis Rich	1 slice (28 g)	35	10	0
pastrami	1 slice (28 g)	40	16	9
salami (Louis Rich)	1 slice (28 g)	45	25	9
Cotted Salami (Louis Rich)	1 slice (28 g)	90	50	18
Turkey Roll				
light and dark meat	1 slice (28 g)	42	18	5
light meat	1 slice (28 g)	42	18	5

SNACK FOODS

FOOD	AMOUNT	CALORIES		
		TOTAL	FAT	SAT-FAT
BREADSTICKS				
Grissini-style, garlic (Stella D'oro)	3 sticks (15 g)	60	0	0
Thin Bread Sticks (Pepperidge Farm)				
Cheddar cheese	7 sticks (16 g)	70	25	9
CHIPS, CRISPS, ETC.				
Bagel Chips				
Burns & Ricker				
Cinnamon raisin	7 pieces (30 g)	130	30	5
fat-free	7 pieces (30 g)	110	0	0
Garlic				
fat-free	7 pieces (30 g)	100	0	0
Roasted garlic				
bite size	⅔ cup (30 g)	140	40	5
New York Style				
bite size				
Garlic	28 chips (31 g)	140	30	5
Ranch	⅔ cup (28 g)	120	35	5
Rondele				
Cinnamon with honey & raisins	7 pieces (28 g)	130	30	5
Roasted garlic	7 pieces (28 g)	130	30	5
fat-free	9 pieces (30 g)	100	0	0
Banana Chips	⅓ cup (27 g)	140	60	60
Bugles				
Original Baked	1½ cups (30 g)	130	30	5
Original	1⅓ cups (30 g)	160	80	72
Caramel Corn Clusters (Utz)	1⅛ cups (28 g)	142	18	0
Cheese Balls (Utz)	27 balls (28 g)	170	90	18
Cheese Curls				
Utz	30 curls (28 g)	150	90	18
Weight Watchers	1 pkg (14 g)	70	25	9
Cheese Doodles (Wise)				
Crunchy	½ cup (28 g)	150	80	23
Puffed	19 pieces (28 g)	150	70	23
Cheetos	12 pieces (28 g)	160	90	23
Corn Nuts	⅓ cup (28 g)	130	35	9
French Fried Onions (French's)	2 tbsp (7 g)	45	30	9
Fritos	32 chips (28 g)	160	90	14
Bar-B-Q	29 chips (28 g)	150	80	14
Scoops	11 chips (28 g)	160	90	9
Jax (Bachman)	25 pieces (30 g)	150	70	9
Onion Rings (Wise)	39 rings (28 g)	140	50	14
Pita Chips (Pechter's)				
Original	2 chips (14 g)	80	45	9
Sesame Seed	2 chips (14 g)	80	45	9
Toasted Garlic	2 chips (14 g)	70	40	9

SNACK FOODS

| FOOD | AMOUNT | CALORIES | | |
		TOTAL	FAT	SAT-FAT
Plantain Chips (Goya)	38 pieces (30 g)	170	**100**	18
Potato Chips				
Lay's				
Baked	32 g	130	**15**	0
Bar-B-Q	15 chips (28 g)	150	**90**	27
Classic	20 chips (28 g)	150	**90**	27
Sour Cream & Onion	17 chips (28 g)	160	**100**	27
Wavy Lay's				
Original	11 chips (28 g)	150	**90**	23
Wow	20 chips (28 g)	75	**0**	0
Pringles				
Original	14 crisps (28 g)	160	**90**	27
Ridges	12 crisps (28 g)	150	**90**	23
Right Crisps	16 crisps (28 g)	140	**60**	18
Sour Cream & Onion	14 crisps (28 g)	160	**90**	23
fat-free	16 crisps (28 g)	70	**0**	0
Ruffles (Frito-Lay)				
Cheddar & sour cream	11 chips (28 g)	160	**90**	27
Ranch	13 chips (28 g)	150	**80**	NA
The Works!	14 chips (28 g)	160	**100**	23
Wow	17 chips (28 g)	75	**0**	0
Utz	20 chips (28 g)	150	**80**	18
Baked Potato Crisps	12 chips (28 g)	110	**15**	0
Bar-B-Q Ripple Cut	20 chips (28 g)	150	**90**	23
reduced fat	22 chips (28 g)	140	**60**	14
Grandma Utz's Handcooked	20 chips (28 g)	140	**70**	14
Kettle Classics	20 chips (28 g)	150	**80**	14
Ripple Cut	20 chips (28 g)	150	**90**	23
reduced fat	24 chips (28 g)	140	**60**	14
Sour Cream & Onion, Ripple Cut	20 chips (28 g)	160	**90**	27
Potato Sticks (French's)	¾ cup (30 g)	180	**110**	18
Terra Chips				
mixed vegetables	28 g	140	**70**	9
Tortilla Chips				
Doritos	11 chips (28 g)	140	**70**	9
3Ds (all flavors)	27 pieces (28 g)	140	**60**	14
Doritos Wow	11 chips (28 g)	90	**10**	0
Guiltless Gourmet	18 chips (28 g)	110	**15**	0
Utz White Corn Tortillas	12 chips (28 g)	140	**60**	9
Baked Tortilla	8 chips (28 g)	120	**15**	0
Nacho Tortilla	12 chips (28 g)	140	**60**	9
Tostitos	6 chips (28 g)	130	**50**	9
Baked Tostitos	9 chips (28 g)	110	**5**	0
Baked, Salsa & Cream Cheese				
flavor, bite size	16 chips (28 g)	120	**25**	5

SNACK FOODS

FOOD	AMOUNT	CALORIES TOTAL	FAT	SAT-FAT
Veggie Rings (Good Health)				
Potato Onion	28 g	140	**60**	5
Veggie Stix (Good Health)				
Mixed Vegetables	28 g	140	**60**	5
CRACKERS				
Austin				
Cheese Crackers on Cheese	6 (39 g)	200	**100**	24
Cheese Crackers & Creamy Peanut				
Butter	6 (39 g)	200	**100**	18
Cheese Peanut Butter Cracker				
Sandwiches	4 (26 g)	140	**70**	14
Cream Cheese & Chives	6 (39 g)	190	**90**	23
Toasty Crackers & Peanut Butter	6 (39 g)	190	**90**	18
Toasty Peanut Butter Cracker				
Sandwiches	4 (26 g)	140	**60**	14
Wheat 'n Cheddar	6 (39 g)	200	**100**	27
Delicious				
Snack Crackers	8 (30 g)	140	**60**	9
Cheddar Cheese	28 (30 g)	150	**60**	18
Garden Vegetable	13 (31 g)	150	**60**	14
Devonsheer				
Melba Rounds				
Garlic	5 pieces (15 g)	60	**10**	0
Onion	5 pieces (15 g)	50	**0**	0
Plain	5 pieces (15 g)	50	**0**	0
Sesame	3 pieces (14 g)	50	**10**	0
12-Grain	5 pieces (15 g)	50	**0**	0
Vegetable	5 pieces (15 g)	50	**0**	0
Melba Toast				
Plain	3 pieces (14 g)	50	**0**	0
Sesame	3 pieces (14 g)	50	**10**	0
Herr's				
Sandwiches				
Cheese in Cheese	6 (39 g)	200	**100**	23
Cheese Peanut Butter	6 (39 g)	200	**100**	18
Toast Peanut Butter	1 pkg (39 g)	190	**90**	18
Keebler				
Club				
Original	4 (14 g)	70	**25**	9
reduced fat	5 (16 g)	70	**20**	0
Sandwich Crackers				
Cheese & Peanut Butter	1 package (38 g)	190	**80**	18
Club & Cheddar	1 package (36 g)	190	**100**	23
Toast & Peanut Butter	1 package (38 g)	190	**80**	18

SNACK FOODS

FOOD	AMOUNT	CALORIES		
		TOTAL	**FAT**	**SAT-FAT**
Keebler (cont.)				
Munch 'ems				
Cheddar	41 (30 g)	130	**40**	9
Mesquite BBQ	41 (30 g)	140	**40**	9
Original	41 (30 g)	130	**40**	9
Ranch	41 (30 g)	130	**40**	9
Sour Cream & Onion	41 (30 g)	140	**40**	9
Toasteds				
Buttercrisp	5 (16 g)	80	**30**	9
Onion	5 (16 g)	80	**30**	5
Rye	9 (29 g)	140	**60**	NA
Sesame	5 (16 g)	80	**30**	5
Wheat	5 (16 g)	80	**25**	5
Town House				
Original	5 (16 g)	80	**40**	9
reduced fat	6 (15 g)	70	**20**	5
Wheatables				
Ranch	29 (30 g)	130	**35**	9
Savory Original	26 (30 g)	150	**60**	18
reduced fat	29 (30 g)	130	**30**	9
White Cheddar	27 (30 g)	130	**35**	9
Zesta Saltines				
Fat-free	5 (14 g)	50	**0**	0
Original	5 (15 g)	60	**20**	5
Kraft Handi-Snacks				
Cheez 'n Breadsticks	1 unit (31 g)	120	**60**	27
Cheez 'n Crackers	1 unit (27 g)	110	**60**	27
Cheez 'n Pretzels	1 unit (29 g)	100	**45**	27
Nacho Stix 'n Cheez	1 unit (31 g)	110	**60**	27
Lu				
Le Petite Beurre Butter Biscuits	4 crackers (33 g)	150	**35**	27
Manischewitz				
Matzo				
American	1 matzo (28 g)	110	**15**	5
Egg 'n Onion	1 matzo (28 g)	100	**10**	0
Whole Wheat	1 matzo (28 g)	110	**5**	0
Milk Lunch				
New England Biscuits	4 crackers (32 g)	140	**35**	9
Safeway Snack Crackers				
Bacon-Flavored	11 crackers (30 g)	150	**60**	14
Cheddar Cheese	28 crackers (30 g)	150	**60**	18
Chicken-Flavored	10 crackers (31 g)	160	**80**	18
Garden Vegetable	13 crackers (31 g)	150	**60**	14
Onion	11 crackers (30 g)	140	**50**	14
Ranch	10 crackers (30 g)	160	**80**	14
Sesame Cheddar	13 crackers (31 g)	150	**70**	14

SNACK FOODS

		CALORIES		
FOOD	AMOUNT	TOTAL	FAT	SAT-FAT
Safeway Snack Crackers (cont.)				
Sesame Wheat Snack	13 crackers (31 g)	150	60	NA
Snack Crackers	10 crackers (30 g)	140	45	9
Sour Cream 'n Chives	9 crackers (31 g)	160	80	18
Wheat	15 crackers (30 g)	140	50	14
reduced fat	16 crackers (30 g)	120	30	5
Woven Wheats	7 crackers (31 g)	140	45	9
Nabisco				
Air Crisps				
Cheese Nips	32 crackers (30 g)	130	35	9
Potato Barbecue	22 crisps (28 g)	120	35	5
Pretzel	23 crisps (28 g)	110	0	0
Ritz	24 crackers (30 g)	140	45	9
Ritz Sour Cream & Onion	23 crackers (30 g)	140	40	9
Wheat Thins Ranch	23 pieces (30 g)	140	40	9
Better Cheddars	22 crackers (30 g)	150	70	2
reduced fat	24 crackers (30 g)	140	50	14
Cheese Nips	29 crackers (30 g)	150	60	14
reduced fat	31 crackers (30 g)	130	35	9
Chicken in a Biskit	12 crackers (30 g)	160	80	14
Harvest Crisps				
5-grain	13 crackers (31 g)	130	30	5
Garden Vegetable	15 crackers (30 g)	130	30	5
Italian Herb	13 crackers (31 g)	130	30	5
Premium Saltines				
Fat-Free	5 crackers (15 g)	60	0	0
Low Sodium	5 crackers (14 g)	60	15	0
Original	5 crackers (14 g)	60	15	0
Unsalted Tops	5 crackers (14 g)	60	15	0
With Multigrain	5 crackers (14 g)	60	15	0
Rice Crackers	½ cup (30 g)	110	0	0
Ritz Bits				
Cheese Sandwiches	14 sandwiches (31 g)	170	90	23
Peanut Butter Sandwiches	14 sandwiches (31 g)	150	70	14
Ritz Crackers	5 crackers (16 g)	80	35	5
reduced fat	5 crackers (15 g)	70	15	0
Whole Wheat	5 crackers (15 g)	70	20	0
SnackWell's Snack Crackers				
French Onion	38 crackers (30 g)	130	25	5
Ranch	38 crackers (30 g)	130	25	5
Salsa Cheddar	32 crackers (30 g)	120	15	0
Wheat Crackers	5 crackers (15 g)	70	15	0
Sociables	7 crackers (15 g)	80	35	5
Sweet Crispers				
Caramel	18 crisps (31 g)	140	25	5
Chocolate	18 crisps (31 g)	130	25	5

SNACK FOODS

FOOD	AMOUNT	CALORIES		
		TOTAL	FAT	SAT-FAT
Nabisco (cont.)				
Cinnamon	18 crisps (31 g)	130	25	0
Honey	18 crisps (31 g)	130	20	0
Triscuit Wafers	7 wafers (31 g)	140	45	9
Deli-style Rye	7 wafers (32 g)	140	45	9
Garden Herb	6 wafers (28 g)	130	40	9
Reduced Fat	8 wafers (32 g)	130	25	5
Thin Crisps	15 crackers (30 g)	130	45	9
Uneeda Biscuit	2 crackers (15 g)	60	15	0
Vegetable Thins	14 crackers (31 g)	160	80	14
Waverly Crackers	5 crackers (15 g)	70	30	5
Wheat Thins				
Multigrain	17 crackers (30 g)	130	35	5
Original	16 crackers (29 g)	140	50	9
Reduced Fat	18 crackers (29 g)	120	35	5
Wheatsworth Stone-Ground Wheat				
crackers	5 crackers (16 g)	80	30	5
Pepperidge Farm				
Distinctive				
Butter Thins	4 crackers (15 g)	70	25	9
Hearty Wheat	3 crackers (16 g)	80	30	0
Quartet	4 crackers (15 g)	70	20	5
Sesame	3 crackers (14 g)	70	25	0
Three-Cracker	4 crackers (15 g)	70	20	0
Goldfish				
Cheddar Cheese	55 pieces (30 g)	140	50	14
Extra Cheddar Cheese	51 pieces (30 g)	140	50	14
Nacho	51 pieces (30 g)	140	60	9
Original	55 pieces (30 g)	140	60	18
Parmesan Cheese	60 pieces (30 g)	140	50	14
Pizza-Flavored	55 pieces (30 g)	140	60	14
Pretzel	43 pieces (30 g)	120	25	5
Sour Cream & Onion	51 pieces (30 g)	150	60	9
Snack Sticks				
Pumpernickel	15 sticks (31 g)	120	15	0
Sesame	8 sticks (29 g)	130	50	5
Three-Cheese	8 sticks (29 g)	140	50	18
Ry Krisp				
Natural	2 crackers (15 g)	60	0	0
Seasoned	2 crackers (14 g)	60	10	0
SnackWell's Crackers: *see under* Nabisco				
Sunshine				
Cheez-It				
Big Cheez-It				
reduced fat	15 crackers (30 g)	140	40	9
Heads and Tails	37 crackers (30 g)	140	50	14

SNACK FOODS

FOOD	AMOUNT	CALORIES		
		TOTAL	FAT	SAT-FAT
Sunshine (cont.)				
Hot & Spicy	27 crackers (30 g)	160	**80**	18
Nacho	28 crackers (30 g)	150	**60**	14
reduced fat	29 crackers (30 g)	140	**40**	9
Sandwich crackers				
Cheese	1 pkg (36 g)	200	**110**	23
Peanut Butter	1 pkg (38 g)	190	**90**	18
White Cheddar	27 crackers (30 g)	160	**80**	18
Hi-Ho, all flavors	4 crackers (14 g)	70	**35**	9
Krispy Saltines				
fat-free	5 crackers (14 g)	50	**0**	0
Mild Cheddar	5 crackers (15 g)	60	**20**	5
Original	5 crackers (14 g)	60	**10**	0

FROZEN SNACKS

FOOD	AMOUNT	TOTAL	FAT	SAT-FAT
Anchor				
Stuffed Jalapeños Cream Cheese				
Poppers	6 pieces (136 g)	360	**200**	90
Farm Rich				
Double Cheese Pizza Dippers	3 sticks (90 g)	210	**80**	36
Italian Four Cheese Sticks	2 sticks (45 g)	150	**80**	27
Giorgio Pierogies (lowfat)				
Potato & Cheddar Cheese–Filled				
Pierogies	3 (132 g)	220	**25**	14
Potato & Onion–Filled Pierogies	3 (132 g)	230	**25**	9
Hanover				
Baked Soft Pretzels	1 pretzel (61 g)	160	**0**	0
Inland Valley Munchskin Meals				
Cheese & Bacon Potato Skins	2 topped potato skins (113 g)	250	**140**	63
J & J Snack Foods				
Cinnamon Raisin Minis	2 pretzels (57 g) + 1 icing pkt (7 g)	190	**15**	0
SuperPretzel	1 pretzel (64 g)	170	**9**	0
Mrs. T's Pierogies (lowfat)				
Potato & Cheddar Cheese–Filled				
Pasta Pockets	3 (120 g)	180	**20**	9
Potato & Onion–Filled Pasta Pockets	3 (120 g)	180	**15**	0

FRUIT SNACKS

FOOD	AMOUNT	TOTAL	FAT	SAT-FAT
Fruit by the Foot				
all flavors	1 roll (21 g)	80	**10**	5
Fruit Roll-ups				
all flavors	2 rolls (28 g)	110	**10**	0

SNACK FOODS

FOOD	AMOUNT	CALORIES		
		TOTAL	FAT	SAT-FAT
Mrs. T's Pierogies (lowfat)				
Potato & Cheddar Cheese–Filled				
Pasta Pockets	3 (120 g)	180	20	9
Potato & Onion–Filled Pasta Pockets	3 (120 g)	180	15	0
FRUIT SNACKS				
Fruit by the Foot				
all flavors	1 roll (21 g)	80	10	5
Fruit Roll-ups				
all flavors	2 rolls (28 g)	110	10	0
GRANOLA BARS, BREAKFAST BARS, AND POWER BARS				
Balance				
Almond Brownie	1 bar (50 g)	190	50	14
Chocolate	1 bar (50 g)	190	50	27
Honey Peanut	1 bar (50 g)	200	50	23
Boulder Bar				
Apple Cinnamon	1 bar (71 g)	190	10	0
Original Chocolate	1 bar (71 g)	190	10	0
Clif				
Chocolate Chip	1 bar (68 g)	250	27	5
Crunchy Peanut Bar	1 bar (68 g)	250	36	9
Real Berry	1 bar (68 g)	250	18	5
Kellogg's				
Nutrigrain Lowfat Cereal Bar				
Apple Cinnamon	1 bar (37 g)	140	25	5
Blueberry	1 bar (37 g)	140	25	5
Rice Crispies Treats				
Chocolate Chip	1 bar (22 g)	90	25	9
Crispy Marshmallow Squares	1 bar (22 g)	90	20	5
Kudos				
Chocolate Chip	1 bar (28 g)	120	40	23
with Snickers Chunks	1 bar (23 g)	100	30	9
with M&M's	1 bar (23 g)	90	25	9
Mountain Lift	1 bar (60 g)	220	40	36
Nature Valley Oats 'n Honey	1 bar (21 g)	90	30	5
Power Bar				
Banana	1 bar (65 g)	230	20	5
Chocolate	1 bar (65 g)	230	20	5
Malt Nut	1 bar (65 g)	230	25	5
Mocha	1 bar (65 g)	230	25	10
Oatmeal Raisin	1 bar (65 g)	230	25	5
Wild Berry	1 bar (65 g)	230	25	5
Quaker				
Cap'n Crunch's				
Crunch Berries Treats	1 bar (22 g)	90	20	5
Peanut Butter Crunch Treats	1 bar (22 g)	90	25	5

SNACK FOODS

		CALORIES		
FOOD	AMOUNT	TOTAL	FAT	SAT-FAT
Quaker (cont.)				
Chewy				
Chocolate Chip	1 bar (28 g)	120	**35**	14
Cookies 'n Cream	1 bar (28 g)	110	**25**	5
Peanut Butter & Chocolate Chunk	1 bar (28 g)	120	**25**	9
Fruit & Oatmeal, all flavors	1 bar (37 g)	140	**25**	0
Lowfat, all flavors	1 bar (28 g)	110	**20**	5
Safeway Healthy Advantage Cereal Bars				
all flavors	1 bar (37 g)	140	**25**	5
SnackWell's (Nabisco)				
Fat-Free Cereal Bars, all flavors	1 bar (37 g)	120	**0**	0
Granola Bars, all flavors	1 bar (28 g)	120	**25**	5
Sunfelt				
Almond	1 bar (28 g)	130	**60**	18
Chocolate Chip	1 bar (35 g)	160	**60**	27
Oatmeal Raisin or Raisin	1 bar (35 g)	150	**50**	18
Oats and Honey	1 bar (28 g)	120	**45**	18
JERKY AND PORK RINDS				
Beef Jerky				
Giant Jerk (Slim Jim)	1 (16 g)	70	**35**	18
Hickory Smoked (Pemmican)	1 bag (35 g)	90	**10**	5
Pork Rinds				
Utz Pork Cracklins	½ oz (14 g)	90	**70**	27
LUNCH PACKS				
Lunchables (Oscar Mayer)				
with dessert & drink				
96% Fat-Free Ham & Cheddar	1 pkg (164 g)	390	**100**	45
Beef Tacos	1 pkg (161 g)	470	**120**	54
Bologna & American Cheese	1 pkg (107 g)	530	**240**	117
Cheese & Salsa Nachos	1 pkg (135 g)	550	**220**	54
Lean Ham & American Cheese	1 pkg (107 g)	460	**180**	81
Lean Turkey Breast & American				
Cheese	1 pkg (107 g)	440	**170**	81
Lean Turkey Breast & Cheddar	1 pkg (107 g)	440	**140**	63
Pizza (3 extra-cheesy pizzas)	1 pkg (136 g)	460	**140**	72
Pizza (3 pepperoni-flavored				
sausage pizzas)	1 pkg (136 g)	460	**140**	72
Pizza Dunks (4 soft breadsticks)	1 pkg (143 g)	510	**130**	72
Pizza Swirls	1 pkg (130 g)	480	**160**	90
without drink				
Beef Tacos	1 pkg (152 g)	310	**100**	45
Bologna & American Cheese +				
Chocolate Chip Cookie	1 pkg (118 g)	480	**300**	117
Cheese & Salsa Nachos	1 pkg (125 g)	380	**190**	41
Lean Ham & Cheddar	1 pkg (128 g)	360	**200**	99

SNACK FOODS

FOOD	AMOUNT	CALORIES		
		TOTAL	FAT	SAT-FAT
Lunchables (Oscar Mayer) (cont.)				
Lean Ham & Cheddar + Vanilla				
Sandwich Cookie	1 pkg (129 g)	420	200	81
Lean Turkey Breast & American				
Cheese + Fudge Cookie	1 pkg (119 g)	360	170	81
Lean Turkey Breast & Cheddar	1 pkg (128 g)	350	180	99
Pizza (3 extra-cheesy pizzas)	1 pkg (128 g)	300	120	63
Pizza (3 pepperoni-flavored				
sausage pizzas)	1 pkg (128 g)	310	130	63
Safeway Snacks				
Bologna & American Cheese +				
Peanut Butter Cookies	1 pkg (112 g)	370	230	90
Fat-Free Ham & Swiss + Chocolate				
Chip Cookies	1 pkg (112 g)	350	170	72
Fat-Free Turkey Breast & Cheddar +				
Chocolate Chip Cookies	1 pkg (112 g)	350	170	72
NUTS AND SEEDS (*see also* **NUTS AND SEEDS,** page 439)				
Colossal Pistachios	¼ cup without shells	190	130	18
Honey Nut Crunch	3 tbsp 27 g)	150	70	14
Roasted Salted Cashews	¼ cup (33 g)	210	140	27
Roasted Salted Sunflower Kernels	2 tbsp (28 g)	170	140	18
POPCORN				
Air-popped, no added fat	1 cup popped	30	0	0
Commercially popped				
Bachman All Natural				
Air-popped Lite	5 cups (30 g)	120	15	0
Cheese Popcorn	3 cups (30 g)	160	80	NA
with white cheddar cheese	2½ cups (30 g)	160	80	9
Boston's				
Caramel Popcorn, fat-free	⅔ cup (30 g)	100	0	0
Lite Popcorn	4 cups (30 g)	140	50	5
White Cheddar (40% less fat)	2¾ cups (29 g)	140	50	14
Crunch 'n Munch				
Almond Supreme	½ cup (30 g)	140	40	0
Toffee fat-free	¾ cup (28 g)	110	0	0
Toffee Popcorn with Peanuts	⅔ cup (31 g)	140	35	9
Fiddle Faddle				
Caramel Popcorn w/peanuts	¾ cup (30 g)	140	50	27
fat-free	1 cup (30 g)	110	0	0
Olde Tyme air-popped buttery				
popcorn	3⅛ cups (28 g)	140	70	5
Smartfood				
White Cheddar	1¾ cups (28 g)	160	90	18
reduced fat	3 cups (30 g)	140	50	14

SNACK FOODS

FOOD	AMOUNT	CALORIES		
		TOTAL	FAT	SAT-FAT
Commercially popped (cont.)				
Weight Watchers (Smart Snackers)				
Butter flavor	1 pkg (19 g)	90	**20**	0
Butter Toffee	1 pkg (26 g)	110	**25**	9
Caramel	1 pkg (26 g)	100	**10**	0
White Cheddar	1 pkg (19 g)	90	**35**	9
Wise				
Original Butter Popcorn	3 cups (28 g)	150	**90**	18
White Cheddar Popcorn	2 cups (28 g)	160	**100**	23
Microwave				
Jolly Time				
Blast O Butter	3½ cups popped	150	**100**	23
Healthy Pop	5 cups popped	90	**0**	0
Light	5 cups popped	120	**50**	9
Newman's Own Oldstyle Picture				
Show	3½ cups popped	170	**100**	18
Orville Redenbacher's				
Butter	4½ cups popped	170	**110**	23
Natural flavor	1 cup popped	30	**18**	0
Reden Budders	4 cups popped	170	**110**	23
Smart Pop, butter	5 cups popped	90	**20**	0
Pop Secret				
Butter	4 cups popped	180	**110**	27
Video Club Generic				
Butter flavor Light	5 cups (39 g unpopped)	170	**60**	9
Natural	4½ cups (39 g unpopped)	200	**110**	23
Movie Theater Popcorn				
Popped in coconut oil	kid's (5 cups)	300	**180**	126
	small (7 cups)	398	**243**	171
	med. (11 cups)	647	**387**	279
	med. (16 cups)	901	**540**	387
	large (20 cups)	1161	**693**	495
Popped in coconut oil with butter topping	kid's (5 cups)	472	**333**	198
	small (7 cups)	632	**450**	261
	med. (11 cups)	910	**639**	369
	med. (16 cups)	1221	**873**	504
	large (20 cups)	1642	**1134**	657
Popped in canola oil	small (7 cups)	361	**198**	63
	medium (11 cups)	627	**342**	108
	large (16 cups)	850	**468**	144

SNACK FOODS

FOOD	AMOUNT	CALORIES		
		TOTAL	FAT	SAT-FAT
TOASTER PASTRIES				
Kellogg's Pop Tarts				
Apple cinnamon	1 pastry (52 g)	210	**50**	9
Blueberry	1 pastry (52 g)	200	**45**	9
Brown sugar cinnamon	1 pastry (50 g)	210	**60**	9
Frosted blueberry or cherry	1 pastry (52 g)	200	**45**	9
Frosted brown sugar cinnamon	1 pastry (50 g)	210	**60**	14
Frosted chocolate fudge	1 pastry (52 g)	200	**45**	9
Frosted raspberry	1 pastry (52 g)	210	**45**	9
Frosted strawberry	1 pastry (52 g)	200	**45**	9
S'Mores	1 pastry (52 g)	200	**50**	9
Strawberry	1 pastry (52 g)	200	**50**	9
Wild berry	1 pastry (54 g)	210	**50**	14
Wild Tropical Blast	1 pastry (54 g)	210	**45**	18
Wild Watermelon	1 pastry (54 g)	210	**50**	14
Kellogg's Low-fat Pop Tarts				
Blueberry	1 pastry (52 g)	190	**25**	5
Frosted brown sugar cinnamon	1 pastry (50 g)	190	**25**	5
Frosted chocoate fudge	1 pastry (52 g)	180	**25**	5
Frosted strawberry	1 pastry (52 g)	190	**25**	5
Safeway				
Frosted strawberry	1 pastry (52 g)	200	**60**	18
Toastem Pop-Ups				
Frosted chocolate fudge	1 pastry (52 g)	200	**45**	9
Frosted wild berry	1 pastry (52 g)	200	**45**	9
PRETZELS				
Combos				
Cheddar Cheese Pretzel	⅓ cup (28 g)	130	**45**	9
Pizzeria Pretzel	⅓ cup (28 g)	130	**40**	5
Snyder's of Hanover				
Honey Mustard & Onion	⅓ cup (28 g)	140	**60**	9
Oat Bran	3 pretzels (28 g)	100	**5**	0
Old Tyme	3 pretzels (30 g)	120	**10**	0
Old Tyme Stix	28 stix (30 g)	110	**10**	0
Sourdough Hard Pretzel, Fat-free	1 pretzel (28 g)	100	**0**	0
Sourdough Nibblers, Fat-Free	16 nibblers (30 g)	120	**0**	0
Ultra-Thin, Fat-Free	11 pretzels (30 g)	110	**0**	0
Unsalted Mini, Fat-Free	20 minis (30 g)	110	**0**	0
Snyder's of Hanover Nibblers				
Garlic Bread	13 pieces (30 g)	130	**20**	5
Honey Mustard & Onion	13 pieces (30 g)	130	**25**	0
Utz				
Sourdough Hard Pretzels, Fat-Free	1 pretzel (23 g)	90	**0**	0
Sourdough Nuggets	10 pretzels (28 g)	100	**0**	0
Sourdough Specials	4 pretzels (27 g)	110	**15**	0
Stix Pretzels	12 stix (28 g)	110	**5**	0

SNACK FOODS

FOOD	AMOUNT	CALORIES		
		TOTAL	FAT	SAT-FAT
Nibs	½ cup (30 g)	110	15	0
Thin (Rold Gold)	10 pretzels (28 g)	110	0	0
RICE, CORN, AND POPCORN CAKES				
Corn Cakes				
Quaker				
Butter	1 cake (9 g)	35	0	0
Caramel Corn	1 cake (13 g)	50	0	0
Popcorn Cakes				
Orville Redenbacher's Mini Cakes				
Caramel	6 cakes (15 g)	60	0	0
Chocolate Peanut Crunch	6 cakes (15 g)	60	10	0
Nacho	8 cakes (15 g)	60	5	0
Peanut Caramel Crunch	6 cakes (16 g)	60	5	0
Orville Redenbacher's Cakes				
Butter	2 cakes (17 g)	60	10	0
Caramel	1 cake (11 g)	40	0	0
Milk Chocolate	1 cake (10 g)	40	5	0
Rice Cakes				
Quaker				
all flavors	1 cake (13 g)	35–50	0	0
SNACK MIXES				
California Mix	¼ cup (33 g)	130	45	14
Chex Mix (Ralston)				
Bold 'n Zesty	½ cup (30 g)	140	50	9
Cheddar	½ cup (30 g)	130	45	9
Traditional	⅔ cup (30 g)	130	35	5
Cranberry Nut & Fruit Mix	3 tbsp (26 g)	110	45	9
Doo Dads Snack Mix (Nabisco)	½ cup (32 g)	150	60	9
Fiesta Fun Mix	½ cup	300	180	27
Goldfish				
Honey Mustard	½ cup	180	90	14
Nutty Deluxe	½ cup	180	80	14
Original	½ cup (35 g)	170	70	14
Roasted Peanuts	½ cup	170	70	14
Savory	½ cup (32 g)	150	60	9
Seasoned	½ cup	170	70	14
Nut & Fruit Mix	3 tbsp (28 g)	120	45	9
Oriental Party Mix	⅓ cup (31 g)	170	100	14
Party Mix				
Oriental	½ cup	300	180	27
Pastamore	½ cup	260	100	18
Sesame Walnut	½ cup	300	180	27
Smokehouse	½ cup	260	160	18
Cheez-It (Sunshine)				
Nacho	½ cup (30 g)	130	40	9

SNACK FOODS

FOOD	AMOUNT	CALORIES TOTAL	CALORIES FAT	CALORIES SAT-FAT
Cheez-It (Sunshine) (cont.)				
Party Mix	½ cup (30 g)	140	**45**	9
Reduced Fat	½ cup (30 g)	130	**30**	5
Snak-ens Snack Mix				
Chicago Style Pizza	½ cup (30 g)	140	**45**	9
Mustard	½ cup (30 g)	120	**20**	0
Original	½ cup (34 g)	170	**80**	14
Swiss Mix	3 tbsp (29 g)	130	**50**	23
Trail Mix	½ cup	300	**160**	27
Deluxe Super	½ cup	300	**120**	45
Tropical	½ cup	300	**120**	72
VENDING MACHINE FOOD (LANCE)				
Cakes				
Brownies	1¾ oz/pkg	200	**81**	9
Dunking Sticks	5½ oz/pkg	380	**180**	54
Fig Cake	2⅛ oz/pkg	210	**27**	9
Oatmeal Cake	2 oz/pkg	240	**99**	27
Raisin Cake	2 oz/pkg	230	**90**	27
Candy				
Chocolaty Peanut Bar	2 oz/pkg	320	**162**	54
Peanut Bar	1¾ oz/pkg	260	**126**	27
Chips, etc.				
Cheese Balls	1⅛ oz/pkg	190	**117**	27
Corn Chips				
BBQ	1¾ oz/pkg	260	**144**	36
Plain	1¾ oz/pkg	270	**153**	27
Crunchy Cheese Twists	1½ oz/pkg	260	**144**	36
Gold-N-Chee	1⅜ oz/pkg	180	**81**	18
6-pack tray	6 oz/pkg	780	**432**	54
Jalapeño Cheese Tortilla Chips	1⅛ oz/pkg	160	**72**	18
Nacho Tortilla Chips	1⅛ oz/pkg	160	**72**	18
Potato Chips				
Baked	1⅛ oz	130	**15**	0
BBQ	1⅛ oz/pkg	190	**108**	27
Cajun style	2 oz/pkg	320	**180**	36
Handcooked	35 chips (50 g)	260	**140**	45
Plain	1⅛ oz/pkg	190	**135**	36
Sour cream & onion	1⅛ oz/pkg	190	**108**	27
Cookies				
Apple-Cinnamon Cookies	2 oz/pkg	240	**72**	18
Apple-Oatmeal Cookies	1.65 oz/pkg	190	**63**	18
Blueberry Cookies	2 oz/pkg	240	**72**	18
Bonnie Sandwich	1 3/16 oz/pkg	160	**63**	18
Choc-O-Lunch	1 5/16 oz/pkg	180	**63**	18
	4½ oz/pkg	585	**203**	41
Choc-O-Mint	1¼ oz/pkg	180	**90**	27

SNACK FOODS

		CALORIES		
FOOD	**AMOUNT**	**TOTAL**	**FAT**	**SAT-FAT**
Cookies (cont.)				
Coated Graham	1⁵⁄₁₆ oz/pkg	200	**90**	36
Fig Bar	1½ oz/pkg	150	**18**	9
Fudge/Chocolate Chip Cookies	2 oz/pkg	260	**90**	36
Malt	1¼ oz/pkg	190	**99**	18
Nekot	1½ oz/pkg	210	**90**	18
Nut-O-Lunch	4½ oz/pkg	630	**243**	81
Oatmeal Cookies	2 oz/pkg	260	**90**	18
Peanut Butter Creme-filled Wafer	1¾ oz/pkg	240	**90**	27
Soft Chocolate Chip Cookies	2 oz/pkg	260	**90**	36
Strawberry Cookies	2 oz/pkg	240	**72**	18
Van-O-Lunch	1⁵⁄₁₆ oz/pkg	180	**63**	18
	4½ oz/pkg	630	**162**	41
Crackers				
Captain's Wafers with Cream Cheese & Chives	1⁵⁄₁₆ oz/pkg	170	**81**	18
Cheese-on-Wheat	1⁵⁄₁₆ oz/pkg	180	**81**	18
Golden Toast Cheese (Cheetos)	6 crackers (45.3 g)	240	**130**	36
Lanchee	1¼ oz/pkg	180	**99**	18
Nacho Cheesier (Doritos)	6 crackers (45.3 g)	240	**120**	36
Nip-Chee	1⁵⁄₁₆ oz/pkg	130	**81**	18
Peanut Butter Wheat	1⁵⁄₁₆ oz/pkg	190	**99**	18
Rye-Chee	1⁷⁄₁₆ oz/pkg	190	**81**	18
Spicy Gold-N-Chee	10 oz/pkg	1400	**540**	180
Thin Wheat Snacks	10 oz/pkg	1600	**720**	180
Toast Peanut Butter (Peter Pan)	6 crackers (41 g)	210	**100**	23
Toastchee	1⅜ oz/pkg	190	**99**	18
Toasty	1¼ oz/pkg	180	**90**	18
Nut products				
Cashews	1⅛ oz/pkg	190	**135**	27
long tube	2½ oz/pkg	400	**288**	54
Peanuts				
Honey toasted	1⅜ oz/pkg	230	**153**	27
Roasted (shell)	1¾ oz/pkg	190	**135**	27
Salted	1⅛ oz/pkg	190	**135**	27
tube	3 oz/pkg	480	**360**	72
Pistachios	1⅛ oz/pkg	180	**126**	18
Pie				
Pecan Pie	3 oz/pkg	350	**135**	27
Popcorn				
Cheese	⅞ oz/pkg	130	**72**	9
Plain	1 oz/pkg	160	**90**	18
Pork Skins				
BBQ	½ oz/pkg	80	**45**	18
Plain	½ oz/pkg	80	**45**	18
Pretzel Twist	1½ oz/pkg	150	**9**	0

SNACK FOODS

		CALORIES		
FOOD	AMOUNT	TOTAL	FAT	SAT-FAT
MISCELLANEOUS SNACKS				
Cajun Hot Snacks	⅓ cup (34 g)	180	**110**	14
Yogurt Pretzels	6 pieces (40 g)	150	**80**	72
Yogurt Raisins	3 tbsp (35 g)	150	**50**	45

SOUPS

If you are keeping track of total fat calories and your soup is made with whole milk, add 94 fat calories and 188 total calories per can. With 2% milk, add 56 fat calories and 150 total calories per can. If you are keeping track of saturated fat and your soup is made with whole milk, add 56 sat-fat calories per can. With 2% milk, add 34 sat-fat calories per can.

		CALORIES		
FOOD	AMOUNT	TOTAL	FAT	SAT-FAT
CONDENSED				
Prepared with water				
Campbell's				
Bean with Bacon	1 cup prepared	180	**45**	18
Beef Broth	1 cup prepared	15	**0**	0
Beef Noodle	1 cup prepared	70	**25**	9
Broccoli Cheese 98% fat-free	1 cup prepared	80	**25**	14
Cheddar Cheese	1 cup prepared	130	**70**	32
Chicken Alphabet	1 cup prepared	80	**20**	9
Chicken and Stars	1 cup prepared	70	**20**	5
Chicken Broth	1 cup prepared	30	**20**	5
Chicken Gumbo	1 cup prepared	60	**15**	5
Chicken Noodle	1 cup prepared	70	**20**	9
Chicken Noodle (Healthy Request)	1 cup prepared	70	**20**	5
Chicken NoodleO's	1 cup prepared	80	**25**	9
Chicken Rice (Healthy Request)	1 cup prepared	60	**25**	9
Chicken Vegetable	1 cup prepared	80	**20**	5
Chicken Vegetable (Healthy Request)	1 cup prepared	80	**20**	5
Chicken with Rice	1 cup prepared	70	**25**	9
Chicken with White & Wild Rice	1 cup prepared	70	**20**	5
Chicken Won Ton	1 cup prepared	45	**10**	0
Consomme Beef	1 cup prepared	25	**0**	0
Cream of Asparagus	1 cup prepared	110	**60**	18
Cream of Broccoli	1 cup prepared	100	**50**	23

SOUPS

FOOD	AMOUNT	CALORIES		
		TOTAL	FAT	SAT-FAT
Campbell's (cont.)				
Cream of Broccoli 98% fat-free	1 cup prepared	80	25	9
Cream of Celery	1 cup prepared	110	60	23
Cream of Celery (Healthy Request)	1 cup prepared	70	20	5
Cream of Celery 98% fat-free	1 cup prepared	70	25	9
Cream of Chicken	1 cup prepared	130	70	27
Cream of Chicken 98% fat-free	1 cup prepared	80	25	14
Cream of Chicken (Healthy Request)	1 cup prepared	70	20	9
Cream of Chicken & Mushroom	1 cup prepared	130	80	23
Cream of Chicken with Herbs	1 cup prepared	80	35	14
Cream of Mushroom	1 cup prepared	110	60	23
Cream of Mushroom 98% fat-free	1 cup prepared	70	25	9
Cream of Mushroom (Healthy Request)	1 cup prepared	70	25	9
Cream of Mushroom with Roasted Garlic	1 cup prepared	70	25	9
Cream of Potato	1 cup prepared	90	25	14
Cream of Roasted Chicken (Healthy Request)	1 cup prepared	80	25	9
Cream of Shrimp	1 cup prepared	100	60	18
Double Noodle	1 cup prepared	100	25	9
French Onion	1 cup prepared	70	25	0
Golden Mushroom	1 cup prepared	80	25	9
Green Pea	1 cup prepared	180	25	9
Hearty Pasta & Vegetable (Healthy Request)	1 cup prepared	90	10	5
Herbed Potato (Healthy Request)	1 cup prepared	80	20	9
Homestyle Chicken Noodle	1 cup prepared	70	25	14
Italian Tomato	1 cup prepared	100	5	0
Manhattan Clam Chowder	1 cup prepared	100	25	9
Minestrone	1 cup prepared	100	20	5
New England Clam Chowder	1 cup prepared	100	25	9
New England Clam Chowder 98% fat-free	1 cup prepared	90	20	5
Old-Fashioned Tomato Rice	1 cup prepared	120	20	5
Pepper Pot	1 cup prepared	100	45	18
Split Pea with Ham & Bacon	1 cup prepared	180	30	18
Tomato	1 cup prepared	80	0	0
Tomato (Healthy Request)	1 cup prepared	90	15	5
Tomato Bisque	1 cup prepared	130	25	14
Turkey Noodle	1 cup prepared	80	25	9

SOUPS

FOOD	AMOUNT	CALORIES		
		TOTAL	FAT	SAT-FAT
Campbell's (cont.)				
Vegetable	1 cup prepared	80	**10**	5
Vegetable (Healthy Request)	1 cup prepared	90	**10**	5
Vegetable Beef	1 cup prepared	80	**20**	9
Vegetable Beef (Healthy Request)	1 cup prepared	80	**20**	9
Vegetarian Vegetable	1 cup prepared	90	**10**	0
DEHYDRATED				
Knorr's				
Black Bean	1 package (53 g)	200	**10**	0
Chicken Flavor Vegetable	1 package (30 g)	100	**0**	0
Hearty Lentil	1 package (57 g)	220	**0**	0
Navy Bean	1 package (38 g)	140	**0**	0
Potato Leek	1 package (34 g)	120	**0**	0
Marachan Instant Lunch				
Beef flavor	1 container (64 g)	290	**110**	54
with Shrimp	1 container (64 g)	290	**110**	54
Nissin Top Ramen				
Baked Ramen Noodle Soup (98% fat-free)				
all flavors	½ block (37 g)	140	**10**	0
	1 cup (58 g)	210	**10**	0
Cup Noodles Ramen Noodle Soup				
Chicken flavor	1 container (64 g)	300	**130**	63
Chicken Vegetable flavor	1 container (64 g)	300	**130**	54
Creamy Chicken flavor	1 container (64 g)	300	**120**	54
French Onion flavor	1 container (64 g)	300	**110**	54
Teriyaki Chicken flavor	1 container (64 g)	300	**130**	54
Twin Pack, with Shrimp	1 cup (34 g)	150	**60**	27
Oodles of Noodles, all flavors	½ pkg (43 g)	180–190	**60**	32
Soup Starter (Wyler's)				
Beef Vegetable	⅛ pkg (28 g dry)	90	**5**	0
Chicken Noodle	⅛ pkg (24 g dry)	80	**5**	0
Hearty Beef Stew	⅐ pkg (23 g dry)	80	**0**	0
Hearty Chicken Vegetable	⅐ pkg (23 g dry)	70	**0**	0
HOMEMADE OR RESTAURANT				
Cream of Mushroom Soup	1 cup	170	**155**	98
French Onion Soup	1 cup	350	**125**	65
Gazpacho	1 cup	111	**80**	11
New England Clam Chowder	1 cup	230	**145**	65
Vichyssoise	1 cup	315	**210**	140
READY TO SERVE				
Campbell's				
Chunky Soup				
Beef	10¾ oz (305 g)	200	**45**	14
Beef Pasta	1 cup	150	**25**	9

SOUPS

FOOD	AMOUNT	CALORIES		
		TOTAL	FAT	SAT-FAT
Campbell's (cont.)				
Cheese Tortellini	1 cup	110	20	9
Chicken and Pasta	10¾ oz	150	40	14
Chicken Broccoli Cheese	1 cup	200	110	45
Chicken Corn Chowder	1 cup	250	140	63
Chicken Mushroom				
Chowder	1 cup	210	110	36
Chicken with Rice	1 cup	140	30	9
Clam Chowder,				
Manhattan Style	1 cup	130	35	9
Classic Chicken Noodle	1 cup	130	25	9
Hearty Bean 'n Ham	1 cup	190	20	9
Hearty Chicken with				
Vegetables	1 cup	90	20	5
New England Clam				
Chowder	10¾ oz	300	160	63
Pepper Steak	1 cup	140	25	9
Potato Ham Chowder	1 cup	220	130	72
Sirloin Burger	1 cup	180	60	32
Split Pea 'n Ham	1 cup	190	25	9
Tomato Ravioli	1 cup	150	25	14
Vegetable	10¾ oz	160	35	9
Healthy Request				
Chicken Broth	1 cup	20	0	0
Hearty Chicken Vegetable	1 cup	120	20	5
Home Cookin'				
Bean and Ham	1 cup	180	15	5
Chicken Rice	1 cup	140	15	5
Chicken Vegetable	1 cup	130	35	9
Chicken with Egg Noodles	10¾ oz	110	25	14
Country Mushroom Rice	1 cup	80	5	0
Country Vegetable	1 cup	110	10	0
Cream of Mushroom	1 cup	80	20	9
Creamy Potato	1 cup	180	80	23
Fiesta	1 cup	130	25	5
New England Clam				
Chowder	1 cup	120	30	9
Tomato Garden	1 cup	130	30	9
Vegetable Beef	1 cup	120	20	9
Microwavable Ready-to-Serve Soups (Campbell's)				
Chicken Noodle	10.5 oz	130	35	9
Vegetable Beef	10.5 oz	140	5	0
Manischewitz				
Matzo Ball Soup	1 cup	110	45	18

SWEETS

FOOD	AMOUNT	CALORIES		
		TOTAL	FAT	SAT-FAT
BARS				
Tasty Kake Snack Bars				
Chocolate Chip	1 bar (57 g)	250	110	27
Iced Fudge	1 bar (57 g)	250	90	14
Iced Lemon	1 bar (57 g)	260	90	9
Iced Strawberry	1 bar (57 g)	260	90	9
Oatmeal Raisin	1 bar (57 g)	250	80	23
BROWNIES				
Brownie				
with nuts	1 brownie (40 g)	180	80	18
without nuts	1 brownie (40 g)	160	60	18
Fudge Brownies (Little Debbie)	1 brownie (61 g)	270	120	23
Brownie Bites (Hostess)	3 pieces (37 g)	170	80	18
Nonfat (Entenmann's)	1 brownie (40 g)	110	0	0
BROWNIE MIXES BY BRAND NAME				
Betty Crocker				
Dark Chocolate Supreme	30 g mix	129	15	5
	prep w. eggs & oil	170	70	9
Fudge Brownies	28 g mix	110	15	5
	prep w. eggs & oil	170	70	14
Original Supreme	32 g mix	130	15	5
	prep w. eggs & oil	160	50	9
Sweet Rewards Low-fat				
Fudge Brownie mix	32 g mix	130	25	9
Turtle Supreme	29 g mix	120	20	5
	prep w. eggs & oil	170	70	14
Walnut Supreme	28 g mix	120	30	5
	prep w. eggs & oil	180	80	9
Duncan Hines				
Chewy Fudge Brownie	¼ cup mix (31 g)	130	25	5
	baked	160	60	14
Dark 'n Chunky	¼ cup mix (30 g)	140	30	9
	baked	160	70	14
Double Fudge	¼ cup mix (34 g)	140	25	5
	baked	170	60	9
Milk Chocolate Chunk	¼ cup mix (33 g)	140	35	14
	baked	170	60	14
Pillsbury				
Rich & Moist Fudge Brownie	31 g mix	130	25	5
	baked w. oil & eggs	190	80	15
Thick 'n Fudgy				
Cheesecake Swirl	27 g mix	130	40	14
	baked w. oil & eggs	170	80	25
Chocolate Chunk	27g mix	120	30	14
	baked w. oil & eggs	160	60	18

SWEETS

FOOD	AMOUNT	CALORIES		
		TOTAL	FAT	SAT-FAT
Pillsbury (cont.)				
Double Chocolate	28 g mix	120	**25**	5
	baked w. oil & eggs	150	**50**	10
Walnut	32 g mix	150	**45**	9
	baked w. oil & eggs	190	**90**	14
Washington				
Fudge Brownie	¼ cup mix (31 g)	130	**35**	14
	baked w. oil & eggs	150	**45**	18
BUNS				
Breakfast Buns	1 bun (55 g)	170	**25**	9
Butterfly Buns	1 bun (55 g)	190	**35**	9
Honey Bun (Little Debbie)	1 bun (50 g)	220	**100**	23
Hot Cross Buns	1 bun	168	**56**	16
Iced Honey Bun (Hostess)	1 bun (99 g)	420	**220**	54
Pecan Twirls	1 (28 g)	110	**35**	5
Rum Buns (Hadley Farm)	1 bun (85 g)	290	**80**	18
	1 bun (55 g)	200	**60**	14
Sticky Bun	1 (55 g)	210	**70**	14
Cinnamon Pecan Sticky	1 roll (71 g)	220	**60**	14
Entenmann's Light	1 bun (61 g)	160	**25**	5
CAKES, BAKERY, HOMEMADE, AND RESTAURANT				
Almond Danish Coffee Cake	⅛ cake (57 g)	230	**100**	18
Almond Poppy	¹⁄₁₀ cake (80 g)	320	**160**	27
Angel Food	¹⁄₁₂ cake	125	**0**	0
Angel Food Loaf	2" slice (55 g)	150	**5**	0
Angel Food Ring	⅙ cake (47 g)	130	**5**	0
Apple Danish Coffee Cake	⅛ cake (57 g)	160	**60**	18
Apple Strudel Cake	1 slice (64 g)	190	**90**	27
Baked Alaska	¹⁄₁₂ of cake	263	**112**	60
Banana Nut Loaf	2" slice (76 g)	270	**120**	27
Bavarian Chocolate Cake	2" square (80 g)	340	**180**	63
Black Forest (7" diam)	1 slice (80 g)	330	**170**	41
Blueberry Cheese Coffee Cake	⅛ cake (57 g)	170	**70**	18
Boston Cream Cake	⅙ cake (113 g)	320	**120**	27
Carrot Cake (7" diam)	1 slice (80 g)	300	**130**	36
Cheesecake	¹⁄₁₂ cake	280	**162**	89
	2" wedge (250 g)	820	**540**	342
Blueberry-Topped Cheesecake	⅙ cake (113 g)	350	**180**	81
French Cheesecake	4" wedge (125 g)	370	**200**	54
Cherry Puddin' Cake	⅛ cake (74 g)	290	**130**	23
Chocolate Crunch Ring	⅛ cake (71 g)	310	**140**	36
Chocolate Fudge (7" diam)	1 slice (80 g)	300	**140**	32
Chocolate Marble Loaf	⅕ cake (80 g)	340	**150**	32

SWEETS

FOOD	AMOUNT	CALORIES		
		TOTAL	FAT	SAT-FAT
CAKES, BAKERY, HOMEMADE, AND RESTAURANT (cont.)				
Chocolate Sheet Cake with				
Vanilla Icing	1 slice (80 g)	320	160	36
Cinnamon Stix	1 stick (57 g)	200	60	14
Creme Cakes				
Blueberry	1 slice (80 g)	280	120	23
Chocolate	1 slice (80 g)	300	140	27
Maple Nut	1 slice (80 g)	310	140	23
Strawberry	1 slice (80 g)	290	120	23
Vanilla	1 slice (80 g)	300	140	23
Crumb Cakes				
Apple Cinnamon Walnut	1 slice (80 g)	320	140	31
Blueberry	1 slice (80 g)	320	140	31
Cupcake, low fat	1 (80 g)	340	140	36
Creme-filled Chocolate	2 cakes (64 g)	200	25	9
Creme-filled Vanilla	2 cakes (64 g)	200	25	9
Devil's Food Fudge Cake	⅙ cake (85 g)	340	140	36
Devil's Food Layer Cake				
w/white icing	2½" wedge (80 g)	360	170	45
Fruitcake	1 slice (125 g)	470	170	32
German Apple Strudel	⅛ cake (53 g)	140	60	18
German Chocolate Cake				
(10" diam)	1/16 cake	521	277	27
(7" diam)	1 slice (80 g)	300	140	36
Golden Coconut (7" diam)	1 slice (80 g)	320	160	36
Hazelnut Torte	1/16 torte	315	187	56
Ladyfingers	12 (85 g)	280	35	14
Lemon Crunch Ring	⅛ cake (71 g)	270	110	23
Lemon Supreme (7" diam)	1 slice (80 g)	320	160	36
Marble Cake (7" diam)	1 slice (80 g)	330	160	36
Pecan Cinnamon Ring	⅛ cake (71 g)	300	130	23
Pecan Danish Ring	⅛ cake (57 g)	230	120	27
Pecan Twirls Sweet Rolls	2 twirls (56 g)	220	80	9
Pineapple Upside-Down Cake				
(7" diam)	1 slice (80 g)	210	80	14
Pound cake, not iced	2" slice (80 g)	300	140	45
Strawberry Cheese Danish				
Coffee Cake	⅛ cake (57 g)	170	80	18
Walnut Danish Ring	⅛ cake (55 g)	230	120	18
Yellow Layer Cake				
with white icing	2½" wedge (80 g)	350	170	45
with chocolate icing	2½" wedge (80 g)	320	140	36
CAKES AND SNACK CAKES BY BRAND NAME				
Entenmann's				
All Butter Loaf	⅙ cake (57 g)	210	80	45
All Butter French Crumbcake	⅛ cake (50 g)	210	90	45
Apple Puffs	1 puff (85 g)	260	110	27

SWEETS

FOOD	AMOUNT	CALORIES		
		TOTAL	FAT	SAT-FAT
Entenmann's (cont.)				
Cheese Coffee Cake	⅛ cake (48 g)	160	**60**	23
Cheese Crumb Babka	⅛ danish (48 g)	160	**60**	23
Cheese-Filled Crumb Coffee Cake	⅛ cake (57 g)	200	**90**	32
Cinnamon Filbert Ring	⅕ danish (60 g)	260	**150**	27
Cinnamon Rugelach	1 piece (21 g)	100	**60**	NA
Crumb Coffee Cake	⅒ cake (57 g)	250	**110**	27
Raspberry Danish Twist	⅛ danish (53 g)	220	**100**	32
Rugelach				
all flavors	1 piece (19 g)	90	**45**	27
Entenmann's Light				
Apple Spice Cake	⅕ cake (79 g)	200	**0**	0
Banana Crunch Cake	⅕ cake (85 g)	220	**0**	0
Banana Loaf	⅙ cake (76 g)	190	**0**	0
Blueberry Crunch Cake	⅙ cake (76 g)	180	**0**	0
Chocolate Crunch Cake	⅕ cake (79 g)	210	**0**	0
Chocolate Loaf Cake	⅕ cake (85 g)	210	**0**	0
Cinnamon Apple Coffee Cake	⅑ cake (54 g)	120	**0**	0
Cinnamon Apple Twist	⅛ danish (53 g)	140	**0**	0
Cherry Cheese Pastry	⅑ pastry (54 g)	130	**0**	0
Crumb Delight	⅑ cake (57 g)	210	**60**	9
Fudge Brownie	⅒ brownie (40 g)	110	**0**	0
Fudge-Iced Chocolate Cake	⅙ cake (85 g)	190	**0**	0
Golden Chocolatey Chip Loaf	⅕ cake (85 g)	220	**0**	0
Golden Loaf Cake	⅛ cake (48 g)	130	**0**	0
Lemon Twist	⅛ danish (53 g)	130	**0**	0
Louisiana Crunch Cake	⅙ cake (76 g)	210	**0**	0
Marble Loaf	⅛ cake (50 g)	130	**0**	0
Mocha-Iced Chocolate Cake	⅙ cake (85 g)	200	**0**	0
Pineapple Crunch Cake	⅙ cake (76 g)	190	**0**	0
Raspberry Cheese Pastry	⅑ cake (54 g)	140	**0**	0
Raspberry Twist	⅛ danish (53 g)	140	**0**	0
Hostess				
Baseballs	1 cake (46 g)	150	**30**	9
Cinnamon Crumb Cakes, low-fat	1 cake (28 g)	90	**5**	0
Cup Cakes				
Chocolate	1 cake (50 g)	180	**50**	23
low-fat	1 cake (46 g)	140	**15**	5
Orange	1 cake (43 g)	160	**45**	18
HoHos	1 cake (29 g)	130	**55**	36
King Dons	1 cake (40 g)	170	**80**	45
Sno Balls	1 cake (50 g)	180	**50**	23
Suzy Q's	1 cake (58 g)	220	**80**	36
Twinkies	1 cake (43 g)	150	**45**	18
low-fat	1 cake (43 g)	130	**15**	5

SWEETS

FOOD	AMOUNT	CALORIES TOTAL	FAT	SAT-FAT
Krispy Kreme				
Apple Danish	1 pastry (90 g)	380	**210**	54
Cherry Danish	1 pastry (92 g)	370	**180**	45
Cream Cheese Danish	1 pastry (96 g)	410	**240**	72
Honey Bun	1 bun (96 g)	410	**220**	54
Little Debbie				
Apple Streusel Coffee Cake	2 cakes (60 g)	230	**70**	14
Chocolate Cup Cakes	1 cake (45 g)	180	**80**	18
Coffee Cakes	1 cake (30 g)	115	**30**	7
Devil Squares	1 cake (31 g)	135	**55**	14
Oatmeal Lights	1 wrap (38 g)	130	**50**	5
Snack Cakes	1 cake (36 g)	155	**70**	32
Strawberry Shortcake Rolls	1 roll (61 g)	230	**70**	18
Swiss Cake Rolls	1 cake (31 g)	130	**55**	9
Zebra Cakes	1 cake (37 g)	165	**75**	16
Pepperidge Farm				
Cream Cheese Carrot	$\frac{1}{9}$ cake (80 g)	320	**180**	41
Devil's Food Cake	$\frac{1}{6}$ slice (80 g)	290	**122**	NA
Three-Layer Cake	$\frac{1}{8}$ cake (69 g)	250	**110**	27
Sara Lee				
Banana Sundae Layer Cake	$\frac{1}{10}$ cake (81 g)	270	**120**	90
Butter Streusel Coffee Cake	$\frac{1}{6}$ cake (54 g)	220	**110**	54
Chocolate Swirl Cake	$\frac{1}{4}$ cake (83 g)	330	**140**	72
Double Chocolate Layer Cake	$\frac{1}{8}$ cake (79 g)	260	**120**	99
Flaky Coconut Layer Cake	$\frac{1}{8}$ cake (81 g)	280	**130**	108
French Cheesecake	$\frac{1}{5}$ cake (133 g)	410	**230**	144
German Chocolate Layer Cake	$\frac{1}{8}$ cake (83 g)	280	**130**	99
Mint Chocolate Mousse	$\frac{1}{5}$ mousse (122 g)	440	**250**	189
Original Cream Cheesecake	$\frac{1}{4}$ cake (121 g)	350	**160**	81
Pecan Coffee Cake	$\frac{1}{6}$ cake (54 g)	230	**110**	41
Pound Cake, all butter	$\frac{1}{6}$ cake (76 g)	320	**150**	81
Strawberry French Cheese Cake	$\frac{1}{6}$ cake (123 g)	320	**130**	81
Strawberry Shortcake	$\frac{1}{8}$ cake (71 g)	180	**70**	45
Vanilla Layer Cake	$\frac{1}{8}$ cake (80 g)	250	**120**	90
Tastykake				
Cinnamon Sweet Rolls	1 cake (60 g)	190	**30**	9
Cup Cakes				
Banana Creamies	1 cake (43 g)	170	**60**	14
Butter Cream–Iced Chocolate	2 cakes (64 g)	250	**70**	18
Chocolate Creamies	1 cake (43 g)	180	**70**	18
Chocolate Cup Cakes	3 cakes (92 g)	310	**80**	14
Creme Filled Chocolate	2 cakes (64 g)	230	**70**	9
Vanilla Creamies	1 cake (43 g)	190	**80**	14
Honey Bun	1 cake (92 g)	360	**150**	27

SWEETS

FOOD	AMOUNT	CALORIES		
		TOTAL	FAT	SAT-FAT
Tastykake (cont.)				
Juniors				
Chocolate Junior	1 cake (94 g)	330	**110**	18
Coconut Junior	1 cake (94 g)	310	**170**	36
Koffee Kake Junior	1 cake (71 g)	270	**180**	14
Kandy Kakes				
Chocolate Kandy Kakes	3 cakes (57 g)	250	**110**	63
Peanut Butter Kandy Kakes	3 cakes (57 g)	280	**130**	63
Koffee Kakes				
Chocolate	3 cakes (99 g)	380	**130**	23
Creme Filled Koffee Kakes	2 cakes (57 g)	240	**80**	14
Kreme Krimpies	3 cakes (85 g)	340	**110**	14
Krimpets				
Butterscotch Krimpets	3 cakes (85 g)	310	**70**	14
Jelly Krimpets	3 cakes (85 g)	280	**40**	9
Strawberries Krimpets	3 cakes (85 g)	310	**70**	9
Marshmallow Treats	1 cake (57 g)	210	**35**	9
Pound Kake	1 cake (85 g)	320	**120**	45
Tropical Delights				
Coconut Tropical Delights	2 cakes (57 g)	190	**80**	41
Guava Tropical Delights	2 cakes (57 g)	190	**60**	36
Papaya Tropical Delights	2 cakes (57 g)	190	**60**	36
Pineapple Tropical Delights	2 cakes (57 g)	190	**60**	36
Weight Watchers				
Chocolate Eclair	1 eclair (59 g)	150	**35**	9
Chocolate Raspberry Royale	1 dessert (99 g)	190	**30**	9
New York–Style Cheesecake	1 cake (70 g)	150	**45**	23
CAKE MIXES BY BRAND NAME				
Any brand				
Angel Food	$\frac{1}{12}$ cake (36 g)	140	**0**	0
Betty Crocker				
Angel Food				
fat-free	38 g mix	140	**0**	0
Easy	¼ loaf or 3 cupcakes (44 g mix)	170	**0**	0
Lemon Bars	29 g mix	130	**30**	9
	prep with eggs	140	**40**	9
Pound Cake	57 g mix	250	**60**	27
	prep with eggs	270	**70**	27
Super Moist				
Butter Recipe Chocolate	43 g mix	190	**40**	14
	prep with eggs, butter, frosting	270	**120**	63

SWEETS

FOOD	AMOUNT	CALORIES		
		TOTAL	FAT	SAT-FAT
Betty Crocker (cont.)				
Butter Recipe Yellow	43 g mix	170	**20**	9
	prep with eggs, butter, frosting	260	**100**	54
Carrot	51 g mix	200	**30**	9
	prep with eggs, butter, frosting	320	**140**	23
Chocolate Fudge	43 g mix	170	**25**	9
	prep with eggs, butter, frosting	270	**110**	23
Devil's Food	43 g mix	180	**35**	14
	prep with eggs, butter, frosting	240	**100**	36
Double Chocolate Swirl	43 g mix	170	**25**	9
	prep with eggs, butter, frosting	270	**110**	23
French Vanilla	43 g mix	170	**30**	9
	prep with eggs, butter, frosting	240	**90**	18
Lemon	43 g mix	170	**30**	9
	prep with eggs, butter, frosting	240	**90**	18
Yellow	43 g mix	170	**30**	9
	prep with eggs, butter, frosting	250	**90**	23
Stir 'n Bake				
Carrot Cake	61 g mix	250	**60**	14
Coffee Cake	47 g mix	200	**50**	14
Devil's Food	58 g mix	240	**70**	18
Super Moist Light				
Devil's Food	52 g mix	210	**30**	14
	prep with eggs & frosting	230	**40**	18
Sweet Rewards reduced fat				
Devil's Food	43 g mix	160	**15**	5
	prep with oil & eggs	200	**45**	10
Yellow	43 g mix	160	**10**	5
	prep with oil & eggs	200	**40**	15
Duncan Hines				
Angel Food	¼ cup mix (38 g)	140	**0**	0
Moist Deluxe				
Butter Recipe Golden	52 g mix	230	**50**	18
	prep with eggs, butter, topping	320	**140**	63

SWEETS

FOOD	AMOUNT	CALORIES		
		TOTAL	FAT	SAT-FAT
Duncan Hines (cont.)				
Devil's Food	⅓ cup mix (43 g)	180	**40**	14
	prep with eggs, oil, topping	290	**130**	27
White	⅓ cup mix (43 g)	170	**30**	14
	prep with eggs, oil, topping	190	**50**	9
all other flavors	⅓ cup mix	180	**30**	14
	prep with eggs, oil, topping	250	**100**	18
Pillsbury				
Chocolate Chip Streusel				
Coffee Cake	50 g mix	210	**50**	18
	prep with oil & eggs	270	**110**	23
Cinnamon Streusel Coffee Cake	47 g mix	190	**45**	14
	prep with oil & eggs	260	**100**	23
Moist Supreme (Jell-O pudding in the mix)				
Butter Recipe	43 g mix	170	**25**	9
	prep w. eggs & butter	260	**110**	54
Devil's Food	43 g mix	180	**35**	14
	prep w. oil & eggs	270	**130**	27
Lemon	52 g mix	210	**35**	14
	prep w. oil & eggs	300	**120**	27
Yellow	43 g mix	180	**35**	14
	prep w. oil & eggs	240	**90**	23
CAKE DECORATIONS				
Dessert Decorations (Betty Crocker)				
Alphabet & Numbers	5 pieces (4 g)	20	**15**	5
Animal Shapes	3 pieces (4 g)	20	**15**	5
Happy Birthday Pieces	2 pieces (4 g)	20	**15**	5
Lace Decors	4 pieces (4 g)	20	**15**	5
Leaves	3 pieces (4 g)	20	**15**	5
CAKE FROSTING BY BRAND NAME				
Betty Crocker Rich & Creamy frosting				
Chocolate	2 tbsp (33 g)	130	**45**	14
Coconut Pecan	2 tbsp	150	**70**	27
Cream Cheese	2 tbsp (34 g)	140	**45**	14
Dark Chocolate	2 tbsp (36 g)	150	**50**	14
French Vanilla	2 tbsp (34 g)	140	**45**	14
Rainbow Chip	2 tbsp (36 g)	160	**60**	27
Vanilla	2 tbsp (34 g)	140	**45**	14

SWEETS

FOOD	AMOUNT	CALORIES		
		TOTAL	FAT	SAT-FAT
Betty Crocker Soft Whipped frosting				
Chocolate	2 tbsp (24 g)	100	**45**	18
Cream Cheese	2 tbsp (24 g)	100	**40**	14
Fluffy Lemon	2 tbsp (24 g)	110	**45**	14
Fluffy White	2 tbsp (24 g)	100	**40**	14
Strawberry	2 tbsp (24 g)	110	**45**	14
Vanilla	2 tbsp (24 g)	100	**40**	14
Betty Crocker Sweet Rewards reduced-fat frosting				
Chocolate	2 tbsp (33 g)	120	**20**	9
Vanilla	2 tbsp (33 g)	120	**20**	5
Cake Mate Decorating Icing				
all colors	1 tsp (6 g)	30	**10**	0
Duncan Hines Homestyle Frosting				
Vanilla	2 tbsp (32 g)	140	**50**	14
all other flavors	2 tbsp (32 g)	130	**45**	14
Washington Frosting Mix				
Creamy Fudge	¼ cup mix (26 g)	110	**15**	5
	prep w. margarine	150	**50**	10
Creamy White	¼ cup mix (26 g)	110	**15**	5
	prep w. margarine	150	**50**	10
CANDY				
3 Musketeers	1 bar (60.4 g)	260	**70**	36
Miniatures	7 pieces (41 g)	170	**45**	23
After Eight	5 pieces (49 g)	170	**50**	32
Almond Joy	1 bar (49 g)	240	**120**	72
Snack size	2 bars (38 g)	190	**90**	63
Andes				
Crème de menthe thins	8 pieces (38 g)	210	**120**	108
Mint Parfait Thins	8 pieces (38 g)	210	**120**	99
Baby Ruth	1 bar (59.5 g)	280	**110**	63
Fun size	2 bars (42 g)	190	**80**	45
Butterfinger	1 bar (60 g)	280	**100**	54
Fun size	2 bars (42 g)	200	**70**	36
Butterscotch				
Brach's	3 pieces (18 g)	70	**0**	0
Callard & Bowser	3 pieces (18 g)	60	**10**	5
Candy Corn	26 pieces (39 g)	140	**0**	0
Caramels				
Chocolate Chew (Riesen)	5 pieces (40 g)	180	**60**	27
Classic (Hershey's)	6 pieces (37 g)	160	**45**	41
Classic (Kraft)	6 pieces (37 g)	160	**50**	41
Creams (Goetze's)	3 pieces (34 g)	130	**30**	9
Milk Maid (Brach's)	4 pieces (39 g)	150	**40**	9
Milkfuls (Storck)	6 pieces (40 g)	170	**25**	14
Carob Peanut Clusters	1 piece (28 g)	150	**90**	36

SWEETS

FOOD	AMOUNT	CALORIES		
		TOTAL	FAT	SAT-FAT
Carob Raisins	40 pieces (41 g)	160	45	36
Chocolate-covered peanuts	15 pieces (40 g)	220	120	54
Chocolate-covered peanut clusters	3 pieces (43 g)	230	130	63
Chocolate-covered fudge mix	14 pieces (40 g)	190	70	36
Chocolate Mint Pattie (Brach's)	3 pieces (36 g)	140	26	18
Dots	12 pieces (43 g)	150	0	0
Dove Chocolate Bar	1 bar (37 g)	200	110	63
Dove Promises, all flavors	7 pieces (42 g)	220–230	120	72
Fondant (mints, candy corn, other)	1 oz	105	0	0
French Burnt Peanuts	28 pieces (40 g)	190	80	9
Fruit Roll-ups, all flavors	2 rolls (28 g)	110	10	0
Goldenberg's Peanut Chews	3 pieces (37 g)	270	120	27
Good & Plenty	33 pieces (40 g)	130	0	0
Gumdrops	1 oz	100	0	0
Gummy Bears	10 pieces (40 g)	140	0	0
Halvah (Joyva)				
Chocolate-covered	½ bar (57 g)	380	210	45
Chocolate-flavored	½ bar (57 g)	390	230	36
Marble	½ bar (57 g)	390	230	36
Hard candies	1 oz	110	0	0
	1 piece (5.6 g)	18	0	0
Heath Sensations	⅓ bag (43 g)	220	120	63
Hershey's Chocolate				
Cookies 'n Creme	1 bar (43 g)	230	110	54
Hugs	8 pieces (38 g)	210	110	54
Kisses	8 pieces (39 g)	210	110	72
with almonds	8 pieces (38 g)	210	120	63
Milk Chocolate	1 bar (43 g)	230	120	81
with almonds	1 bar (41 g)	230	130	63
Sweet Escapes				
Caramel & Peanut Butter	1 bar (20 g)	70	25	9
Chocolate-Toffee	1 bar (39 g)	190	70	45
Crispy Caramel Fudge	1 bar (20 g)	80	20	9
Miniatures	5 pieces (42 g)	230	130	72
Symphony	1 bar (42 g)	240	140	72
Triple Chocolate Wafer	1 bar (39 g)	160	45	23
	1 bar (20 g)	80	25	14
Hot Tamales	19 pieces (40 g)	150	0	0
Jellybeans	14 pieces (39 g)	140	0	0
Jordan Almonds (Brach's)	10 pieces (41 g)	180	50	0
Jujyfruits	15 pieces (40 g)	160	0	0
Junior Mints	16 pieces (40 g)	160	25	18
Kit Kat	1 bar (42 g)	220	100	63
Snack	3 bars (47 g)	240	110	72
Licorice Sticks	4 pieces (37 g)	120	5	0

SWEETS

		CALORIES		
FOOD	AMOUNT	TOTAL	FAT	SAT-FAT
M&M's				
Almond	¼ cup (42 g)	230	110	36
Peanut Butter	¼ cup (42 g)	220	110	72
Peanut	¼ cup (42 g)	220	100	41
Plain	¼ cup (42 g)	210	80	54
Malted Milk Balls	17 pieces (40 g)	180	60	60
Maple Nut Goodlies (Brach's)	7 pieces (39 g)	190	80	9
Mars Bar	1 bar (50 g)	240	110	36
Marshmallows (Kraft)	5 pieces (34 g)	110	0	0
Mary Janes	6 pieces (40 g)	160	40	0
Mighty Malts malted milk balls	10 pieces (42 g)	200	60	60
Mike and Ike	19 pieces (40 g)	150	0	0
Milk Chocolate–Covered Jots	39 pieces (40 g)	190	60	36
Milk Chocolate Peanut Jots	17 pieces (40 g)	200	90	27
Milk Duds	13 pieces (40 g)	170	50	36
Milky Way	1 bar (58 g)	270	90	45
Fun size	2 bars (40 g)	180	60	32
Lite	1 bar (45 g)	170	50	23
Miniatures	5 pieces (41 g)	180	60	32
Mr. Goodbar	1 bar (49 g)	270	150	63
Mounds Bar	1 bar (53 g)	250	120	99
Snack size	2 bars (38 g)	180	90	72
Necco Mints	2 pieces (6 g)	24	0	0
Nerds	1 box (11 g)	40	0	0
Nestlé				
100 Grand	1 bar (43 g)	200	70	45
Nestle Crunch	1 bar (44 g)	230	100	63
Fun size	4 bars (40 g)	210	100	63
Nips				
Caramel	2 pieces (14 g)	60	10	9
Chocolate Parfait	2 pieces (14 g)	60	15	9
Coffee	2 pieces (14 g)	50	10	14
NutRageous	1 bar (54 g)	290	150	45
Nonpareils (dark chocolate)	17 pieces (41 g)	200	80	54
Pastel Mints (Petite)	¼ cup (40 g)	210	100	18
Payday	1 bar (52 g)	250	120	18
Snack size	2 bars (40 g)	190	90	32
Peanut brittle	½ cup (40 g)	180	45	9
Peanut Butter Cups (Estee)	5 candies (38 g)	200	110	63
Pretzel Flipz (Nestle)	9 pieces (28 g)	130	50	45
Raisinets	¼ cup (45 g)	200	70	41
Raisins, chocolate-covered	34 pieces (40 g)	170	60	45
Reese's				
Miniatures	5 pieces (39 g)	210	110	41
Peanut Butter Cups	2 cups (45 g)	250	130	45
Pieces	50 pieces (39 g)	190	70	41
Sticks	1 pkg (42 g)	220	120	54

SWEETS

FOOD	AMOUNT	CALORIES		
		TOTAL	**FAT**	**SAT-FAT**
Rolo	7 pieces (42 g)	200	**80**	45
Russell Stover				
Almond Delights	2 pieces (40 g)	210	**110**	45
Assorted Caramels	3 pieces (40 g)	190	**80**	45
Assorted Chocolates	1 box (57 g)	300	**120**	72
	3 pieces (40 g)	190	**70**	45
Assorted Creams	3 pieces (40 g)	180	**60**	36
Assorted Whips	2 pieces (40 g)	210	**60**	36
Bars				
Almond Delight Bar	1 bar (57 g)	290	**150**	63
Caramel Bar	1 bar (46 g)	230	**100**	63
French Chocolate Mint	1 bar (42 g)	240	**140**	63
Mint Dream	1 bar (32 g)	160	**70**	45
Pecan Delight Bar	1 bar (57g)	310	**180**	63
Pecan Roll	1 bar (50 g)	260	**160**	18
Caramels	3 pieces (40 g)	170	**70**	45
Cherry Blimps	2 pieces (40 g)	180	**80**	36
Chocolate Truffle Golf Balls	1 ball (40 g)	200	**110**	72
Dark Chocolate Assortment	3 pieces (40 g)	190	**70**	45
French Chocolate Mints	4 pieces (40 g)	220	**130**	81
Home-Fashioned Favorites	3 pieces (40 g)	170	**60**	45
Milk Chocolate Assortment	3 pieces (40 g)	190	**80**	45
Nut, Chewy and Crispy				
Centers	3 pieces (40 g)	200	**90**	45
Toffee Sticks	3½ sticks (40 g)	230	**140**	72
Skittles (all flavors)	¼ cup (42 g)	170	**15**	0
	1 bag (61.5 g)	250	**25**	5
Snickers	1 bar (59 g)	280	**130**	45
Fun size	2 bars (40 g)	190	**90**	32
Toffee				
Brach's	3 pieces (18 g)	80	**20**	9
Butter Toffee (Farley's)	3 pieces (16 g)	70	**10**	5
English Toffees (Callard &				
Bowser)	2 pieces (17 g)	80	**35**	23
Licorice Toffees (Callard &				
Bowser)	2 pieces (17 g)	80	**30**	31
Tootsie Roll				
Midgies	6 pieces (40 g)	160	**25**	5
Pops	1 pop (17 g)	60	**0**	0
Twix	2 cookies (50 g)	280	**130**	45
Miniatures	3 pieces (29 g)	150	**60**	23
Villa Cherries (Brach's)	2 pieces (38 g)	150	**30**	18
Werther's				
Chocolates	10 pieces (40 g)	220	**120**	63
Original	3 pieces (15 g)	60	**10**	9

SWEETS

| FOOD | AMOUNT | CALORIES | | |
		TOTAL	FAT	SAT-FAT
Whitman's				
Bars				
Cookies 'N Cream	1 bar (28 g)	150	**80**	63
Sampler				
Assorted Chocolates	4 pieces (50 g)	250	**110**	63
Assorted Creams	3 pieces (40 g)	180	**70**	45
Dark Chocolates	3 pieces (40 g)	200	**90**	54
Truffles	3 pieces (40 g)	200	**100**	63
Whoppers	17 pieces (40 g)	180	**65**	63
Yogurt-covered				
Almonds	11 pieces (42 g)	210	**120**	63
Peanuts	17 pieces (41 g)	210	**120**	54
Pretzels	6 pieces (40 g)	150	**80**	72
Raisins (Harmony)	30 pieces (41 g)	180	**70**	54
York Peppermint Patties	3 patties (41 g)	160	**25**	18
COOKIES AND BARS BY BRAND NAME				
Assorted, no brand name				
Biscotti	1 (30 g)	270	**20**	5
Chocolate-Covered Pretzels	8 pieces (30 g)	140	**45**	27
White Chocolate–Covered				
Pretzels	8 pieces (30 g)	140	**45**	27
Danish Butter Cookies	4 (30 g)	160	**45**	45
French Roulettes				
Chocolate	4 (45 g)	225	**155**	36
Cinnamon	4 (33 g)	190	**130**	18
Original	4 (33 g)	190	**130**	18
Mundel Bread	2 pieces (30 g)	130	**60**	9
Archway				
Chocolate Chip 'n Toffee	1 (28 g)	130	**60**	18
Frosty Lemon	1 (26 g)	110	**40**	14
Gingersnaps	5 (32 g)	150	**5**	14
Oatmeal	1 (25 g)	110	**35**	9
Apple-Filled	1 (25 g)	100	**30**	5
Date-Filled	1 (28 g)	100	**30**	5
Iced	1 (28 g)	120	**45**	14
Raisin	1 (26 g)	110	**30**	9
Ruth's Golden	1 (28 g)	120	**45**	9
Strawberry-Filled	1 (25 g)	100	**30**	14
Old-Fashioned Molasses	1 (26 g)	100	**25**	5
Old-Fashioned Windmill	1 (20 g)	90	**30**	5
Rocky Road	1 (28 g)	130	**50**	14
Delicious				
Animal Crackers	9 (28 g)	130	**45**	14
Applesauce Oatmeal	3 (306 g)	140	**40**	14
Assorted Sandwich	3 (30 g)	150	**50**	14

SWEETS

FOOD	AMOUNT	CALORIES		
		TOTAL	FAT	SAT-FAT
Delicious (cont.)				
Banana Ramas	2 (25 g)	120	40	18
Butterfinger	3 (28 g)	130	50	23
Butter Thins	10 (29 g)	110	45	18
Chocolate Chip	2 (28 g)	130	40	9
Chocolate Chip Thins	10 (29 g)	110	45	18
Coconut Bars	3 (28 g)	140	60	27
Duplex Sandwich	3 (30 g)	150	50	14
English Toffee Heath	3 (36 g)	170	80	36
Fig Bars, lowfat	2 (37 g)	130	27	5
Fruit Bars (all flavors)	2 (29 g)	90	0	0
Ginger Snaps	4 (29 g)	130	30	5
Graham				
Cinnamon	2 crackers (30 g)	130	30	5
Honey	2 crackers (30 g)	130	30	5
Jelly Tops	5 (28 g)	140	60	14
Land O Lakes Frosted Butter	2 (27 g)	120	50	36
Lemon Sandwich	3 (30 g)	150	50	14
Oatmeal	2 (28 g)	120	45	9
Iced	2 (28 g)	130	40	9
Shortbread Cookies	4 (29 g)	140	50	27
Skippy Peanut Butter	3 (28 g)	150	90	18
Strawberry Sandwich	3 (30 g)	150	50	14
Sugar	2 (28 g)	140	50	9
Sugar Wafers	4 (30 g)	140	54	27
Vanilla Sandwich	3 (30 g)	150	50	14
Vanilla Wafers	8 (28 g)	130	40	9
Entenmann's				
Chocolate Chip	4 (28 g)	130	60	18
Chocolate Chip & Pecans	4 (28 g)	140	70	18
Chocolate Chunk	1 (16 g)	80	35	14
Chocolate Sandwich	3 (33 g)	150	60	14
Oatmeal Macaroon	3 (33 g)	150	60	18
Oatmeal Raisin	4 (28 g)	130	45	9
Peanut Butter Chocolate Chunk	1 (16 g)	80	40	14
Vanilla Sandwich	3 (33 g)	160	60	14
Entenmann's Light Cookies				
Chocolatey Chip	2 (30 g)	120	35	14
Oatmeal Raisin	2 (30 g)	100	0	0
Entenmann's Soft Bake Cookies				
Chocolate Chip	1 (20 g)	100	45	18
Milk Chocolate Chip	1 (20 g)	100	45	18
Original Recipe Chocolate Chip	3 (30 g)	150	60	18
White Chocolate Macadamia				
Nut	1 (20 g)	100	50	18

SWEETS

FOOD	AMOUNT	TOTAL	FAT	SAT-FAT
			CALORIES	
Estee				
Chocolate Chip	4 (31 g)	150	60	18
Chocolate Sandwich	3 (34 g)	160	50	14
Creme Wafer				
all flavors	5 (33 g)	155	75	14
Original Sandwich	3 (34 g)	160	50	9
Peanut Butter Sandwich	3 (34 g)	160	60	14
Vanilla Sandwich	3 (34 g)	160	50	9
Famous Amos				
Chocolate Chip & Pecans	4 (28 g)	140	70	18
Chocolate Chip	4 (28 g)	130	60	18
Chocolate Chunk	1 (16 g)	80	35	14
Chocolate Sandwich	3 (33 g)	150	60	14
Oatmeal Macaroon	3 (33 g)	160	60	18
Oatmeal Raisin	4 (28 g)	130	45	9
Peanut Butter Chocolate Chunk	1 (16 g)	80	40	14
Vanilla Sandwich	3 (33 g)	160	60	14
Fifty 50				
Chocolate Chip	4 (32 g)	170	90	NA
Coconut	4 (32 g)	160	90	27
Duplex Sandwich	3 (36 g)	160	60	14
Hearty Oatmeal	4 (32 g)	140	50	14
Grandma's				
Fudge Chocolate Chip	1 (39 g)	170	60	18
Molasses	1 (39 g)	160	35	14
Keebler				
Animal				
Iced	1 (32 g)	150	45	9
Sprinkled	1 (32 g)	150	40	9
Chips Deluxe	1 (15 g)	80	40	14
with Peanut Butter	1 (16 g)	80	40	18
Chocolate Chewy	2 (28 g)	130	60	18
Chocolate Lover's	1 (17 g)	90	45	23
Coconut	2 (16 g)	80	45	18
Rainbow	1 (16 g)	80	35	18
Soft 'n Chewy	1 (16 g)	80	30	9
Classic Collection				
Chocolate Fudge Creme	1 (17 g)	80	30	9
French Vanilla Creme	1 (17 g)	80	30	9
Cookie Stix				
Butter Cookies	4 (27 g)	130	45	18
Chocolate Chip	4 (27 g)	130	45	14
Sugar Cookies	5 (27 g)	150	50	14
E. L. Fudge				
Butter-flavored Sandwich	2 (25 g)	120	50	9
Fudge Sandwich	2 (25 g)	120	50	9
Summer	2 (25 g)	120	50	9

SWEETS

FOOD	AMOUNT	CALORIES		
		TOTAL	FAT	SAT-FAT
Keebler (cont.)				
Fudge Shoppe				
Deluxe Grahams	3 (27 g)	140	60	41
Fudge Sticks	3 (29 g)	150	70	41
Fudge Stripes	3 (32 g)	160	70	41
reduced fat	3 (27 g)	130	40	18
Grasshopper	4 (30 g)	150	60	41
Grahams	1 (16 g)	80	45	9
reduced fat	1 (16 g)	80	30	5
Chocolate	8 (31 g)	130	35	9
Cinnamon Crisp	8 (31 g)	130	25	9
low-fat	8 (28 g)	110	10	5
Honey	8 (31 g)	140	40	9
low-fat	9 (28 g)	120	15	5
Sandies				
Pecan Shortbread	1 (16 g)	80	45	9
reduced fat	1 (16 g)	80	30	5
Simply Shortbread	1 (15 g)	80	40	18
Snackin' Grahams				
Cinnamon	21 (29 g)	130	25	9
Honey	33 (30 g)	130	25	9
Soft Batch Chocolate Chip	1 (16 g)	80	35	9
Vanilla Wafers	8 (31 g)	150	60	18
reduced fat	8 (31 g)	130	30	5
Little Debbie				
Figaroos				
low-fat	1 (43 g)	150	23	5
Fudge Rounds	1 cake (34 g)	140	50	14
Fudge Macaroons	1 (29 g)	140	70	36
Lemon Creme Wafers	1 (20 g)	100	45	9
Marshmallow Pies	1 (39 g)	160	50	27
Marshmallow Supremes	1 (32 g)	130	45	9
Muffin Loaves	1 (55 g)	220	90	14
Nutty Bars	2 (57 g)	310	160	27
Oatmeal Creme Pies	1 (38 g)	170	60	14
Oatmeal Lights	1 (38 g)	130	20	5
Peanut Butter Bars	2 (54 g)	270	140	27
Peanut Butter Naturals	1 wrap (44 g)	230	120	23
Star Crunch	1 (31 g)	140	50	14
Lu				
Fondant	4 (32 g)	170	80	72
Le Chocolatier	3 (28 g)	150	70	63
Le Pim's Orange	2 (25 g)	90	25	9
Le Truffé	4 (33 g)	170	80	63
Murray				
Assortment	5 (27 g)	130	60	14
Butter	8 (30 g)	130	40	9

SWEETS

FOOD	AMOUNT	CALORIES		
		TOTAL	FAT	SAT-FAT
Murray (cont.)				
Chocolate Chips	8 (30 g)	140	45	14
Ginger Snaps	5 (30 g)	140	40	9
Lemon Cremes	3 (28 g)	140	50	14
Sugar Wafers	5 (28 g)	150	70	18
Vanilla Cremes	3 (28 g)	140	50	14
Vanilla Wafers	8 (28 g)	120	25	9
Murray Sugar Free				
Chocolate Chip	3 (31 g)	140	60	27
Chocolate Sandwich	3 (28 g)	120	50	14
Shortbread	8 (28 g)	120	40	9
Nabisco				
Apple Newtons, fat-free	2 (29 g)	100	0	0
Barnum's Animal Crackers	12 (31 g)	140	35	5
Cameo Creme Sandwich	2 (28 g)	130	40	9
Chips Ahoy!	3 (32 g)	160	70	23
Chewy	3 (36 g)	170	70	23
Chunky	1 (16 g)	80	35	14
Munch Size	6 (32 g)	160	70	18
Reduced Fat	3 (31 g)	140	45	14
Snack Bars	1 (37 g)	150	45	18
Chocolate Teddy Grahams	24 (30 g)	140	40	9
Cinnamon Teddy Grahams	24 (30 g)	140	40	9
Cranberry Newtons, fat-free	2 (29 g)	100	0	0
Famous Chocolate Wafers	5 (32 g)	140	35	14
Fig Newtons	2 (31 g)	110	20	0
Fat-Free	2 (29 g)	100	0	0
Fudge Striped Shortbread	3 (32 g)	160	70	14
Ginger Snaps	4 (28 g)	120	25	5
Grahams	4 (28 g)	120	25	5
Honey Maid Grahams				
Chocolate	8 (28 g)	120	25	5
Cinnamon	8 (28 g)	120	20	0
Honey	8 (28 g)	120	25	0
Low-fat	8 (28 g)	110	15	0
Oatmeal Crunch	8 (28 g)	120	20	0
Lorna Doone Shortbread	4 (29 g)	140	60	9
Mallomars	2 (26 g)	120	45	23
Marshmallow Twirls	1 (30 g)	130	50	9
Mystic Mint Sandwich	1 (17 g)	90	40	9
Newtons Cobblers	1 (22 g)	70	0	0
Nilla Wafers	8 (32 g)	140	40	9
Nutter Butter				
Bites	10 (30 g)	150	60	9
Chocolate	2 (28 g)	130	45	9
Peanut Butter Sandwich	2 (28 g)	130	50	9
Peanut Creme Patties	5 (31 g)	160	80	14

SWEETS

| FOOD | AMOUNT | CALORIES | | |
		TOTAL	FAT	SAT-FAT
Nabisco (cont.)				
Oatmeal	1 (17 g)	80	**30**	5
Iced Oatmeal	1 (17 g)	80	**25**	0
Oreos				
Brownie Bars	1 (37 g)	150	**50**	14
Chocolate Sandwich	3 (33 g)	160	**60**	14
Double Stuf Chocolate				
Sandwich	2 (28 g)	140	**60**	14
Fudge Covered Oreos	1 (21 g)	110	**50**	14
Raspberry, fat-free	2 (29 g)	10	**0**	0
Reduced Fat	3 (32 g)	130	**30**	9
SnackWell's (*see* listing, page 367)				
Social Tea Biscuits	6 (28 g)	120	**30**	5
Vanilla Sandwich	3 (35 g)	160	**45**	9
Pepperidge Farm				
Bordeaux	4 (28 g)	130	**50**	23
Brussels	3 (30 g)	150	**60**	27
Chessmen	3 (26 g)	120	**70**	27
Chocolate Chip Blondie (fat-free)	1 blondie (40 g)	120	**0**	0
Chocolate Chunk Classic Cookies				
Chesapeake	1 (26 g)	140	**70**	23
Chocolate Chunk Pecan	1 (26 g)	140	**70**	23
Milk Chocolate				
Macadamia	1 (26 g)	130	**60**	23
Montauk Milk Chocolate				
Chunk	1 (26 g)	130	**60**	23
Nantucket Chocolate Chunk	1 (26 g)	140	**60**	23
Sausalito Milk Chocolate				
Macadamia Chocolate				
Chunk	1 (26 g)	140	**70**	23
Tahoe White Chocolate				
Macadamia Chocolate				
Chunk	1 (26 g)	140	**70**	27
Chocolate Laced Pirouettes	5 (33 g)	180	**90**	23
Fruitful				
Apricot Raspberry Cup	3 (32 g)	140	**50**	18
Raspberry Tart	2 (30 g)	120	**25**	9
Strawberry Cup	3 (32 g)	140	**50**	18
Fudge Dipped Brownie				
(reduced fat)	1 (48 g)	190	**40**	9
Fudge Striped Chocolate				
Chunk Cookies	1 (18 g)	80	**20**	14
Geneva	3 (31 g)	160	**80**	32
Lido	1 (17 g)	90	**45**	14
Milano	3 (34 g)	180	**90**	32
Double Chocolate	2 (27 g)	140	**70**	27
Endless Chocolate	3 (34 g)	180	**90**	45

SWEETS

FOOD	AMOUNT	CALORIES TOTAL	FAT	SAT-FAT
Pepperidge Farm (cont.)				
Milk Chocolate	3 (33 g)	170	**80**	32
Mint	2 (25 g)	130	**70**	32
Orange	2 (25 g)	130	**70**	32
Old-Fashioned				
Chocolate Chip	3 (28 g)	140	**60**	23
Ginger Man	4 (28 g)	130	**35**	9
Hazelnut	3 (32 g)	160	**70**	18
Lemon-Nut Crunch	3 (31 g)	170	**80**	18
Shortbread	2 (26 g)	140	**70**	23
Sugar	3 (30 g)	140	**60**	14
Santa Fe Oatmeal Raisin	1 (26 g)	120	**45**	9
Soft Baked				
Chocolate Chunk	1 (26 g)	130	**60**	23
reduced fat	1 (26 g)	110	**35**	18
Milk Chocolate Macadamia	1 (26 g)	130	**60**	23
Oatmeal Raisin	1 (26 g)	110	**40**	9
reduced fat	1 (26 g)	100	**25**	5
Rippin' Good				
Assorted Creme Wafers	3 (28 g)	140	**60**	14
Butter Thins	10 (29 g)	110	**45**	18
Chocolate Chip	3 (32 g)	150	**60**	18
Chocolate Chip Sandwich	2 (31 g)	150	**60**	18
Chocolate Chip Thins	10 (29 g)	110	**45**	18
Chocolate Sandwich	3 (34 g)	160	**60**	14
Coconut Bars	3 (26 g)	130	**50**	23
Cookie Jar Assortment	3 (33 g)	150	**60**	18
Duplex Sandwich	3 (34 g)	160	**50**	14
Ginger Snaps	5 (28 g)	130	**40**	9
Granola & Peanut Butter				
Sandwich	2 (31 g)	150	**50**	14
Iced Spice	3 (32 g)	130	**25**	5
Lemon Crisp	3 (32 g)	160	**70**	14
Lemon Sandwich	3 (34 g)	160	**50**	14
Macaroon Sandwich	2 (31 g)	150	**60**	23
Oatmeal	3 (32 g)	150	**50**	14
Iced	3 (36 g)	150	**40**	9
Striped	2 (28 g)	150	**70**	36
Peanut Butter Sandwich	2 (31 g)	150	**60**	14
Shortbread Cookies	4 (29 g)	140	**50**	27
Strawberry Sandwich	3 (34 g)	160	**50**	14
Striped Dainties	3 (28 g)	150	**70**	36
Sugar	3 (32 g)	150	**60**	14
Toffee 'n Creme Sandwich	2 (31 g)	150	**60**	14
Vanilla Sandwich	3 (34 g)	160	**50**	14
Vanilla Wafers	5 (28 g)	120	**35**	9

SWEETS

FOOD	AMOUNT	CALORIES TOTAL	FAT	SAT-FAT
SnackWell's (Nabisco)				
Caramel Delights	1 (18 g)	70	20	5
Chocolate Chip	13 (29 g)	130	35	14
Chocolate Sandwich	2 (26 g)	110	25	5
Creme Sandwich	2 (26 g)	110	25	5
Devil's Food	1 (16 g)	50	0	0
Double Chocolate Chip	13 (30 g)	130	35	14
Golden Devil's Food	1 (16 g)	50	0	0
Mint Creme	2 (25 g)	110	30	9
Oatmeal Raisin	2 (30 g)	120	30	5
Peanut Butter Chip	13 (29 g)	120	35	9
Stella D'oro				
Almond Toast Cookie	2 (29 g)	110	20	5
Anginetti Cookies	4 (31 g)	140	35	5
Anisette Sponge Cookies	2 (27 g)	90	10	0
Anisette Toast Cookies	3 (35 g)	130	10	0
Biscotti				
Chocolate Chunk	1 (22 g)	90	25	9
French Vanilla	1 (22 g)	90	20	5
Breakfast Treats Cookies	1 (23 g)	100	30	9
Lady Stella Cookie Assortment	3 (28 g)	130	45	14
Sunshine				
Ginger Snaps	7 (29 g)	130	40	9
Golden Fruit				
Cranberry Biscuits	1 (20 g)	80	20	0
Raisin Biscuits	1 (20 g)	80	15	5
Hydrox Chocolate Sandwich				
Cremes	3 (31 g)	150	60	18
Oatmeal, Country Style	2 (24 g)	120	45	9
Peanut Butter Sugar Wafers	4 (32 g)	170	80	18
Sugar Wafers	3 (26 g)	130	60	14
Vanilla Wafers	7 (31 g)	150	60	14
Vienna Fingers	2 (29 g)	140	50	14
reduced fat	2 (29 g)	130	40	9
Twix				
Chocolate Caramel	1 (29 g)	140	60	23
Weight Watchers				
Apple Raisin Bar	1 (21 g)	70	20	5
Chocolate Chip	2 (30 g)	140	45	18
Chocolate Sandwich	3 (31 g)	140	35	9
Oatmeal Raisin	2 (30 g)	120	15	0
Vanilla Sandwich	3 (31 g)	140	25	9
COOKIES AND BARS, MIXES				
Betty Crocker				
Chocolate Chip	3 tbsp mix (28 g)	120	30	14
	2 cookies	160	70	23

SWEETS

FOOD	AMOUNT	CALORIES		
		TOTAL	FAT	SAT-FAT
COOKIES AND BARS, MIXES (cont.)				
Double Chocolate Chunk	3 tbsp mix (28 g)	120	**25**	14
	2 cookies	150	**60**	18
Oatmeal Chocolate Chip	3 tbsp mix (28 g)	120	**30**	14
	2 cookies	160	**70**	18
Peanut Butter	3 tbsp mix (28 g)	120	**35**	5
	2 cookies	160	**70**	14
Sugar	3 tbsp mix (28 g)	120	**25**	9
	2 cookies	170	**70**	18
COOKIES, READY-TO-MAKE				
Pillsbury				
Chocolate Chip	28 g dough	130	**50**	23
reduced fat	28 g dough	110	**25**	14
with walnuts	28 g dough	140	**60**	18
Cookies with M&M's	28 g dough	130	**50**	18
Double Chocolate Chip &				
Chunk	28 g dough	130	**50**	18
Cookie mixes, refrigerated				
Nestlé Toll House				
Chocolate Chip	2 tbsp (32)	140	**50**	18
DANISH PASTRY				
Almond	1 (100 g)	420	**190**	41
Apple-Filled	1 (110 g)	350	**110**	36
Blueberry-Filled	1 (100 g)	360	**150**	27
Cheese	1 (110 g)	380	**170**	45
Cherry Cheese	1 (100 g)	360	**140**	45
Cherry-Filled	1 (100 g)	320	**100**	27
Coconut	1 (100 g)	400	**150**	45
Custard-Filled	1 (100 g)	350	**140**	36
Danish Ring				
Pecan	⅛ ring (57 g)	230	**100**	23
Walnut	⅛ ring (55 g)	240	**120**	23
Danish Twist (Entenmann's)				
Cinnamon	⅙ ring (61 g)	260	**130**	27
Raspberry	⅙ ring (53 g)	220	**100**	27
Lemon-Filled	1 (100 g)	350	**140**	31
Orange Danish (Pillsbury,				
ready-to-make)	1 (41 g)	140	**50**	NA
Pecan	1 (100 g)	400	**180**	41
DONUTS				
Bakery type				
Apple Raisin Rosebud	1 (55 g)	220	**90**	23
Blueberry Cake	1 (56 g)	250	**100**	23
Blueberry-Filled	1 (65 g)	250	**120**	27
Carrot Cake	1 (80 g)	340	**180**	45

SWEETS

| FOOD | AMOUNT | CALORIES | | |
		TOTAL	FAT	SAT-FAT
Bakery type (cont.)				
Cherry Cake	1 (56 g)	250	100	27
Chocolate Chip	1 (70 g)	310	140	41
Chocolate Creme-Filled	1 (65 g)	290	150	41
Chocolate-Iced Chocolate Cake	1 (65 g)	270	110	31
Chocolate-Iced Yellow Cake	1 (55 g)	230	90	27
Cinnamon Rosebud	1 (64 g)	260	110	36
Custard-Creme Filled	1 (65 g)	240	130	63
Glazed Yeast Raised	1 (55 g)	240	130	36
Honey Wheat	1 (80 g)	340	150	36
Lemon Custard–Filled	1 (65 g)	190	140	36
Old-Fashioned	1 (62 g)	270	140	36
Orange Glazed Cake	1 (65 g)	310	160	41
Sour Cream	1 (80 g)	340	160	36
Spicy Apple–Filled	1 (65 g)	250	130	36
Entenmann's				
Crumb-Topped Donuts	1 (60 g)	260	110	27
Devil's Food Crumb Donuts	1 (60 g)	250	120	36
Rich Frosted Donuts	1 (57 g)	280	170	54
Old-Fashioned Donuts	1 (62 g)	270	140	36
Sour Cream Donuts	1 (80 g)	340	160	36
Hostess				
Cinnamon Donettes	4 (61 g)	240	90	36
Frosted Donettes	3 (43 g)	200	110	63
Frosted Donuts	1 (47 g)	330	160	72
Plain Donuts	1 (47 g)	150	80	36
Powdered Donettes	3 (43 g)	180	70	27
Powdered Donuts	1 (47 g)	230	160	72
Krispy Kreme				
Enrobed Knibbles	5 pieces (54 g)	270	150	72
Glazed Donuts	1 (52 g)	200	100	27
Glazed Knibbles	3 pieces (49 g)	220	120	27
Mini Crullers	3 (56 g)	230	90	27
Powdered Sugar Knibbles	3 pieces (48 g)	220	120	36
Little Debbie				
Donut Sticks	1 (47 g)	220	110	42
TastyKake				
Cinnamon Donut	1 (48 g)	190	90	14
Donut Holes				
Chocolate glazed	5 (54 g)	230	130	23
Glazed	3 (39 g)	190	100	23
Orange glazed	5 (54 g)	230	130	18
Sweet Sprinkles	4 (56 g)	250	120	27
Plain Donut	1 (41 g)	160	80	14
Powdered Sugar	1 (48 g)	190	80	14
Rich Frosted Donut	1 (58 g)	250	130	54

SWEETS

| FOOD | AMOUNT | CALORIES | | |
		TOTAL	FAT	SAT-FAT
DUMPLINGS, TURNOVERS, AND STRUDEL				
Apple Dumpling (Pepperidge Farm)	1 dumpling (85 g)	290	**99**	23
Apple-Filled Pastry	1 pastry (64 g)	190	**45**	9
Apple Fritter	1 fritter (70 g)	300	**130**	32
Apple Strudel	1 piece (64 g)	200	**90**	27
Apple Turnover (Pepperidge Farm)	1 turnover (89 g)	330	**130**	27
Apricot-Filled pastry	1 roll (64 g)	200	**50**	9
Apricot Strudel	1 piece (64 g)	220	**100**	27
Custard-Filled Pastry	1 (64 g)	190	**40**	9
Peach Dumpling (Pepperidge Farm)	1 dumpling (85 g)	320	**99**	23
Toaster Strudel				
Pillsbury (all flavors)	1 (54 g)	180	**60**	14
FROZEN DESSERTS				
Frozen custard				
Kohr Brothers				
Light, Vanilla & Chocolate	4 fl oz	130	**50**	36
FROZEN NOVELTIES				
Ben & Jerry's Peace Pops				
Cookie Dough	1 (108 g)	420	**230**	126
Dole Juice Bars				
Fruit 'n Juice, all flavors	1	70	**0**	0
Fruit Juice Bar, all flavors	1	45	**0**	0
Dove Bars				
Dark Chocolate Chocolate	1 bar (79 g)	260	**150**	90
French Vanilla Bite-Size	5 bars (92 g)	330	**190**	117
Milk Chocolate & Vanilla	1 bar (77 g)	260	**150**	99
Milk Chocolate with Almonds & Vanilla Ice Cream	1 bar (80 g)	280	**170**	99
Eskimo Pie				
Chocolate-coated Vanilla Ice Cream Bar	1 (49 g)	120	**70**	54
Vanilla Cone with no-sugar Choc & Peanut topping	1 (74 g)	210	**110**	72
Vanilla Ice Cream Sandwich, no sugar	1 (65 g)	160	**40**	18
Good Humor				
Chocolate Eclair	1 bar (59 g)	170	**70**	27
Dark & Milk Chocolate	1 bar (57 g)	180	**110**	72
Strawberry Shortcake	1 bar (59 g)	170	**70**	27
Toasted Almond	1 bar (88 mL)	180	**80**	36
Fudgsicle	1 (43 g)	60	**5**	5
fat-free	1 (43 g)	60	**0**	0

SWEETS

FOOD	AMOUNT	CALORIES		
		TOTAL	FAT	SAT-FAT
Good Humor (cont.)				
King Cone	1 (136 mL)	300	90	54
Original Ice Cream Bar	1 (89 mL)	190	90	72
Popsicle (Twister)	1 (52 mL)	45	0	0
Premium Sundae Cone	1 (136 mL)	290	120	63
Strawberry Shortcake	1 bar (88 mL)	160	70	27
Toasted Almond	1 bar (88 mL)	180	80	36
Häagen-Dazs Ice Cream Bars				
Cookies & Cream Crunch	1 (88 g)	320	200	117
Mint Dark Chocolate	1 (84 g)	290	180	108
Strawberry & White Chocolate	1 (80 g)	270	170	108
Vanilla & Almonds	1 (87 g)	320	210	108
Vanilla and Milk Chocolate	1 (100 g)	330	220	126
Klondike				
Almond	1 piece (96 g)	310	190	117
Big Bear Ice Cream Cookie Sandwich	1 (85 g)	290	110	72
Big Bear Vanilla Ice Cream Sandwich	1 (78 g)	200	60	27
Caramel Crunch	1 piece (96 g)	290	150	117
Choco Taco	1 bar (91 g)	310	150	90
Chocolate	1 piece (92 g)	280	170	117
Krispy Krunch	1 piece (96 g)	300	170	126
Neapolitan	1 piece (91 g)	280	170	126
Original	1 piece (93 g)	290	180	126
Reduced Fat, no sugar added	1 piece (78 g)	190	90	63
Vanilla (Original)	1 piece (93 g)	290	180	126
Milky Way				
Ice Cream Bar, Dark	1 (69 g)	220	120	81
Low-Fat Milk Shake	1 cup (237 mL)	220	30	NA
Mrs. Fields Cookie Ice Cream Sandwich	1 (116 g)	395	185	117
Nestlé				
Bon Bons	8 pieces (93 g)	350	230	144
Cool Creations				
Tiger Tails	1 pop (69 g)	60	0	0
Crunch				
reduced fat	1 bar (51 g)	150	80	54
Vanilla	1 bar (62 g)	200	130	99
Drumstick Sundae Cones				
Chocolate	1 (99 g)	320	150	90
Vanilla	1 (99 g)	340	170	99
reduced fat	1 (97 g)	300	130	45
Vanilla Caramel	1 (103 g)	360	180	117
Drumstick Supreme Cones				
Cappucccino	1 (89 g)	270	120	81

SWEETS

| FOOD | AMOUNT | CALORIES | | |
		TOTAL	FAT	SAT-FAT
Nestlé (cont.)				
Strawberry	1 (88 g)	230	**90**	54
Triple Chocolate	1 (89 g)	260	**120**	63
Snickers				
Ice Cream Bar	1 (52 g)	200	**110**	72
snack bar	1 (50 g)	180	**100**	54
Ice Cream Cone	1 (87 g)	290	**130**	72
Trix				
Pops	1 (53 g)	40	**0**	0
Tropicana Orange Cream Bar	1 (71 g)	80	**10**	5
Weight Watchers Smart Ones				
Chocolate Chip Cookie				
Dough Sundae	1 dessert (75 g)	190	**40**	18
Chocolate Mousse	1 dessert (77 g)	190	**45**	18
Chocolate Treat	1 bar (87 g)	100	**5**	0
Double Fudge Brownie Parfait	1 parfait (109 g)	190	**25**	18
Orange Vanilla Treat	2 bars (80 g)	70	**10**	5
Strawberry Parfait Royale	1 parfait (104 g)	180	**20**	9
Vanilla Sandwich	1 (65 g)	150	**25**	9

FROZEN YOGURT—FREEZER COMPARTMENT, GROCERY STORE

FOOD	AMOUNT	TOTAL	FAT	SAT-FAT
Ben & Jerry's Frozen Yogurt				
Cherry Garcia (low-fat)	½ cup	170	**30**	18
Chocolate Chip Cookie Dough	½ cup	210	**35**	23
Chocolate Fudge Brownie	½ cup	180	**20**	9
Coffee Almond Fudge	½ cup	180	**40**	9
Vanilla Heath Bar Crunch	½ cup	210	**50**	23
Breyers Frozen Yogurt				
Natural Vanilla	½ cup	120	**25**	14
Colombo Nonfat Shoppe-Style Frozen Yogurt				
chocolate flavors	½ cup	130	**0**	0
all other flavors	½ cup	110	**0**	0
Häagen-Dazs Frozen Yogurt				
Vanilla	½ cup	140	**0**	0
Vanilla Fudge	½ cup	160	**0**	0
Vanilla-Raspberry Swirl	½ cup	130	**0**	0
Fat-Free Frozen Yogurt				
Vanilla	½ cup	140	**0**	0
Vanilla-Raspberry Swirl	½ cup	140	**0**	0
Kemp's Frozen Yogurt				
Chocolate	½ cup	110	**25**	18
Fudge Marble	½ cup	110	**0**	0
Mint Fudge	½ cup	110	**0**	0
Strawberry	½ cup	90	**0**	0
Vanilla	½ cup	110	**25**	18
Safeway Select Fat Free Frozen Yogurt				
all flavors	½ cup	80–90	**0**	**0**

SWEETS

FOOD	AMOUNT	CALORIES		
		TOTAL	FAT	SAT-FAT
FROZEN YOGURT—YOGURT OR ICE CREAM SHOP				
Colombo *(These figures are for 1 fl oz. Ask the server for the number of ounces in your serving.)*				
Lite (nonfat)	1 fl oz	25	**0**	0
Low-fat	1 fl oz	28	**4**	2
Peanut butter low-fat	1 fl oz	30	**6**	1
ICBIY				
Nonfat	small (6¾ fl oz)	135	**0**	0
	medium (9⅓ fl oz)	187	**0**	0
	large (12 fl oz)	240	**0**	0
Original	small (6¾ fl oz)	182	**43**	NA
	medium (9⅓ fl oz)	251	**59**	NA
	large (12 fl oz)	324	**76**	NA
TCBY				
Nonfat	small (5 fl oz)	138	**0**	0
	medium (7 fl oz)	193	**0**	0
	large (9 fl oz)	248	**0**	0
Original	small (5 fl oz)	163	**38**	23
	medium (7 fl oz)	228	**53**	32
	large (9 fl oz)	293	**68**	41
ICE CREAM, BY BRAND NAMES				
Ben & Jerry's				
Ice Cream				
Butter Pecan	½ cup	310	**220**	99
Cherry Garcia	½ cup	240	**140**	90
Chocolate Chip Cookie Dough	½ cup	270	**150**	81
Chocolate Fudge Brownie	½ cup	260	**110**	63
Chubby Hubby	½ cup	350	**210**	99
Chunky Monkey	½ cup	280	**170**	90
Coffee with Heath Toffee Crunch	½ cup	280	**170**	90
Cool Britannia	½ cup	260	**140**	90
New York Super Fudge Chunk	½ cup	290	**190**	99
Peanut Butter & Jelly	½ cup	280	**150**	81
Wavy Gravy	½ cup	330	**210**	99
Vanilla Caramel Fudge	½ cup	280	**150**	90
All Natural Ice Cream				
Chocolate Chip Cookie Dough	½ cup	300	**140**	90
Chocolate Fudge Brownie	½ cup	280	**130**	90
New York Super Fudge Chunk	½ cup	320	**190**	108
Phish Food	½ cup	300	**120**	90
Totally Nuts	½ cup	310	**190**	99
Low-fat Ice Cream				
Blackberry Cobbler	½ cup	180	**30**	18

SWEETS

FOOD	AMOUNT	CALORIES		
		TOTAL	FAT	SAT-FAT
Ben & Jerry's (cont.)				
Blond Brownie Sundae	½ cup	190	25	14
Coconut Cream Pie	½ cup	160	25	14
S'mores	½ cup	190	20	9
Sweet Cream & Cookies	½ cup	170	25	18
Vanilla & Chocolate Mint				
Patty	½ cup	180	25	18
Breyers				
Ice Cream				
Butter Pecan	½ cup	180	110	54
Cherry Vanilla	½ cup	150	70	45
Chocolate	½ cup	160	80	54
Chocolate Chip	½ cup	170	90	63
Chocolate Chip Dough	½ cup	180	90	54
Coffee	½ cup	150	80	54
French Vanilla	½ cup	160	90	54
Mint Chocolate Chip	½ cup	170	90	63
Peanut Butter & Fudge				
Swirls	½ cup	180	80	41
Strawberry	½ cup	130	60	41
Vanilla	½ cup	150	80	54
Viennetta				
Cappuccino & Vanilla	1 slice (68 g)	190	100	63
Chocolate	1 slice (68 g)	190	100	72
Vanilla	1 slice (68 g)	190	100	63
Edy's				
Grand Ice Cream				
Butter Pecan	½ cup	160	90	45
Cherry Chocolate Chip	½ cup	150	70	45
Chocolate Chip Dough	½ cup	170	80	45
Cookie Jar	½ cup	180	80	54
Double Fudge Brownie	½ cup	170	80	45
French Vanilla	½ cup	160	90	45
Rocky Road	½ cup	170	90	45
Vanilla Bean	½ cup	140	70	45
Ice Cream				
Baby Ruth Baseball Sundae	½ cup	170	70	45
Girl Scouts Thin Mint	½ cup	170	90	54
Godzilla Vanilla	½ cup	160	70	45
Homemade Ice Cream				
Banana Cream Pie	½ cup	130	50	27
Vanilla	½ cup	140	60	36
Light Ice Cream				
Almond Praline	½ cup	110	35	18
Cheesecake Chunk	½ cup	120	45	27

SWEETS

FOOD	AMOUNT	CALORIES		
		TOTAL	FAT	SAT-FAT
Edy's (cont.)				
Chiquita 'n Chocolate	½ cup	110	45	23
Chocolate Fudge Mousse	½ cup	110	25	18
French Silk	½ cup	120	35	23
Rocky Road	½ cup	120	40	23
Vanilla	½ cup	100	25	18
Häagen-Dazs				
Ice Cream				
Butter Pecan	½ cup	310	210	99
Chocolate	½ cup	270	160	99
Coffee	½ cup	270	160	99
Dulce de Leche Caramel	½ cup	290	150	90
Macadamia Brittle	½ cup	300	180	99
Rum Raisin	½ cup	270	160	90
Strawberry	½ cup	250	150	90
Vanilla	½ cup	270	160	99
Vanilla Swiss Almond	½ cup	310	190	99
Low-fat Ice Cream				
Chocolate	½ cup	170	25	14
Strawberry	½ cup	150	20	9
Vanilla	½ cup	170	25	14
Healthy Choice Low-Fat Ice Cream				
Cappuccino Chocolate Chunk	½ cup	120	20	9
Chocolate Chunk	½ cup	120	20	9
Fudge Brownie	½ cup	120	20	9
Praline & Caramel	½ cup	130	20	5
Rocky Road	½ cup	140	20	9
Vanilla	½ cup	100	20	9
Lucerne Ice Cream				
Almond & Caramel	½ cup	170	90	45
Cappuccino Chip	½ cup	150	70	45
Cherry Blossom	½ cup	140	70	45
Chocolate	½ cup	140	80	45
Chocolate Chip	½ cup	150	80	45
Chocolate Marble	½ cup	140	60	36
Coffee	½ cup	140	70	45
French Vanilla	½ cup	150	70	45
Golden Nut Sundae	½ cup	160	70	45
Mint Chocolate Chip	½ cup	150	80	45
Neapolitan	½ cup	140	70	14
Rocky Road	½ cup	160	80	45
Swiss Chocolate Cherry	½ cup	140	60	36
Tin Roof Sundae	½ cup	160	70	45
Lucerne Low-fat Ice Cream				
Neapolitan	½ cup	100	20	14

SWEETS

| FOOD | AMOUNT | CALORIES | | |
		TOTAL	FAT	SAT-FAT
Newman's Own Ice Cream				
Milk Chocolate Mud Bath	½ cup	190	90	63
Obscene Vanilla Bean	½ cup	170	90	63
Pistol Packin' Praline Pecan	½ cup	200	100	63
Safeway Select				
Fat-Free Ice Cream				
all flavors	½ cup	70–90	0	0
Health Advantage Low-fat Ice Cream				
Coffee Latte Chocolate Swirl	½ cup	100	10	5
Cookies 'n Cream	½ cup	100	20	9
Rocky Road	½ cup	110	20	5
Vanilla	½ cup	90	15	9
Light Ice Cream				
Chocolate Chip Cookie				
Dough	½ cup	130	50	27
Cookies 'n Cream	½ cup	130	50	27
Rocky Road	½ cup	130	45	23
Vanilla	½ cup	120	40	27
Starbucks Coffee				
Biscotti Bliss	½ cup	260	120	63
Chocolate Chocolate Fudge	½ cup	290	150	72
Coffee Almond	½ cup	250	117	63
Coffee Almond Fudge	½ cup	260	120	63
Espresso Swirl	½ cup	220	90	54
Frappuccino	1 bar (80 g)	110	20	9
Italian Roast	½ cup	230	110	63
Java Chip	½ cup	250	117	63
Starbucks Low-fat Ice Cream				
Latte	½ cup	170	25	14
Mocha Mambo	½ cup	170	25	14
ICE CREAM CONES				
Cake Cone	1 (4.5 g)	20	0	0
Oreo Chocolate Cone	1 (13 g)	50	5	0
Sugar Cone	1 (13 g)	50	0	0
Waffle Cone	1 (20 g)	80	10	0
ICE CREAM TOPPINGS				
Hershey's				
Candy Bar Sprinkles	2 tbsp	140	45	27
Chocolate Chips	1 oz	140	72	45
Coconut	2 tbsp	58	37	33
Mrs. Richardson				
Hot Fudge	2 tbsp	140	60	54
Caramel	2 tbsp	130	0	0
Parlor Perfect				
Confetti Sprinkles	2 tbsp	110	20	5
Cookie 'n Nut Crunch	2 tbsp	80	30	9

SWEETS

FOOD	AMOUNT	TOTAL	CALORIES FAT	SAT-FAT
Parlor Perfect (cont.)				
Ice Cream Critters	2 tbsp	90	**15**	14
Praline Nut Crunch	2 tbsp	100	**40**	18
Shell Topping				
Chocolate	2 tbsp	210	**150**	72
Chocolate Fudge	2 tbsp	200	**120**	72
Heath	2 tbsp	230	**150**	63
Hershey's Krackel	2 tbsp	190	**130**	54
Reese's Chocolate & Peanut				
Butter	2 tbsp	220	**150**	72
Sundae Syrup				
all flavors	2 tbsp	110	**0**	0
Walnut	2 tbsp	170	**80**	9
Syrup				
Chocolate	2 tbsp	100	**0**	0
Smuckers				
Butterscotch, Caramel	2 tbsp	130	**0**	0
Dove Dark Chocolate	2 tbsp	140	**45**	14
Dove Milk Chocolate	2 tbsp	130	**35**	14
Fruit, all flavors	2 tbsp	90–110	**0**	0
Hot Fudge	2 tbsp	140	**35**	9
Fat-Free	2 tbsp	90	**0**	0
SHERBET				
Safeway Select Sherbet				
all flavors	½ cup	120	**15**	9
SORBET				
Ben & Jerry's				
Devil's Food Chocolate	½ cup	160	**15**	9
Doonesberry	½ cup	130	**0**	0
Lemon Swirl	½ cup	120	**0**	0
Purple Passion Fruit	½ cup	120	**0**	0
Edy's Whole Fruit				
all flavors	½ cup	140	**0**	0
Häagen-Dazs				
all flavors	½ cup	120	**0**	0
Chocolate	2 tbsp	100	**0**	0
MUFFINS, BAKERY				
Almond Poppy Seed	1 (127 g)	320	**120**	23
Apple Walnut	1 (127 g)	320	**120**	23
Banana Walnut	1 (113 g)	440	**200**	31
Banana Walnut (Hostess)	3 minis (34 g)	160	**80**	9
Blueberry	1 (127 g)	290	**90**	23
Blueberry (Entenmann's)	1 (57 g)	120	**0**	0
Blueberry (Hostess)	3 minis (34 g)	150	**70**	9
Blueberry (Sara Lee)	1 (64 g)	220	**100**	18
Blueberry (Weight Watchers)	1 (71 g)	160	**0**	0

SWEETS

FOOD	AMOUNT	CALORIES		
		TOTAL	FAT	SAT-FAT
MUFFINS, BAKERY (cont.)				
Bran	1 (127 g)	320	**90**	18
Chocolate Chocolate Chip				
(Weight Watchers)	1 (71 g)	190	**20**	9
Cinnamon Apple (Hostess)	3 minis (34 g)	160	**80**	14
Corn	1 (127 g)	330	**90**	23
Corn (Sara Lee)	1 (64 g)	260	**130**	27
Country Corn Muffin	1 (113 g)	420	**210**	31
Lemon-Flavored Poppyseed	1 (113 g)	450	**180**	27
Oat Bran	1 (127 g)	330	**100**	31
Strawberry	1 (127 g)	300	**90**	23
Low-fat Muffins				
Blueberry (Entenmann's)	1 (57 g)	120	**0**	0
Muffin Tops				
Blueberry	1 (113 g)	260	**80**	18
Bran	1 (113 g)	270	**70**	18
Corn	1 (113 g)	290	**80**	18
MUFFINS (MIXES BY BRAND NAME)				
Betty Crocker				
Banana Nut	3 tbsp mix (37 g)	140	**25**	5
	1 muffin prepared	170	**50**	10
Double Chocolate	¼ cup mix (43 g)	190	**60**	27
	1 muffin prepared	200	**70**	27
Lemon Poppy Seed	¼ cup mix (37 g)	150	**15**	5
	1 muffin prepared	190	**60**	15
Twice the Blueberries (low-fat)	¼ cup mix (39 g)	120	**15**	5
	1 muffin prepared	140	**35**	10
Wild Blueberry	¼ cup mix (40 g)	140	**15**	5
	1 muffin prepared	170	**50**	13
Betty Crocker Corn Bread or				
Muffin Mix	⅙ pkg (31 g mix)	110	**10**	0
	1 muffin prepared	160	**50**	14
Betty Crocker Sweet Rewards Fat-Free Muffin Mix				
Wild Blueberry	3 tbsp mix (36 g)	120	**0**	0
	1 muffin prepared	120	**0**	0
Duncan Hines Muffin Mix				
Chocolate Chip	¼ cup mix (42 g)	180	**70**	27
	1 muffin prepared	190	**70**	27
Cranberry Orange	¼ cup mix (34 g)	150	**40**	9
	1 muffin prepared	150	**45**	9
Jiffy Muffin Mix				
Blueberry	¼ cup mix (38 g)	160	**45**	18
	1 muffin prepared	190	**60**	27
Corn	¼ cup mix (38 g)	160	**35**	14
	1 muffin prepared	180	**50**	14
Raspberry	¼ cup mix (38 g)	170	**60**	23
	1 muffin prepared	180	**70**	25

SWEETS

| FOOD | AMOUNT | CALORIES | | |
		TOTAL	FAT	SAT-FAT
Mrs. Crutchfield's Fat-Free Muffin Mix				
All flavors	¼ cup mix (40 g)	150	0	0
Raga Muffin Mix				
Blueberry	¼ cup mix (40 g)	160	40	18
	1 muffin prepared	170	50	20
All other flavors	¼ cup mix (40 g)	160	40	18
	1 muffin prepared	170	40	18
PIES—BAKERY, HOMEMADE, OR RESTAURANT				
Apple	⅙ pie (104 g)	280	120	36
Boston Cream Pie	1/12 pie	370	153	83
Cherry	⅙ pie (104 g)	310	120	32
Cherry Beehive Pie				
(Entenmann's)	⅕ pie (130 g)	270	0	0
Coconut Custard	¼ pie (139 g)	410	200	81
Dutch Apple	⅙ pie (104 g)	290	110	27
Key Lime	⅛ pie (113 g)	390	150	54
Meringues				
Chocolate	3" wedge (130 g)	320	110	27
Coconut	3" wedge (130 g)	340	130	36
Lemon	⅙ pie (113 g)	290	120	36
Peach	⅙ pie (104 g)	300	100	23
Pecan	⅙ pie (113 g)	440	200	45
Pumpkin	⅙ pie (109 g)	290	100	31
Sweet Potato Pie	⅙ pie (104 g)	270	80	23
SNACK PIES, BY BRAND NAME				
Hostess Fruit Pies				
Apple	1 pie (128 g)	480	200	81
Blueberry	1 pie (128 g)	480	190	90
Cherry	1 pie (128 g)	470	200	99
Lemon	1 pie (128 g)	500	220	99
Tastykake				
Apple Pie	1 pie (113 g)	270	100	9
Blueberry Pie	1 pie (113 g)	320	100	23
Cherry Pie	1 pie (113 g)	290	100	9
Coconut Creme Pie	1 pie (113 g)	370	190	36
French Apple Pie	1 pie (120 g)	360	110	27
Lemon Pie	1 pie (113 g)	300	120	14
Peach Pie	1 pie (113 g)	300	100	22
Strawberry Pie	1 pie (106 g)	310	100	27
Tasty-Klair Pie	1 pie (113 g)	410	180	45
PIES, FROZEN				
Marie Callender's				
Apple Cobbler	¼ cobbler (120 g)	350	160	36
Berry Cobbler	¼ cobbler (120 g)	390	170	45
Peach Cobbler	¼ cobbler (120 g)	370	160	27

SWEETS

FOOD	AMOUNT	CALORIES		
		TOTAL	FAT	SAT-FAT
Mrs. Smith's				
Blackberry Cobbler	⅛ cobbler (113 g)	250	**80**	36
Oven Bake & Serve Pie				
Apple	⅛ pie (131 g)	310	**130**	23
reduced fat	⅙ pie (123 g)	210	**70**	14
Cherry	⅛ pie (131 g)	310	**120**	23
Coconut Custard	⅕ pie (142 g)	280	**110**	45
Dutch Apple Crumb	⅛ pie (131 g)	350	**130**	27
Hearty Pumpkin	⅛ pie (131 g)	240	**70**	14
Pumpkin Custard	⅛ pie (131 g)	230	**70**	18
Restaurant Classics				
Cookies & Cream	⅑ pie (120 g)	390	**180**	117
French Silk Chocolate	⅑ pie (126 g)	560	**360**	216
Key Lime, Authentic	⅑ pie (123 g)	420	**170**	108
Special Recipe				
Deep Dish Apple	⅒ pie (139 g)	370	**150**	27
Deep Dish Cherry	⅒ pie (139 g)	340	**120**	23
Deep Dish Cherry-Berry	⅒ pie (139 g)	360	**140**	27
Deep Dish Peach	⅒ pie (139 g)	330	**120**	23
Thaw-and-Serve Pie				
Banana Cream	¼ pie (108 g)	290	**130**	36
Boston Cream	⅛ pie (69 g)	180	**60**	18
Chocolate Cream	¼ pie (108 g)	330	**150**	36
Coconut Cream	¼ pie (114 g)	340	**170**	45
Lemon Cream	¼ pie (108 g)	300	**140**	36
Sara Lee				
Apple	⅛ pie (131 g)	340	**140**	32
Chocolate Cream	¼ pie (108 g)	330	**150**	36
Coconut Cream	⅕ pie (136 g)	480	**280**	NA
Lemon Meringue	⅙ pie (142 g)	350	**100**	23
PIE CRUSTS				
Graham cracker crumbs	3 tbsp (18 g)	80	**18**	5
Graham Cracker (Keebler				
Ready Crust)	⅛ 9" crust (21 g)	110	**45**	9
reduced fat	⅛ 9" crust (21 g)	100	**30**	9
2 Extra Servings	⅒ 10" crust	130	**60**	14
Hershey's Chocolate (Keebler				
Ready)	⅛ 9" crust (21 g)	110	**45**	9
Oreo (Nabisco)	⅙ 9" crust	140	**60**	14
2 Regular 9" Crusts				
Bel-Air	⅛ 9" crust (18 g)	80	**45**	23
Mrs. Smith's	⅛ 9" crust (18 g)	80	**45**	9
2 Deep-Dish 9" Crusts				
Bel-Air	⅛ 9" crust (21 g)	100	**60**	32
Mrs. Smith's	⅛ 9" crust (25 g)	110	**60**	14

SWEETS

FOOD	AMOUNT	CALORIES		
		TOTAL	FAT	SAT-FAT
PUDDINGS—REFRIGERATOR CASE OR SHELF				
Banana				
Kozy Shack	4 oz (113 g)	130	30	18
Butterscotch				
Hunt's Snack Pack	3.5 oz (99 g)	130	40	9
Swiss Miss	3.5 oz (99 g)	130	45	9
Cheesecake (Jell-O)				
Blueberry	3.5 oz (99 g)	140	40	23
Strawberry	3.5 oz (99 g)	150	40	23
Chocolate				
Hunt's Snack Pack	3.5 oz (99 g)	140	50	14
fat-free	3.5 oz (99 g)	90	0	0
Jell-O	4 oz (113 g)	160	45	18
fat-free	4 oz (113 g)	100	0	0
Kozy Shack	4 oz (113 g)	140	30	18
Kraft Handi-Snacks	3.5 oz (99 g)	130	45	14
fat-free	3.5 oz (99 g)	90	0	0
Swiss Miss	3.5 oz (99 g)	150	60	14
Chocolate/Vanilla Swirls (Jell-O)	4 oz (113 g)	160	45	18
fat-free	1 snack (113 g)	100	0	0
Double Chocolate Fudge				
Healthy Choice	3.5 oz (99 g)	110	20	5
Flan				
Kozy Shack	4 oz (113 g)	150	35	18
French Vanilla				
Healthy Choice	3.5 oz (99 g)	110	20	5
Rice				
Kozy Shack	4 oz (113 g)	130	30	18
Tapioca				
Hunt's Snack Pack	3.5 oz (99 g)	130	35	14
Swiss Miss	4 oz (113 g)	140	30	18
fat-free	3.5 oz (99 g)	90	0	0
Vanilla				
Hunt's Snack Pack	3.5 oz (99 g)	130	45	14
fat-free	3.5 oz (99 g)	80	0	0
Kozy Shack	6 oz (170 g)	195	45	27
Kraft Handi-Snacks	3.5 oz (99 g)	140	40	14
Swiss Miss	3.5 oz (99 g)	140	45	9
PUDDINGS—RESTAURANT				
Caramel Bavarian Cream	½ cup	246	128	73
Chocolate Mousse	½ cup	324	199	115
Creme Caramel	1 cup	303	125	27
Custard, baked	1 cup	305	125	61

SWEETS

FOOD	AMOUNT	CALORIES		
		TOTAL	FAT	SAT-FAT
SPREADS				
Nutella	2 tbsp	160	**80**	9
Milky Way				
Chocolate & Hazelnut	2 tbsp	170	**90**	27
SUGARS, SYRUPS, ETC.				
Honey	1 tbsp	65	**0**	0
Jams, Jellies, and Preserves	1 tbsp	55	**0**	0
Molasses	1 tbsp	43	**0**	0
Sugar				
Brown, firmly packed	1 tbsp	51	**0**	0
	½ cup	410	**0**	0
White				
Granulated	1 tsp	16	**0**	0
	½ cup	385	**0**	0
Powdered, sifted	1 cup	385	**0**	0
Syrups (*see also* **ICE CREAM TOPPINGS**)				
Chocolate-flavored (Hershey's)	2 tbsp	100	**0**	0
Corn	1 tbsp	61	**0**	0
Maple	1 tbsp	61	**0**	0
MISCELLANEOUS SWEETS				
Apple Fritter	1 (70 g)	300	**130**	31
Apple Tart (French)	⅛ tart	265	**100**	65
Baklava (Apollo)	4½ pieces (125 g)	540	**280**	45
Baklava	1 piece (28 g)	140	**72**	0
Carob Chips	1 oz (2⅔ tbsp)	140	**63**	52
Chocolate				
Baking, unsweetened	1 oz	145	**135**	81
Chocolate Chips	1 oz	140	**72**	45
semi-sweet	30 chips (15 g)	70	**35**	23
Mini Baking Bits (M&M's)	1 tbsp (14 g)	70	**35**	18
Hershey's				
Milk chocolate chips	1 tbsp (15 g)	80	**40**	23
Reduced-fat baking chips	1 tbsp (16 g)	60	**20**	31
Reese's Peanut Butter Chips	1 tbsp (15 g)	80	**35**	36
Nestlé				
Milk chocolate morsels	1 tbsp (14 g)	70	**40**	23
Chocolate Eclairs	1 (57 g)	220	**110**	90
Custard cream puffs	1	303	**163**	63
Escalloped Apples (Stouffer's)	⅔ cup (158 g)	180	**25**	0
Gelatin dessert	½ cup	70	**0**	0
Jell-O, all flavors	½ cup	90	**0**	0
Madeleines	1	90	**50**	30
Puff Pastry, frozen (Pepperidge Farm)				
Sheets	⅙ sheet (41 g)	200	**100**	23
Shells	1 shell (47 g)	230	**130**	27
Tiramisu	2" × 2" piece	395	**220**	130

VEGETABLES AND VEGETABLE PRODUCTS

FOOD	AMOUNT	CALORIES		
		TOTAL	FAT	SAT-FAT
See also **FROZEN, MICROWAVE, AND REFRIGERATED FOODS.**				
Alfalfa seeds, sprouted, fresh	1 cup	10	**0**	0
Artichoke				
fresh	1 medium	65	**0**	0
	1 large	83	**0**	0
cooked	1 medium	53	**0**	0
hearts				
canned in water	½ cup	35	**0**	0
marinated, undrained	½ cup	190	**135**	18
Asparagus				
fresh	½ cup	15	**0**	0
	4 spears	13	**0**	0
cooked	½ cup	22	**0**	0
	4 spears	15	**0**	0
Baked beans, canned				
Brown Sugar & Bacon				
(Campbell's)	½ cup	170	**25**	9
Plain or vegetarian	½ cup	117	**5**	2
in tomato sauce				
(Campbell's)	½ cup	130	**20**	9
Pork 'n Beans (Hanover)	½ cup	120	**15**	5
with beef	½ cup	160	**42**	20
with franks	½ cup	184	**76**	27
with pork	½ cup	134	**18**	7
and sweet sauce	½ cup	141	**17**	7
and tomato sauce	½ cup	124	**12**	5
Bamboo shoots				
fresh	1 cup	41	**0**	0
cooked	1 cup	15	**0**	0
canned	1 cup	25	**0**	0
Beans				
Black				
dry	1 cup	661	**25**	6
boiled	1 cup	227	**8**	2
Fermented Black	1 tbsp	35	**10**	0
Great Northern				
dry	1 cup	621	**19**	6
boiled	1 cup	210	**7**	2
canned	1 cup	300	**9**	3
Kidney				
dry	1 cup	613	**14**	2
boiled	1 cup	225	**8**	1
canned	1 cup	208	**7**	1
Kidney, California red				
dry	1 cup	607	**0**	0
boiled	1 cup	219	**0**	0

VEGETABLES AND VEGETABLE PRODUCTS

		CALORIES		
FOOD	AMOUNT	TOTAL	FAT	SAT-FAT
Beans (cont.)				
Kidney, Red				
dry	1 cup	619	**18**	3
boiled	1 cup	225	**8**	1
canned	1 cup	216	**8**	1
Kidney, Royal Red				
dry	1 cup	605	**7**	1
boiled	1 cup	218	**3**	0
Lima, Baby				
fresh	1 cup	216	**6**	1
boiled	1 cup	188	**5**	1
Lima, Large				
fresh	1 cup	176	**11**	3
boiled	1 cup	208	**6**	1
canned	1 cup	186	**4**	1
Navy				
dry	1 cup	697	**24**	6
boiled	1 cup	259	**9**	2
canned	1 cup	296	**10**	3
Pink				
dry	1 cup	721	**21**	6
boiled	1 cup	252	**7**	2
Pinto				
dry	1 cup	656	**20**	4
boiled	1 cup	235	**8**	2
canned	1 cup	186	**7**	1
Refried				
canned (Del Monte)	1 cup	260	**32**	10
Mexican restaurant	¾ cup	375	**146**	60
Snap (includes green, Italian, and yellow)				
fresh	1 cup	34	**0**	0
cooked	1 cup	44	**0**	0
canned	1 cup	36	**0**	0
Soy				
dry	1 cup	774	**334**	48
boiled	1 cup	298	**139**	20
Soy products				
Aka Miso	1 tbsp	30	**10**	0
Miso	1 cup	565	**150**	22
Shiro Miso	1 tbsp	30	**10**	0
Tofu	1 piece (2½ x 2¾ x 1")	88	**50**	7
White, small				
dry	1 cup	723	**23**	4
boiled	1 cup	253	**10**	1
Yellow				
fresh	1 cup	676	**46**	12
boiled	1 cup	254	**17**	4

VEGETABLES AND VEGETABLE PRODUCTS

		CALORIES		
FOOD	**AMOUNT**	**TOTAL**	**FAT**	**SAT-FAT**
Beets				
fresh	1 cup slices	60	0	0
	2 beets	71	0	0
cooked	1 cup slices	52	0	0
	2 beets	31	0	0
canned, drained	1 cup	54	0	0
Black-eyed or cowpeas, cooked	1 cup	190	0	0
Broadbeans				
fresh	1 cup	511	21	3
boiled	1 cup	186	6	1
canned	1 cup	183	5	0
Broccoli				
fresh	1 cup chopped	24	0	0
	1 spear	42	0	0
cooked	1 cup chopped	46	0	0
	1 spear	53	0	0
Brussels sprouts, cooked	1 cup	60	0	0
	1 sprout	8	0	0
Cabbage				
fresh	1 cup shredded	16	0	0
	1 head	215	0	0
cooked	1 cup shredded	32	0	0
	1 head	270	0	0
Cabbage, Chinese				
fresh	1 cup shredded	9	0	0
cooked	1 cup shredded	20	0	0
Cabbage, red				
fresh	1 cup shredded	19	0	0
cooked	1 cup shredded	32	0	0
Cabbage, Savoy				
fresh	1 cup shredded	19	0	0
cooked	1 cup shredded	35	0	0
Carob flour	1 tbsp	14	0	0
	1 cup	185	0	0
Carrots				
fresh	1	31	0	0
	1 cup shredded	48	0	0
cooked	1 cup sliced	70	0	0
Carrot juice	1 cup	98	0	0
Cauliflower, cooked or fresh	3 flowerets	13	0	0
	1 cup pieces	24	0	0
Celery, fresh	1 stalk	6	0	0
	1 cup diced	18	0	0
Chard, Swiss				
fresh	1 cup chopped	6	0	0
	1 lcaf	9	0	0
cooked	1 cup chopped	35	0	0

VEGETABLES AND VEGETABLE PRODUCTS

		CALORIES		
FOOD	AMOUNT	TOTAL	FAT	SAT-FAT
Chickpeas or garbanzos				
dry	1 cup	729	109	11
boiled	1 cup	269	38	4
canned	½ cup (120 g)	110	18	3
Chili with beans, canned	1 cup	286	126	54
Coleslaw (see also **FAST FOODS**)				
made with mayonnaise	1 cup	171	161	34
Collard greens, cooked	1 cup chopped	27	0	0
Corn				
Cooked	1 ear	70	7	1
	1 cup kernels	130	15	3
baby corn nuggets (Haddon House)	½ cup (132 g)	30	13	9
canned, cream style	1 cup	186	10	1
popcorn (see **SNACKS**)				
Cucumber, fresh	1 cucumber	39	0	0
	1 cup slices	14	0	0
Dandelion greens				
fresh	1 cup chopped	25	0	0
cooked	1 cup chopped	35	0	0
Eggplant				
fresh	1 eggplant	27	0	0
cooked	1 cup cubes	27	0	0
Endive, fresh	1 cup chopped	8	0	0
	1 head	86	0	0
Garlic, fresh	1 clove	4	0	0
Kale				
fresh	1 cup chopped	33	0	0
cooked	1 cup chopped	41	0	0
Kohlrabi				
fresh, diced	1 cup	41	0	0
cooked, drained	1 cup	40	0	0
Leeks				
fresh	1	76	0	0
	¼ cup chopped	16	0	0
cooked	1	38	0	0
	¼ cup chopped	8	0	0
Lentils				
dry	1 cup	649	17	2
boiled	1 cup	231	7	1
Lettuce, fresh				
butterhead, Boston	1 head (5-inch)	21	0	0
	1 outer or 2 inner leaves	2	0	0
crisphead, iceberg	1 head (6-inch)	70	0	0
	1 wedge (¼ head)	20	0	0
	1 cup chopped	5	0	0
loose leaf, romaine	1 cup chopped	10	0	0

VEGETABLES AND VEGETABLE PRODUCTS

		CALORIES		
FOOD	**AMOUNT**	**TOTAL**	**FAT**	**SAT-FAT**
Mushrooms				
fresh, sliced, chopped	1 cup, pieces	20	0	0
	1 lb	127	0	0
cooked	1 cup, pieces	42	0	0
canned	1 cup, pieces	38	0	0
Mushrooms, shiitake				
dried	4 mushrooms	44	0	0
cooked	4 mushrooms	40	0	0
	1 cup pieces	80	0	0
Mustard Greens	1 cup chopped	14	0	0
Okra				
fresh	8 pods	36	0	0
	1 cup slices	38	0	0
cooked	8 pods	27	0	0
	1 cup slices	50	0	0
Onions				
fresh	1 cup chopped	54	0	0
cooked	1 cup chopped	58	0	0
fried onion rings, frozen	7 rings	285	168	54
Onions, green, fresh	1 cup chopped	26	0	0
Parsley, fresh	10 sprigs	3	0	0
Parsnips				
fresh	1 cup slices	100	0	0
cooked	1 cup slices	126	0	0
Peas, green				
fresh	1 cup	118	4	0
cooked	1 cup	134	0	0
Peas, split				
fresh	1 cup	671	21	0
boiled	1 cup	231	7	0
Peas and carrots, canned	1 cup	96	6	0
Peas and onions, canned	1 cup	122	8	0
Peppers				
hot chili, fresh	1	18	0	0
	½ cup chopped	30	0	0
jalapeño	½ cup chopped	17	0	0
sweet, raw	1	18	0	0
	½ cup chopped	12	0	0
sweet, cooked	1	18	0	0
	½ cup chopped	12	0	0
Potatoes				
Au gratin	1 cup	320	167	104
Baked in skin	8 oz	145	0	0
	1 lb	325	0	0
	1 (2⅓ x 4¾ inch)	173	0	0

VEGETABLES AND VEGETABLE PRODUCTS

		CALORIES		
FOOD	AMOUNT	TOTAL	FAT	SAT-FAT
Potatoes (cont.)				
Boiled in skin	5 oz	104	0	0
	1 cup diced or sliced	118	0	0
	1 lb	345	0	0
Boiled, pared before cooking	8 oz	146	0	0
	5 oz	88	0	0
	1 cup diced or sliced	101	0	0
	1 lb	295	0	0
Raw, without skin	4 oz	88	0	0
Fried, Frozen (*see also* **FROZEN, MICROWAVE, AND REFRIGERATED FOODS**)				
French fries (*see also* **FAST FOODS**)				
Act II Microwave	1 box (88 g)	240	110	23
Frozen, other preparations				
Hash brown	½ cup	170	81	38
Mashed				
with whole milk	½ cup	81	6	3
with whole milk and butter	½ cup	111	40	22
Potato Chips (*see* **SNACK FOODS**)				
Potato Pancakes	1 pancake	495	113	31
Potato Salad	½ cup	180	92	16
Potato Sticks (*see* **SNACK FOODS**)				
Scalloped, from dry mix	1 cup	230	99	25
Pumpkin, cooked	1 cup mashed	49	0	0
Radishes, fresh	10	7	0	0
	½ cup slices	10	0	0
Sauerkraut, canned	1 cup	44	0	0
Shallots, fresh	1 tbsp chopped	7	0	0
Spinach				
fresh	1 cup chopped	6	0	0
	10 oz pkg	46	0	0
cooked	1 cup	41	0	0
Spinach souffle, made with whole milk, eggs, cheese, butter	1 cup	218	165	64
Squash				
acorn				
raw	1 cup cubes	56	0	0
	1 lb	180	0	0
cooked	1 cup cubes	115	0	0
butternut				
raw	1 cup cubes	63	0	0
	1 lb	203	0	0
cooked	1 cup cubes	83	0	0

VEGETABLES AND VEGETABLE PRODUCTS

		CALORIES		
FOOD	AMOUNT	TOTAL	FAT	SAT-FAT
Squash (cont.)				
spaghetti				
cooked	1 cup	45	0	0
Succotash, cooked	1 cup	222	14	1
Sweet potatoes				
raw with skin	1 lb	343	0	0
baked in skin	1 (5" long,			
	2" diameter)	118	0	0
	½ cup mashed	103	0	0
boiled without skin	1 cup mashed	344	0	0
Tomatoes				
fresh	1	24	0	0
	1 cup chopped	35	0	0
cooked	1 cup	60	0	0
canned in tomato juice	1 cup	67	0	0
crushed	½ cup	30	0	0
Tomato juice, canned	1 cup	42	0	0
Tomato products, canned				
Marinara sauce	1 cup	171	75	11
Paste	1 tbsp	14	0	0
Puree	1 cup	102	0	0
Sauce	1 cup	74	0	0
Spaghetti sauce (*see* **SAUCES, GRAVIES, AND DIPS**)				
Turnips, cooked	1 cup cubes	28	0	0
Vegetable juice cocktail, canned	1 cup	44	0	0
Water chestnuts, canned	1 cup slices	70	0	0
Watercress				
whole	1 cup (10 sprigs)	7	0	0
chopped fine	1 cup	24	0	0
Yam, cooked	1 cup cubes	158	0	0
Zucchini				
raw	1 cup slices	19	0	0
cooked	1 cup slices	28	0	0

MISCELLANEOUS

		CALORIES		
FOOD	AMOUNT	TOTAL	FAT	SAT-FAT
Baking powder	1 tbsp	5	0	0
Carob flour	1 tsp	14	0	0
Cocoa powder	1 tsp	5	0	0
Cocoa powder	1 tbsp	14	5	0
Curry powder	1 tsp	5	0	0

MISCELLANEOUS

FOOD	AMOUNT	CALORIES		
		TOTAL	FAT	SAT-FAT
Garlic powder	1 tsp	10	0	0
Gelatin, dry	1 envelope	25	0	0
Ketchup	1 tbsp	15	0	0
Mustard	1 tsp	5	0	0
Olives, green	4 medium	15	15	2
Olives, ripe	3 small or 2 large	15	15	3
Oregano	1 tsp	5	0	0
Paprika	1 tsp	5	0	0
Pickles				
dill	1 medium	5	0	0
sweet	1	20	0	0
gherkin	1	20	0	0
Vinegar	1 tbsp	0	0	0
Yeast, all types	1 tbsp	20	0	0

Food Tables Index

Appendixes
Glossary
References
Index
Order Forms

Appendix A
The Nitty-Gritty of
Keeping a Food Record

Learning from George's Food Record

Did we say that keeping a food record is essential for success?! Here is a detailed explanation of how to keep a food record using George's food intake. (George uses a handy *Choose to Lose* Passbook.)* Use his example to learn how to keep your own.

To Thine Own Self Be True

To be useful, your food records must be thorough and accurate. Mark down everything that you eat. Be exact. Your body records the exact amount even if you don't write it down. List each ingredient separately. For example, in a turkey sandwich, list bread, turkey, and mayo as separate entries. Make sure the amount is precisely what you ate.

Look up the fat calories right away so you know immediately how much fat you have eaten. Better still — look up the fat calories *before* you eat a food so you know the cost and can decide if you really want to eat it. Don't wait until the end of the day to record your intake. It's quicker to write down each item and the fat-calorie cost *when* you eat it because you are recording fewer items. It's more accurate because, if you wait, you'll forget what you don't want to remember. It's important that you keep a running subtotal so you know the impact of each food on your Fat Budget.

---

* See order form on the last page of this book.

Remember, food records are for you, so you need to be brutally honest. They allow you to see where you need to make changes. They allow you to save up for splurges.

Cool It

Don't have a nervous breakdown over your food records. Your first records may reflect less than a perfect diet. Do not feel guilty. It takes time to make changes. You're learning as you go. As the days and weeks progress and you ease into *Choose to Lose Weight-Loss Plan for Men,* eating a low-fat diet full of lots of nutrient-dense foods will be as natural as breathing.

GEORGE KEEPS HIS FOOD RECORD

Fat Budget: *416*	
Total Calorie Floor: *2080*	**Date:** *1/17/00* **Day:** (circle) S Ⓜ T W T F S

1. George enters his **Fat Budget** of 416. It serves to remind him of his fat-calorie ceiling.
2. He enters his **Total Calorie Floor** of 2080. He knows he must eat *more* than this number of total calories of nutritious foods.
3. He enters the **Date.** Looking back, he can see when the records were kept if he wants to see his progress.
4. He circles the **Day.** He can note patterns. Does he splurge too often on weekends?

Fat Budget: *416* Total Calorie Floor: *2080*			**Date:** *1/17/00* **Day:** (circle) S Ⓜ T W T F S				
Time	**Food**	**Amount**	**#svg F,V G,D or E**	**Total Calories**	**Total Cal Subtotal**	**Fat Calories**	**Fat Cal Subtotal**
8 A.M.	eggs	2		158	158	100	100

5. He enters the **Time: 8 A.M.** Recording the time helps him see his eating patterns. Is he ravenous at dinner because his previous meal was at 9:30 A.M.?

6. Under the heading **Food,** George enters **eggs.**
7. Under **Amount,** he enters **2.** He needs to be specific. One egg has 50 fat calories, but 2 have 100.
8. Because eggs are neither fruit, vegetables, grain, dairy, nor empty calories, George leaves "# svg" (number of servings) blank.
9. He enters **100** fat calories in the **Fat Calories** column for the 2 eggs (50 fat calories × 2). For his first entry, he repeats **100** in the **Fat Cal Subtotal** column.
10. He enters **158** in the **Total Calories** column for the 2 eggs (79 calories × 2). For his first entry, he repeats **158** in the **Total Cal Subtotal** column.

Fat Budget: 416							
Total Calorie Floor: 2080			Date: 1/17/00 Day: (circle) S ⓂT W T F S				
Time	Food	Amount	#svg F,V G,D or E	Total Calories	Total Cal Subtotal	Fat Calories	Fat Cal Subtotal
8 A.M.	eggs	2		158	158	100	100
	shortening	2 tsp		73		73	

11. The eggs were fried in shortening, so he next enters **shortening** under **Food** and **2 tsp** under **Amount.**
12. Because shortening is neither fruit, vegetables, grain, dairy, nor empty calories, George leaves "# svg" blank.
13. He enters **73** in the **Fat Calories** column and **73** in the **Total Calories** column.

Fat Budget: 416							
Total Calorie Floor: 2080			Date: 1/17/00 Day: (circle) S ⓂT W T F S				
Time	Food	Amount	#svg F,V G,D or E	Total Calories	Total Cal Subtotal	Fat Calories	Fat Cal Subtotal
8 A.M.	eggs	2		158	158	100	100
	shortening	2 tsp		73	231	73	173

14. He adds the 73 fat calories to the previous **Fat Cal Subtotal** of 100 and gets a new **Fat Cal Subtotal** of **173.** It is important that with

each food he eats (or considers eating) he sees the effect on his cumulative fat consumption.

15. He adds the 73 total calories to the previous **Total Cal Subtotal** of 158 and gets a new **Total Cal Subtotal** of **231.** It is important that he keep a running total of his total calories so he can see at a glance that his total calorie intake is sufficient. He will continue to enter each food, amount, fat and total calories, and subtotal fat and subtotal total calories as the day progresses.

Fruits (2-4): *0*		**Vegetables (3-5):** *1*		**Grains (6-11):** *2*	**Dairy: (2-3):** *0*		
Aerobic Exercise	Start	Stop	Minutes	Aerobic Exercise	Start	Stop	Minutes

16. At the end of the day George reviews his food records to see how he has met the minimum recommendations of the Food Guide Pyramid (as indicated by the numbers in parentheses). He ate no fruit, so he enters **0** for fruit. He enters **1** vegetable for his baked potato. He ate **2** slices of bread, so he enters **2** grains. He consumed no dairy, so he enters **0** dairy.

17. He did not exercise aerobically, so he leaves the aerobic exercise boxes blank.

Appendix B
Determining Fat Budgets
for Women

Table 1. Desirable Weights* for Women Age 25 and Over			
HEIGHT WITHOUT SHOES		FRAME	
FEET	INCHES	SMALL	MEDIUM	LARGE
4	8	92–98	96–107	104–119
4	9	94–101	98–110	106–122
4	10	96–104	101–113	109–125
4	11	99–107	104–116	112–128
5	0	102–110	107–119	115–131
5	1	105–113	110–122	118–134
5	2	108–116	113–126	121–138
5	3	111–119	116–130	125–142
5	4	114–123	120–135	129–146
5	5	118–127	124–139	133–150
5	6	122–131	128–143	137–154
5	7	126–135	132–147	141–158
5	8	130–140	136–151	145–163
5	9	134–144	140–155	149–168
5	10	138–148	144–159	153–173
5	11	142–152	148–163	157–177
6	0	146–156	152–167	161–181
6	1	150–160	156–171	165–185

Courtesy of Metropolitan Life Insurance Company, New York, 1959.
* Without clothing

Table 2. Minimum Total Caloric Intake and Fat Budget for Women Based on Goal Weight and Sex

GOAL WEIGHT	MINIMUM DAILY TOTAL CALORIC INTAKE	FAT BUDGET FAT CALORIES
90	1053	211
95	1111	222
100	1170	234
105	1228	246
110	1287	257
115	1345	269
120	1404	281
125	1462	292
130	1521	304
135	1579	315
140	1638	328
145	1696	339
150	1755	351
155	1813	363
160	1872	374
165	1930	386
170	1989	398
175	2047	409
180	2106	421
185	2164	433
190	2223	445
195	2281	456
200	2340	468

Glossary

Adipose tissue. Tissue in which fat is stored.

Aerobic exercise. Exercise that is steady and repetitive, uses the large muscles, and requires a steady supply of oxygen (in contrast to exercise that requires bursts of activity separated by periods of rest). Examples of aerobic exercise include walking, swimming, running, and biking. Aerobic exercise burns more fat than sports-type activities, which burn more carbohydrate.

Atherosclerosis. A group of diseases characterized by thickening and loss of elasticity of artery walls. This may be due to an accumulation of fibrous tissue, fatty substances (lipids, cholesterol), and/or minerals.

Basal metabolic rate (BMR). The rate at which energy is used when the body is completely at rest to maintain such vital functions as breathing, heart beat, digestion, etc.

Burning or oxidation. The chemical process of combining substances (carbohydrates, fats, proteins in foods) with oxygen, resulting in the release of stored energy.

Calorie. A unit of heat or energy produced by burning (oxidizing) nutrients. Carbohydrates and proteins contain 4 calories per gram, fats 9 calories per gram, and alcohol 7 calories per gram.

Carbohydrate. One of the three major energy-containing nutrients in foods; the others are protein and fat. Carbohydrates are simple (sugars) or complex (starches); each type contains 4 calories per gram.

Cerebrovascular diseases (CVD). Diseases, such as stroke, resulting from interruptions of blood supply to the brain.

Cholesterol. A fatlike substance found in the cell membranes of all animals, including humans. Cholesterol is transported in the bloodstream. Some of it is manufactured by the body, and some comes from the foods of animal origin that we eat. A healthy level of cholesterol for adults is below 200 mg/dL. A higher level is often associated with increased risk of heart disease.

Complex carbohydrate. One of the two major types of carbohydrates. They are found in whole-grain and cereal products and vegetables. In their natural state complex carbohydrates are accompanied by dietary fiber.

Coronary heart disease (CHD). Also known as coronary artery disease and ischemic heart disease. Heart ailments caused by a decreased supply of blood to the heart due to narrowing of the coronary arteries by cholesterol-rich plaque.

Diabetes. Also known as diabetes mellitus. A metabolic disease in which the body is unable to produce or use the hormone insulin to transport glucose from the blood to the cells. Thus, glucose remains in the blood and the body is starved for energy. There are two forms of diabetes: type 1 or juvenile diabetes and type 2 or adult-onset diabetes. Type 1 diabetes results from injury to the pancreas with the consequent inability to form insulin. Type 1 diabetes can occur at any age and requires administration of insulin. Type 2 diabetes, often the consequence of obesity, results in cells that are resistant to insulin.

Dietetic. A term used to describe a food that has been nutritionally altered in some way. "Dietetic" can mean less sodium, less fat, less sugar, or fewer calories. If a food is intended for weight loss, it must meet requirements for "low-calorie" or "reduced-calorie" claims. If not for weight loss, the label must state its special dietary purpose.

Energy. Power to do work. In foods, energy is measured in calories. A "high-energy" food is a high-calorie food. Energy expenditure, as in exercise, is quantified in terms of calories expended or burned.

Fat. One of the three major energy-containing nutrients in foods; the others are carbohydrates and proteins. Fat is an oily substance that is found in many foods, especially oils, dairy products, and meat products. Fat is the major form of storing energy in the body. Fat stores in the adipose tissue total 140,000 calories or more. Fat contains 9 calories per gram.

Fat Budget. The maximum number of calories from ingested fat that are allowed per day on *Choose to Lose Weight-Loss Plan for Men* to reach and maintain ideal weight. Fat Budget is based on 20 percent of BMR.

Fattening. A term that is commonly used to describe any substance that contributes to making a person fat. Many foods (often starchy ones) have been mislabeled "fattening." Truly, the most fattening substance is fat.

Fiber, dietary. A nondigestible form of carbohydrate found in plant products. It can be insoluble, such as wheat fiber, or soluble, such as oat bran, pectin (in fruits), and guar gum (in beans). Both types of fiber provide bulk and moderate the absorption of nutrients. Insoluble fiber helps regularity, whereas soluble fiber reduces blood cholesterol.

Glucose. A simple carbohydrate or sugar found in foods and in the body; the preferred fuel for quick energy and the only fuel used by the brain.

Glycogen. The storage form of carbohydrate in the body; long chains of glucose linked end to end. Glycogen stores, which total about 1200–1500 calories, occur in liver, muscle, and other tissues.

Gram. A metric measure of weight. One ounce equals 28.35 grams. Nutrients are listed in grams on food labels. A gram of fat contains 9 calories; a gram of protein or carbohydrate contains 4 calories.

Hidden fat. Fat in foods that is not visible. Hidden fats include oils used in frying or baking and fat naturally present in foods, such as butter fat in cheese and whole milk, fat marbled throughout beef, or fat in the skin of poultry.

Ideal or desirable weight. Weights associated with general good health and lowest mortality rates.

Insulin. A hormone produced in the pancreas in response to carbohydrate ingestion. Insulin facilitates the transport of sugars from the blood into cells where they are burned for energy.

Lean body mass. The metabolically active tissue in the body, primarily composed of muscle. The greater a person's lean body mass, the higher their metabolic rate and the greater protection they have against weight gain.

"Lite" or "light." A term used to describe certain foods with the implication that they are lower in calories. In fact, lite or light may refer to color, texture, total calories, content of fat, alcohol, carbohydrate, sodium, or even portion size (light breads). The nutrition information on the label should be used to determine how much fat the product contains and thus how it can fit into your Fat Budget.

"Low-fat." A marketing term used to imply the food is acceptable for a weight reduction diet. Since there is no consistent definition of low-fat, foods labeled low-fat may actually contain substantial amounts of fat. To be sure a product can fit into your Fat Budget, consult the fat content on the food label.

Metabolism. The sum of the chemical changes that occur to substances in the body. Much of metabolism is the conversion of food into living tissue and energy.

Monounsaturated fat. One of the three types of naturally occurring fats. Monounsaturated fats in foods help reduce blood cholesterol levels. The richest source of monounsaturated fat is olive oil. Like all other fats, monounsaturated fat has 9 calories per gram.

Nitrites. Substances used to preserve, color, and flavor meat products. In the body, nitrites can be converted into nitrosamines, which have been shown to cause cancer.

Nutrients. Substances in foods (carbohydrates, proteins, and fats) that contain energy and are building blocks for making living tissue. Also includes other substances, such as minerals and vitamins, needed for normal bodily functioning.

Nondairy. A term commonly used for imitation dairy foods that contain no dairy products, such as imitation creamers, sour creams, and whipped toppings. While these products may not contain cholesterol, they do contain fat, often highly saturated fat like coconut oil. Check the nutrition information on the label to determine how much fat is present.

Obesity. Excess accumulation of body fat. Obese is defined as 20% to 40% over ideal weight; massively obese is greater than 40% over ideal weight.

Omega-3 polyunsaturated fats. A type of polyunsaturated fat found in fish and shellfish. It lowers blood triglyceride levels and also reduces blood clotting, thus reducing risk of heart attacks and strokes.

Oxidation. See burning.

Polyunsaturated fat. One of the three types of fat commonly found in foods. Polyunsaturated fat helps to lower blood cholesterol, but in excess it can lower the "good" cholesterol in the blood and has been associated with an increased risk of cancer. The most common sources of polyunsaturated fats are corn, sunflower, and safflower oils. Like all other fats, polyunsaturated fat has 9 calories per gram.

Protein. One of the nutrients in foods that provides energy and building blocks for making essential body constituents such as muscle, enzymes, and cell membranes. Protein has 4 calories per gram.

"Reduced calorie." A term regulated by the Food and Drug Administration that means a product is at least one-third lower in calories than the food with which it is being compared. It does not necessarily mean the product is low in fat. Consult the nutrition information on the label for fat content.

Saturated fat. One of the three types of fat commonly found in foods. Saturated fat has a powerful effect on raising blood cholesterol levels. The most common sources of saturated fats are butterfat, beef, veal, lamb, and chicken fat, cocoa butter, hydrogenated vegetable oil, and the tropical oils (coconut, palm kernel and palm). Like all other fats, saturated fat has 9 calories per gram.

Simple carbohydrate. One of the two major types of carbohydrate, also known as sugar. In contrast to complex carbohydrates, simple carbohydrates are not usually associated with any nutritionally beneficial substances and thus are often called "empty calories."

Strength training. Also called weight training. Use of weights or exercise machines in which muscles exert tension to overcome fixed or variable resistance during muscular contraction.

Stroke. An interrupted supply of blood to some part of the brain due to either blockage or hemorrhage.

Sugar. Any carbohydrate having a sweet taste.

Thermogenesis or thermogenic effect of food. The process of producing heat. Some of the energy stored in the carbohydrates we eat is released as heat upon oxidation.

Trans fats. Man-made fats produced by commercial hydrogenation of polyunsaturated vegetable oils. Trans fats act in the body like saturated fats and raise LDL-cholesterol levels, thus raising risk of heart disease. Found in margarines and processed foods.

Vegetable oil. The fat from plant products. Some vegetable oils are mostly unsaturated and are liquid at room temperature (olive, corn, sunflower) and some are mostly saturated and are solid at room temperature (coconut, palm kernel, palm). All vegetable oils are 100% fat and have 9 calories per gram.

Yo-yo Syndrome. Cycles of weight loss and weight gain resulting in progressive loss of muscle, decrease in metabolic rate, slower weight loss and faster weight gain, and increasing obesity.

References

2. How *Choose to Lose* Works and Why

Acheson, K. J., Y. Schutz, T. Bessard, K. Anantharaman, J. P. Flatt, and E. Jéquier. "Glycogen Storage Capacity and de Novo Lipogenesis During Massive Carbohydrate Overfeeding in Man." *American Journal of Clinical Nutrition* 48 (1988):240–247.

Acheson, K. J., Y. Schutz, T. Bessard, J. P. Flatt, and E. Jéquier. "Carbohydrate Metabolism and De Novo Lipogenesis in Human Obesity." *American Journal of Clinical Nutrition* 45 (1987):78–85.

Astrup, A., S. Toubro, A. Raben, and A. R. Skov. "The Role of Low-Fat Diets and Fat Substitutes in Body Weight Management: What Have We Learned from Clinical Studies?" *Journal of the American Dietetic Association* 97, suppl. (1997):S82–S87.

Barrows, K., and J. T. Snook. "Effect of a High-Protein, Very-Low-Calorie Diet on Resting Metabolism, Thyroid Hormones, and Energy Expenditure in Obese Middle-Aged Women." *American Journal of Clinical Nutrition* 45 (1987):391–398.

Bray, G. A. "Obesity — A Disease of Nutrient or Energy Balance?" *Nutrition Reviews* 45 (1987):33–43.

"Can Eating the 'Right' Food Cut Your Risk of Cancer?" *Tufts University Diet and Nutrition Letter* 6 (1988):2–6.

Donato, K., and D. M. Hegsted. "Efficiency of Utilization of Various Sources of Energy for Growth." *Proceedings of the National Academy of Sciences* 82 (1985):4866–4870.

Dougherty, R. M., A. K. H. Fong, and J. M. Iacono. "Nutrient Content of the Diet When the Fat Is Reduced." *American Journal of Clinical Nutrition* 48 (1988):970–979.

Dreon, D. M., B. Frey-Hewitt, N. Ellsworth, et al. "Dietary Fat: Carbohydrate Ratio and Obesity in Middle-Aged Men." *American Journal of Clinical Nutrition* 47 (1988):995–1000.

Elliott, D. L., L. Goldberg, K. S. Kuehl, and W. M. Bennett. "Sustained Depressions of the Resting Metabolic Rate After Massive Weight Loss." *American Journal of Clinical Nutrition* 49 (1989):93–96.

Flatt, J. P. "Dietary Fat, Carbohydrate Balance, and Weight Maintenance: Effects of Exercise." *American Journal of Clinical Nutrition* 45 (1987):296–306.

———. "Differences in the Regulation of Carbohydrate and Fat Metabolism and Their Implications for Body Weight Maintenance." *Hormones, Thermogenesis, and Obesity.* Edited by Henry Lardy and Frederick Stratman. New York: Elsevier Science Publishing, 1989.

———. "Effect of Carbohydrate and Fat Intake on Postprandial Substrate Oxidation and Storage." *Topics in Clinical Nutrition* 2(2) (1987):15–27.

———. "Importance of Nutrient Balance in Body Weight Regulation." *Diabetes/Metabolism Reviews* 4(6) (1988):571–581.

———. "Metabolic Feedback on Food Intake Among Ad Libitum Fed Mice." *International Journal of Obesity* 9 (1985):A33.

Flatt, J. P., E. Ravussin, K. J. Acheson, and E. Jéquier. "Effects of Dietary Fat on Postprandial Substrate Oxidation and on Carbohydrate and Fat Balances." *Journal of Clinical Investigation* 76 (1985):1019–1024.

Gray, D. S., J. S. Fisler, and G. A. Bray. "Effects of Repeated Weight Loss and Regain on Body Composition in Obese Rats." *American Journal of Clinical Nutrition* 47 (1988):393–399.

Hammer, R. L., C. A. Barrier, E. S. Roundy, J. M. Bradford, and A. G. Fisher. "Calorie-Restricted Low-Fat Diet and Exercise in Obese Women." *American Journal of Clinical Nutrition* 49 (1989):77–85.

Hellerstein, M. K., et al. "Measurement of De Novo Hepatic Lipogenesis in Humans Using Stable Isotopes." *Journal of Clinical Investigations* 87 (1991):1841–1852.

Hultman, E., and L. H. Nilsson. "Factors Influencing Carbohydrate Metabolism in Man." *Nutrition Metabolism* 18, suppl. 1 (1975):45–64.

Jéquier, E. "Carbohydrates as a Source of Energy." *American Journal of Clinical Nutrition* 59, suppl. (1994):682S–685S.

Katch, F., and W. D. McArdle. *Nutrition, Weight Control, and Exercise.* Philadelphia: Lea & Febiger, 1988.

Lissner, L., D. A. Levitsky, B. J. Strupp, et al. "Dietary Fat and the Regulation of Energy Intake in Human Subjects." *American Journal of Clinical Nutrition* 46 (1987):886–892.

Manson, J. E., M. J. Stampfer, C. H. Hennekens, and W. C. Willett. "Body Weight and Longevity." *Journal of the American Medical Association* 257 (1987):353–358.

Mattes, R. D. "Fat Preference and Adherence to a Reduced-Fat Diet." *American Journal of Clinical Nutrition* 57 (1993):373–381.

Mattes, R. D., C. B. Pierce, and M. I. Friedman. "Daily Caloric Intake of Normal-Weight Adults: Response to Changes in Dietary Energy Density of a Luncheon Meal." *American Journal of Clinical Nutrition* 48 (1988):214–219.

Ravussin, E., and P. A. Tataranni. "Dietary Fat and Human Obesity." *Journal of the American Dietetic Association* 97, suppl. (1997):S42–S46.

Romieu, I., W. C. Willett, M. J. Stampfer, G. A. Colditz, et al. "Energy Intake and Other Determinants of Relative Weight." *American Journal of Clinical Nutrition* 47 (1988):406–412.

Schutz, Y., J. P. Flatt, and Eric Jéquier. "Failure of Dietary Fat Intake to Promote Fat Oxidation: A Factor Favoring the Development of Obesity." *American Journal of Clinical Nutrition* 50 (1989):307–314.

Steen, S. N., R. A. Oppliger, and K. D. Brownell. "Metabolic Effects of Repeated

Weight Loss and Regain in Adolescent Wrestlers." *Journal of the American Medical Association* 260 (1988):47–50.

Weiss, L., G. E. Hoffmann, R. Schreiber, H. Andres, E. Fuchs, E. Korber, and H. J. Kolb. "Fatty-Acid Biosynthesis in Man, a Pathway of Minor Importance." *Biological Chemical Hoppe-Seyler* 367 (1986):905–912.

3. Action Plan

Dennison, D. *The DINE System: The Nutritional Plan for Better Health.* St. Louis: C. V. Mosby, 1982.

6. A Celebration of Food

Dougherty, R. M., A. K. H. Fong, and J. M. Iacono. "Nutrient Content of the Diet When the Fat Is Reduced." *American Journal of Clinical Nutrition* 48 (1988):970–979.

Goor, R., and N. Goor. *Eater's Choice: A Food Lover's Guide to Lower Cholesterol,* rev. ed. Boston: Houghton Mifflin, 1995.

James, W. P. T., M. E. J. Lean, and G. McNeill. "Dietary Recommendations After Weight Loss: How to Avoid Relapse of Obesity." *American Journal of Clinical Nutrition* 45 (1987):1135–1141.

7. Fat City

The fat tables are based on data from the following sources:

U.S. Department of Agriculture. *Composition of Foods.* Agriculture Handbook No. 8. Washington, D.C.: Government Printing Office, sec. 1–16, rev. 1976–1989.

————. *Nutritive Value of American Foods in Common Units.* Agriculture Handbook No. 456. Washington, D.C.: Government Printing Office, November 1975.

13. Exercise: An Essential Ingredient

Ballor, D. L., V. L. Katch, M. D. Becque, and C. R. Marks. "Resistance Weight Training During Caloric Restriction Enhances Lean Body Weight Maintenance." *American Journal of Clinical Nutrition* 47 (1988):19–25.

Cooper, Kenneth. *The New Aerobics.* New York: Bantam Books, 1983.

Cooper, Kenneth, and Mildred Cooper. *The New Aerobics for Women.* New York: Bantam Books, 1988.

Hammer, R. L., C. A. Barrier, E. S. Roundy, J. M. Bradford, and A. G. Fisher. "Calorie-Restricted Low-Fat Diet and Exercise in Obese Women." *American Journal of Clinical Nutrition* 49 (1989):77–85.

Hill, J. O., P. B. Sparling, T. W. Shields, and P. A. Heller. "Effects of Exercise and Food

Restriction on Body Composition and Metabolic Rate in Obese Women." *American Journal of Clinical Nutrition* 46 (1987):622–630.

Katch, F., and W. D. McArdle. *Nutrition, Weight Control, and Exercise.* Philadelphia: Lea & Febiger, 1988.

Rippe, J. M., A. Ward., J. P. Porcari, and P. S. Freedson. "Walking for Health and Fitness." *Journal of the American Medical Association* 259 (1988):2720–2724.

U.S. Department of Health and Human Services, Public Health Service. *Exercise and Your Heart.* National Institutes of Health Publication No. 18–1677, 1981.

15. To Your Health

National Center for Health Statistics. *Anthropometric Reference Data and Prevalence of Overweight, United States 1976–1980.* DHHS Publication No. 87-1688. Washington, D.C.: Government Printing Office, 1987.

Pi-Sunyer, F. Xavier. "Health Implications of Obesity." *American Journal of Clinical Nutrition* 53 (1991):1595S–1603S.

U.S. Department of Health and Human Services. "Health Implications of Obesity." *National Institutes of Health Consensus Development Conference Statement.* Vol. 5, no. 9, 1985. National Institutes of Health, Office of Medical Applications of Research, Building 1, Room 216, Bethesda, MD 20205.

U.S. Department of Health and Human Services. *The Surgeon General's Report on Nutrition and Health.* DHHS (PHS) Publication No. 88-50210. Washington, D.C.: Government Printing Office, 1988.

Index

EATER'S CHOICE LOW-FAT COOKBOOK

by Dr. Ron and Nancy Goor
Houghton Mifflin Company, 1999

Eat Your Way to Thinness and Good Health!

320 Scrumptious, Quick and Easy, Low-fat Recipes

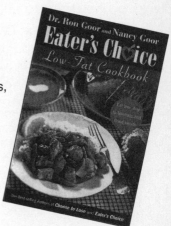

- **Soups,** such as Tortilla Soup, Sour Cherry Soup, Vegetable Soup Provençal, Zucchini Soup
- **Entrées,** such as Cajun Chicken, Chickenburgers, Lemon Chicken, Turkey Mexique, Sweet and Sour Shrimp, Salmon Sublime
- Chili Non Carne, Focaccia, Asparagus Pasta, Calzone, Potato Skins, Spiced Sweet Potatoes, Indian Rice, Onion Flat Bread
- **Low-low-fat desserts,** such as Lemon Cheesecake, Apple Cake, Super Oatmeal Cookies
  . . . and MUCH MORE!

EATER'S CHOICE

A Food Lover's Guide to Lower Cholesterol

by Dr. Ron and Nancy Goor
Houghton Mifflin Company, Fifth Edition, 1999

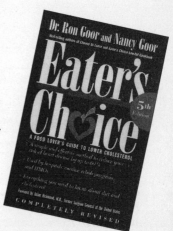

- Everything you need to know about diet, cholesterol, and heart disease, including updated information on trans fats, reversal of coronary heart disease, cholesterol-lowering drugs, etc.
- A simple method to reduce your risk of heart disease by up to 60 percent
- Chapter on children and cholesterol

Both books are available at most bookstores or use order form on next page.

Visit our website: http://www.choicediets.com

PUT **CHOOSE TO LOSE**® TO WORK FOR YOU!

PASSBOOK

The key to losing weight is staying within your Fat Budget. Convenient pocket-size passbook (like a check book) contains everything you need to make keeping track easy:

- Abbreviated FOOD TABLES listing total and fat calories for hundreds of foods
- BALANCE BOOK for keeping food records for two weeks.

SKILL-BUILDER

A step-by-step interactive companion that helps you master the skills needed to lose weight permanently, such as deciphering food labels, modifying recipes, ordering out low-fat, etc.

Books by the Goors to enhance **Choose to Lose**

- Eater's Choice Low-Fat Cookbook (see preceding page)
- Eater's Choice: A Food Lovers Guide to Lower Cholesterol (see preceding page)

. . . and for the woman in your life: • Choose to Lose: A Food Lover's Guide to Permanent Weight Loss

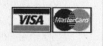

TO ORDER: For quickest delivery: call toll-free 1-888-897-9360 and order by credit card. Or fill out and send order form below with check or money order payable to Choose to Lose.

SHIP TO: Print clearly or type   **O R D E R   F O R M**

Name _____

Address _____

City _____ State _____ Zip _____

ITEM	QUANTITY	PRICE EACH	TOTAL PRICE
Choose to Lose Passbook		$ 4.50	
Choose to Lose Balance Book Refills		.75	
Choose to Lose SKILL-BUILDER*		9.00	
Choose to Lose Weight-Loss Plan for Men		17.00	
Eater's Choice Low-Fat Cookbook		17.00	
Choose to Lose (3rd edition)		18.00	
Eater's Choice (5th edition)		18.00	

*Requires Passbook. At least 2 Refills are useful.

5% tax (MD residents)		
Postage and Handling	2	00
TOTAL ORDER	$	

Send check or money order to:

Choice Diets, Inc.
P.O. Box 2053
Rockville, MD 20847-2053

Prices are subject to change.

Call toll-free 1-888-897-9360 to see if a Choose to Lose Weight Loss/Healthy Eating Program is near you.

1/00